THE EFFECTS OF CHILD ABUSE AND NEGLECT

THE EFFECTS OF CHILD ABUSE AND NEGLECT

Issues and Research

Edited by

RAYMOND H. STARR, JR.
University of Maryland Baltimore County

DAVID A. WOLFE
*Institute for the Prevention of Child Abuse
and The University of Western Ontario*

THE GUILFORD PRESS
London • New York

©1991 The Guilford Press
A Division of Guilford Publications, Inc.
72 Spring Street, New York, NY 10012

Printed in the United States of America

This book is printed on acid-free paper.

Last digit is print number: 9 8 7 6 5 4 3 2 1

Library of Congress Cataloging-in-Publication Data

The Effects of child abuse and neglect : issues and research / edited
  by Raymond H. Starr, Jr., David A. Wolfe
      p.   cm.
    Includes bibliographical references and index.
    ISBN 0-89862-759-1
    1. Child abuse—Research—Methodology.   2. Child abuse—Research—
United States—Methodology.   3. Child abuse—Longitudinal studies.
4. Child abuse—United States—Longitudinal studies.   I. Starr,
Raymond.   II. Wolfe, David A.
    [DNLM: 1. Child Abuse—epidemiology.   2. Longitudinal Studies.
3. Research—methods.   WA 320 E27]
HV715.E34   1991
362.7′6—dc20
DNLM/DLC
for Library of Congress   91-20247
                                                      CIP

To Our Families

Preface

The purpose of this book is to inform professionals and lay persons about research issues and findings relating to our current understanding of both child abuse and neglect. Research in child abuse has expanded dramatically since the first controlled studies were started in the mid-1970s. At the same time, the fields of developmental psychology and clinical child psychology have progressed to the point where the three areas can be seen as merging. This merger has brought both theoretical richness and increasing methodological sophistication, which we have attempted to highlight in this volume.

This increasing sophistication has been accompanied by the realization that child abuse and neglect can only be fully understood through the use of longitudinal research methods. However, the implementation of such studies is difficult, expensive, and time-consuming. Thus, this volume is meant to provide direction to current longitudinal research and to serve as a guide to methodological issues in the conduct of such studies.

The first chapter by Starr, MacLean, and Keating provides a framework within which the importance of longitudinal research for our understanding of child maltreatment and its long-term effects can be understood. It does this through a consideration of the intergenerational transmission of maltreatment and of adult sequelae of childhood abuse and neglect. This chapter is followed by a discussion of three of the first major longitudinal investigations. Byron Egeland, in his chapter, focuses on the value of an at-risk approach to research in this area. He discusses issues he faced in conducting his study and summarizes the findings of his research. The Herrenkohls and their colleagues, in the next chapter, provide a clear statement of the value of structural equations modeling—a relatively new statistical method—in analyzing their longitudinal data. The specific value of this approach is that it allows researchers to carefully delineate the specific outcomes of maltreatment. Peter Vietze and his colleagues, in the next chapter, demonstrate the usefulness of adopting a transactional approach to the longitudinal study of differing forms of maltreatment and discuss the problems involved in using such a strategy.

Following these introductory chapters, the remainder of this volume focuses more specifically on issues of importance in interpreting existing research and in conducting future research. The chapter by Susan Zuravin deals with one of the more complex aspects of working in the area of child maltreament: how do we go about defining it? This is done through an analysis of general issues and of existing definitions. Her discussion is followed by Maureen Black's review of general design issues and of the rationale for conducting longitudinal studies. Jane Gilgun next discusses the value of qualitative data analytic methods for examining the results of longitudinal studies. In particular, she notes that the process involves the use of both qualitative and quantitative mthods for data anlysis in order to determine areas of cross-method congruence. Such a process can be fruitfully used to expand our knowledge of maltreatment.

The remaining five chapters deal with specific measurement issues. Joel Milner discusses basic measurement problems involved in assessing parental personality and psychopathology with a focus on issues of importance in working with maltreating parents. Joan Grusec and Gary Walters next discuss the need to assess parental childrearing belief systems as a fundamental ingredient in understanding maltreatment.

Parent–child interaction styles are key components in understanding the causes of maltreatment and evaluating its consequences. Using parent–child attachment as a basis, Eric Mash describes issues and methods involved in assessing attachment and other domains of parent–child interaction.

The last two chapters deal with the specific effects of maltreatment on children. David Wolfe and Robin McGee discuss the emotional development of maltreated children, and Howard Dubowitz describes the assessment of the effects of maltreatment on child health.

We are indebted to the many individuals who have helped make this volume possible. Raymond Starr would like to thank his wife, Janice, for her emotional support and critical help with certain sections of this book. In addition, he would like to thank his colleagues at the Center for Vulnerable Children at the University of Maryland at Baltimore—Maureen Black, Howard Dubowitz, and Susan Zuravin—for their help in broadly conceptualizing child maltreatment. David Wolfe would like to thank Tricia Thornton (of the Institute for the Prevention of Child Abuse, IPCA) as well as the members of the IPCA's Research Committee who helped with the initial planning of the contents of this volume: Rick Volpe (Chair), Helen Thomas, Gary Walters, Rob McFadden, Nanci Burns, Dennis Raphael, and Michael Thompson. Most importantly, we both want to thank the IPCA and its President/CEO, Ron Luciano, for hosting the research seminar that formed the basis for this book.

Contributors

William A. Altemeier, MD, Department of Pediatrics, Vanderbilt University, Nashville, Tennessee

Maureen Black, PhD, Department of Pediatrics, University of Maryland School of Medicine, Baltimore, Maryland

Howard Dubowitz, MD, MPH, Department of Pediatrics, University of Maryland School of Medicine, Baltimore, Maryland

Byron Egeland, PhD, Institute for Child Development, University of Minnesota, Minneapolis, Minnesota

Brenda P. Egolf, PhD, Psychology Department, Lehigh University, Bethlehem, Pennsylvania

Jane F. Gilgun, PhD, School of Social Work, University of Minnesota, Minneapolis, Minnesota

Joan E. Grusec, PhD, Psychology Department, University of Toronto, Toronto, Ontario, Canada

Ellen C. Herrenkohl, PhD, Psychology Department, Lehigh University, Bethlehem, Pennsylvania

Roy C. Herrenkohl, PhD, Psychology Department, Lehigh University, Bethlehem, Pennsylvania

Daniel P. Keating, PhD, Ontario Institute for Studies in Education, Toronto, Ontario, Canada

Darla J. MacLean, PhD, Psychology Department, Brock University, St. Catharines, Ontario, Canada

Eric J. Mash, PhD, Psychology Department, University of Calgary, Calgary, Alberta, Canada

Robin McGee, PhD, Department of Psychology, University of Western Ontario, London, Ontario, Canada

Joel S. Milner, PhD, Psychology Department, Northern Illinois University, DeKalb, Illinois

Susan O'Connor, MD, Department of Pediatrics, Vanderbilt University, Nashville, Tennessee

Kathryn B. Sherrod, PhD, Department of Psychology, Vanderbilt University, Nashville, Tennessee

Raymond H. Starr, Jr., PhD, Psychology Department, University of Maryland Baltimore County, Baltimore, Maryland

Peter M. Vietze, PhD, New York State Institute for Basic Research in Developmental Disabilities, Staten Island, New York

Gary C. Walters, PhD, Psychology Department, University of Toronto, Toronto, Ontario, Canada

David A. Wolfe, PhD, Institute for the Prevention of Child Abuse, Toronto, Ontario, Canada

Ping Wu, Psychology Department, Lehigh University, Bethlehem, Pennsylvania

Susan J. Zuravin, PhD, University of Maryland at Baltimore School of Social Work, Baltimore, Maryland

Contents

129085

THE EFFECTS OF CHILD ABUSE AND NEGLECT

1

Life-Span Developmental Outcomes of Child Maltreatment

RAYMOND H. STARR, JR.
University of Maryland Baltimore County

DARLA J. MacLEAN
Brock University

DANIEL P. KEATING
Ontario Institute for Studies in Education

A major concern of researchers attempting to understand the causes and correlates of child maltreatment, of clinicians interested in working with perpetrators and victims, and of policy makers desirous of implementing effective prevention programs is the degree to which maltreated children grow up to be either maltreating adults or to exhibit socially deleterious sequelae of abuse and/or neglect. This chapter examines this issue of the long-term effects of child maltreatment on individual development. We organize the available empirical and theoretical literature from a life-span developmental approach. In so doing, we evaluate what we currently know about both developmental origins and sequelae, and seek to identify the key areas in which we need to know more.

As will become clear in the following review of the research literature, much of the available evidence has been generated from a consideration of direct, or "main," effects. Three questions that illustrate this approach are the following:

- Does being maltreated as a child lead to being a maltreating parent? Or even more specifically, does a history of physical or sexual abuse, or neglect lead to that *same* behavior as a parent?

- Does being maltreated as a child lead to identifiable antisocial behaviors, such as delinquency or criminality?
- Do adult victims of child maltreatment exhibit unique patterns of psychological abnormality?

In our research analysis, we suggest that the available evidence does not support a strong finding of such one-to-one correspondence between developmental history and adult behavior. This may be true for at least two reasons. First, despite popular belief, it may be the case that the effects of child maltreatment are either minimal or short-lived, or both. Second, and in our view more likely, it is possible that the effects of maltreatment are rarely as direct and linear as the simple correspondence model would imply. We contrast this simple correspondence theory with an emerging lifespan developmental model, in which the interactive complexities of the self-system and of the ecological context in which the individual develops are acknowledged and studied explicitly.

In the first part of this chapter, we provide a brief overview of a lifespan developmental perspective appropriate for analyzing these questions, drawing on a variety of sources (Baltes, 1987; Belsky & Vondra, 1989; Cicchetti, 1989; Keating & MacLean, 1988; Rutter, 1989; Starr, 1988). Following this, we examine in some detail the available research focusing on long-term effects of maltreatment as they relate to the three questions. In the final section, we bring together the theoretical and empirical issues to suggest fruitful avenues both for future research and for the practical issues of prevention and intervention.

THE LIFE-SPAN DEVELOPMENTAL PERSPECTIVE

Central to the life-span developmental perspective is a conception of the individual as a complex but organized system. This implies several important features. First, it suggests that there is a fundamental organization to the self-system, which undergoes qualitative reorganizations over the course of development. Second, the self-system is composed of interacting subsystems (social, cognitive, affective, behavioral), which are in a dynamic relationship with each other. Third, the self-system does not exist or function independently; it, too, operates in dynamic interaction with an ecological setting, including the family, the community, and the larger society.

In applying this perspective to research on child maltreatment, we need to adopt new approaches to assessing those factors that influence and organize development in order to fully understand the life-span implications of childhood experiences. Thus, rather than seeking specific corresponding target outcomes, such as the tendency of a physically abused child to become a physically abusive parent, we may need to consider a broader range of outcomes. For example, "the adverse experiences in childhood may have no direct effect on parenting. Perhaps their main impact is on personality development . . . " (Rutter, 1989, p. 322). Of course, as Rutter notes, adult personality may have a substantial impact on parenting behaviors, but not necessarily in a way that directly corresponds to earlier experiences in childhood.

Studies of broader classes of outcomes are more likely to reveal the long-term impact of child maltreatment. Aber, Allen, Carlson, and Cicchetti (1989), for example, examined broadly defined measures of competence, security, and adaptation to look at the effects of child maltreatment in preschoolers and early school-age children. Our ability to identify even longer-term sequelae, such as those extending into the adolescent and adulthood years of parenting, will likely be similarly enhanced by a more theoretically guided selection of the types of developmental outcomes to be included in research studies.

A similar level of complexity is introduced in our examination of the characteristics that render individuals more or less vulnerable to the negative effects of child maltreatment. Cicchetti and Rizley (1981) organize risk factors for child maltreatment along two dimensions: one addresses the direction of effect (potentiating factors increase risk, compensating factors reduce risk) and the other emphasizes the temporal duration of these influences (enduring or transient). In principle, when negative factors outweigh positive ones, the risk of negative outcomes becomes a reality. At this point, however, assigning relative weights to specific factors within these categories requires substantially more research than is currently available. As Belsky and Vondra (1989) note, our present knowledge base is derived from main-effects models; evaluating the interactions among factors that are enduring versus transient and potentiating versus compensatory is a goal for the future. The key point here, however, is that the probability of observing direct correspondences at the behavioral level is further reduced.

On the other hand, it is important to recognize that the variety of risk factors just described are themselves often likely to exist in conjunction with each other in the real world. Economic deprivation, psychosocially stressed families, and other risk factors are not entirely independent. Rutter (1989), citing his own work and that of Egeland, Jacobvitz, and Papatola (1984), reports that "the greater the overall burden of poor parenting experienced, the greater the risk of poor parenting provided to the next generation of children" (p. 339).

Further, as Rutter (1989) points out, there is a cumulative effect over time of risk factors, so that children who may be at genetic risk for maladaptive development may also be born into families that maltreat them. The fact of severe maltreatment increases the probability of being

removed from the home, possibly leading to exposure to multiple caretakers, and if return to the home occurs, it is likely to be to a continuing
destabilized situation. In particular, Rutter reports that young women
returning to discordant homes were more likely to become pregnant as
adolescents, and were more likely to engage in poor parenting and to have
unhappy marriages to men with similar psychosocial problems. Thus,
"developmental continuity lies as much in social connections between different forms of adverse environments as in any internal effects on the
child's own personality development. It was striking how one adversity
tended to lead to another" (Rutter, 1989, pp. 339–340).

Recognizing the dynamic complexity of the self-system as it evolves
within a specific ecological context is one step toward formulating a life-
span developmental perspective on child maltreatment. A second step
requires consideration of the developmental sequelae across a span that
includes adulthood. The available evidence for such sequelae, however, is
derived largely from main effects models, which we review below. In the
final section, we will explore the possibilities and difficulties in uniting
these approaches.

MALTREATMENT RESEARCH: ADULT OUTCOMES

Four areas of maltreatment research have implications for life-span developmental theory and research. First, are maltreated children more likely
than nonmaltreated children to become maltreating parents? That is, is
maltreatment intergenerationally transmitted? Second, are maltreated
children more likely to commit criminal acts as adolescents and adults?
Third, what are the broader psychological consequences of maltreatment?
Fourth, given that not all maltreated children display negative outcomes
as adults, can we identify buffers that moderate these effects? This section
of the chapter discusses each area from the view of three types of maltreatment: physical abuse, sexual abuse, and—where data are available—
child neglect.

It is important to note that it is difficult to make exact comparisons
between studies because of differences in samples, methods, and the
definitions of independent and dependent variables. A detailed discussion
of these issues is beyond the scope of this chapter (see Mash & Wolfe,
1991). Where possible, references are provided for materials offering more
detailed analyses of individual topics.

Intergenerational Transmission

The hypothesis of intergenerational transmission of maltreatment is theoretically and intuitively appealing. In an early review, Spinetta and Rigler

(1972), citing numerous references supporting their conclusion, stated that "one basic factor in the etiology of child abuse draws unanimity: Abusing parents were themselves abused or neglected, physically or emotionally, as children" (p. 298). However, their statement is not based upon the results of investigations employing control groups of nonmaltreating parents.

Research

Results of analyses of the validity of the intergenerational hypothesis that have used control or contrast groups suggest that the correspondence between being maltreated as a child and becoming a maltreating adult is far from the one-to-one relationship that has been proposed by some authors (e.g., Blumberg, 1974). Most research has focused on physical abuse and neglect; indeed, studies commonly combine these two forms of maltreatment, making the detailed analysis and interpretation of findings of intergenerational transmission difficult. Another factor complicating our ability to understand intergenerational transmission is that studies have not attempted to assess the validity of different theories about the mechanism underlying this transmission (Bersani & Chen, 1988).

Kaufman and Zigler (1987) summarize this work and conclude that the best estimate is a transmission rate of 30% ± 5% for physical abuse. However, they fail to provide a separate estimate for studies of only physical abuse and include many studies combining abuse and neglect. Although suffering physical abuse as a child should be considered a risk factor for becoming an abusive parent, vast numbers of abused children grow up to eschew violence as a childrearing tactic and, conversely, people who were not abused as children but who suffered other childhood difficulties may become abusive as parents.

There is considerable variation in the reported rate of the intergenerational transmission of physical abuse across studies (Kaufman & Zigler, 1987). These differences are most likely due to differences in study methodology, including the samples studied and the definitions of maltreatment used. This point is illustrated in a study by Hunter and Kilstrom (1979) which found that parents of premature or physically ill infants described being physically abused or neglected as children. A year later 18% of the children of these parents had been abused or neglected compared to 0.5% of children whose parents did not describe maltreatment as children. However, had the researchers used a retrospective rather than a prospective design and interviewed the parents of those children who were abused or neglected at 1 year of age, they would have found a deceptively high intergenerational transmission rate, since 90% of the maltreating parents were themselves maltreated as children.

Interestingly, a much higher rate of intergenerational transmission comes from another prospective study (Egeland et al., 1984). Results indicated that when the children were 2 years old, 44 (16%) of 267 high-risk mothers maltreated their children. Maltreatment included physical abuse (55%), neglect (55%), hostile and rejecting parenting (43%), and psychologically unavailable parenting (43%), with many of the mothers exhibiting multiple parenting deficits. Mothers were interviewed about maltreatment during their own childhood, and 47 reported being physically abused. The authors report that 33 (70%) of these mothers were maltreating their children. Only 16 of these cases (34%) represented clear-cut maltreatment. This percentage drops to 17% when children were evaluated at 6 years of age (Pianta, Egeland, & Erickson, 1989). The authors suggest that the risk of intergenerational transmission decreases as children get older.

Retrospective analyses are a second research approach. One major study found 53% of caretakers who reported using abusive discipline with a child were themselves disciplined by abusive measures during childhood, compared to 38% of parents who stated they were not abusive toward their own children (Herrenkohl, Herrenkohl, & Toedter, 1983). This effect is significant when analysis controls for social desirability, number of children, and family income. One of the most important variables was abuse by the reporting parents' mothers; paternal data were not significant.

Random population surveys represent another way of examining intergenerational transmission. In one of the few studies to examine the intergenerational transmission of physical violence in families, Straus (1979) analyzed the relationship between parental reports of physical punishment as children and the use of potentially physically abusive violence toward their own children. It was found that 18.5% of parents whose mothers had used physical violence on them more than once a year during childhood were abusive toward their own child. This rate compares to 11.8% of parents whose mothers were not violent or used violence once a year. The child abuse rate for parents whose fathers were violent did not differ significantly from the rate of parents whose fathers were not (16.7% for those with frequently violent fathers vs. 13.2% for those with less violent fathers). Interestingly, the intergenerational transmission rate is higher if the parent reported having been physically punished by their opposite sex parent.

Straus (1979) reported other findings suggesting that the climate of violence in the homes of physically abusive parents plays a role in intergenerational transmission. Fathers who saw their fathers hit their mothers were more likely to be abusive as adults. Furthermore, mothers who saw their mothers hit their fathers were more abusive. In addition, a cycle of violence exists within families (Straus, 1983). Violence by husbands toward their wives is positively related to the wife's use of violence with her children. Children subjected to violent childrearing practices are more violent toward their siblings and toward their parents as well (Straus, Gelles, & Steinmetz, 1980).

The research evidence indicates that intergenerational transmission is a factor in the occurrence of physical abuse. However, the relationship is not a simple one. Many factors can lead to an abused child's growing up to be a nonabusive parent and, conversely, children who were never abused can become abusing parents.

Little research has focused on the intergenerational transmission of neglect in spite of its high incidence. The lack of appropriate research is part of what has been called the "neglect of neglect" (Wolock & Horowitz, 1984). Available data limit our ability to estimate the magnitude of this transmission; however, owing to such methodological problems as a lack of a control or comparison group, small samples, and reliance on parental reports of childhood level of care.

Pianta et al. (1989), in one of the few prospective studies, concluded that 9 of the 267 mothers in their larger, prospective longitudinal study were neglected as children. Three of their children were judged to be severely maltreated at age 2, although the type of maltreatment was not specified. Only two of these mothers were judged to be providing adequate child care. As was the case for physical abuse, the incidence of maltreatment declined when the children were assessed at 6 years of age.

The limited research on neglecting families suggests that intergenerational transmission is only present in a minority of cases. In the most complete study, Polansky and his colleagues found about 15% of neglectful mothers had a history of definite neglect during their childhoods (Polansky, Chalmers, Buttenwieser, & William, 1981), but the authors do not discuss the incidence of neglect in their control sample. Data suggest that there are differences with regard to other related variables, including maternal feelings of being unwanted as a child (57% of neglect sample vs. 23% of control mothers) and long-term removal from their natural parents (41% of neglecting vs. 7% of control mothers). Lewis, Jahn, and Bishop (cited in Polansky, 1976) report that the intergenerational transmission rate for neglect is somewhat higher than that reported by Polansky et al. (1981), but still less than 25%.

Two types of indirect evidence also support the conclusion that any intergenerational transmission effect for neglect is weak. First, Giovannoni and Billingsley (1970) found no differences between neglecting and matched control mothers in parental dominance, stability, and structure in their family of origin. Second, research on the long-term maintenance of poverty—a variable linked to neglect—provides conflicting results (Wilson,

1987). The best available evidence indicates that about 60% of people in poverty at a given time represent long-term poor and account for most of the Aid to Families with Dependent Children (AFDC) costs (Bane & Ellwood, 1983, cited in Wilson, 1987). However, the timespan for this analysis was less than a decade, rather than across generations.

Research on the intergenerational transmission of sexual abuse has only recently begun to be performed. As is the case with physical abuse, clinical investigations suggest that intergenerational transmission is common (e.g., DeYoung, 1982; Rosenfeld, 1977; Will, 1983). In one of the earliest controlled studies, Goodwin, McCarthy, and DiVasto (1981) found mothers of 24% of physically and 24% of sexually abused children reported childhood incest experiences, compared with 3% of nonabusing control group mothers. These data agree with the incidence data for other forms of maltreatment reviewed earlier, although they also require further controlled study.

Discussion

Research findings lead to the conclusion that statements concerning the high probability of the transmission of child maltreatment across generations are unwarranted. Given the relative uniformity of the findings of the studies reviewed in this section, it appears likely that the rate of transmission for any of the three forms of maltreatment is even less than the 30% reported by Kaufman and Zigler (1987) for a combination of physical abuse and neglect.

The available research has many inadequacies. Samples are often small; control groups are often not used; prospective intergenerational studies have rarely been performed; maltreatment is often not consistently defined in regard to either assessments of parental background or current child maltreatment; and data for varying types of maltreatment are often combined. However, many of these deficiencies are likely to lead to an overestimation rather than an underestimation of the magnitude of intergenerational transmission. For example, this could be the case with retrospective assessments because the mechanisms underlying reporting bias maximize similarities between self-descriptions and the way others are described (Hastdorf, Richardson, & Dornbusch, 1958).

Professionals' fascination with and emphasis on intergenerational transmission as a direct cause of most child maltreatment is misdirected. In line with an ecological framework (Starr, 1978, 1988) we need to focus on the entire spectrum of childhood experiences as determinants of parenting approaches rather than focus on certain events as critical markers that lead to a predictable outcome. Maltreatment cannot be viewed in a simplistic, mechanistic manner. It occurs in a context where multiple forms of maltreatment—such as physical abuse and neglect—are frequently present in a single family (e.g., American Association for Protecting Children, 1988; Dietrich, Starr, & Weisfeld, 1983; Egeland et al., 1984; Seghorn, Prentky, & Boucher, 1987). The implications of multiple types of maltreatment and of varying family contexts will be discussed in more detail at the end of the next section on other sequelae of maltreatment.

Maltreatment and Later Criminality

Later criminal behavior is one of the most commonly discussed sequelae of child maltreatment. The connection between abuse and maltreatment has been highlighted in televised public service announcements (National Committee on Child Abuse and Neglect, 1978) and in popular print columns (R. S. Welsh, personal communication, April 1977). The critical question remains whether being subject to physical violence or sexual victimization leads children to later delinquency and adult violent crime and to the commission of sex crimes.

Research

The relation between childhood physical abuse and delinquency and adult criminality has been a subject of much concern (see Hunner & Walker, 1981; Lewis, Mallouh, & Webb, 1989; Sandberg, 1989; Widom 1989a). While it is generally acknowledged that an experience of violence during childhood is associated with adult violence (Monahan, 1981), the critical question is the magnitude of this relationship. As is the case with the intergenerational transmission of physical abuse, results of studies using a number of different methodologies indicate that correlations are far from perfect.

Studies of the maltreatment–violence relationship typically have a number of methodological problems. Some of these have been summarized by Widom (1989a): (1) lack of detailed criteria for defining maltreatment, (2) reliance on retrospective data and hearsay information, (3) weak sampling techniques (see also Widom, 1988), (4) use of correlational designs, (5) lack of control groups, (6) a focus on delinquency rather than violent behavior, and (7) a failure to distinguish between abuse and neglect. Thus, studies typically contain mixed samples of abused and neglected children. For example, 92% of Alfaro's (1981) and 67% of Widom's (1989b, 1989c) sample of maltreated children were neglected, 8% of Alfaro's subjects were abused and 14% of Widom's subjects were sexually abused, 8% were physically abused, and 11% were both abused and neglected or were victims of both physical and sexual abuse. Yet a

societal focus on abuse and a neglect of neglect leads to a common interpretation of maltreatment as child abuse (Wolock & Horowitz, 1984) and
increases the likelihood of misinterpreting results of studies such as these.
Thus, Sandberg (1989) labels all maltreatment—including neglect and
psychological abuse—as "child abuse."

Results of retrospective analyses indicate that delinquents are more
likely to be maltreated than are children in low income samples (Gray,
1988). However, Gray's review of nine studies indicates that the strength
of this relationship between maltreatment and delinquency varies considerably, corresponding to variations in the source of information concerning and the definition of maltreatment. Similarly, Widom (1989a), in an
analysis of nine studies, concluded that retrospective studies found an
abuse–delinquency rate ranging from 8% to 26% while the rate for
prospective studies was always less than 20%.

In one interesting, well-controlled, prospective long-term study of
physical abuse, McCord (1983, 1988) analyzed case records of 253 boys
who were between 5 and 13 years old at the start of the study. Record
analyses indicated that 49 of these boys had been abused by their parents.
Follow-up data obtained when the subjects were in middleage indicated
that 39% had been convicted of some crime as juveniles (10%), as adults
(16%), or both (12%), compared to 23% of 101 boys who were classified
as loved by their parents.[*] These data are overestimates of the relationship
between abuse and criminality in the general population since the sample
was selected from children living in deteriorated urban areas where both
crime and abuse are likely to have a higher incidence.

A more relevant question is whether there is a relationship between
abuse and later violent acts (see Widom, 1989a, for a summary of most of
the relevant studies). Results of a limited number of well-controlled studies, while mixed, suggest that a weak transmission cycle is present. Lewis
and her colleagues in a study of 97 incarcerated delinquents found a
significant relationship between the abusive treatment endured during
childhood and the degree of violence involved in the delinquent offense
(Lewis, Shanok, Pincus, & Glaser, 1979). In addition, the more violent
juvenile offenders had been exposed to a greater amount of violence
among other family members. In fact, this latter effect appears to be
stronger; almost 80% of the more violent delinquents had witnessed
"extreme violence," compared to 20% of the less violent delinquents.
However, a multiple regression analysis indicated that experiencing childhood abuse was not a significant predictor of the degree of delinquent

* Widom (1989a), in her analysis of the aforementioned McCord (1983) study, omitted data
for subjects who were criminals both as adolescents and as adults. If these data are included,
the percentage of abused youth who were later delinquent increases to 22%—higher than the
20% maximum rate for the prospective studies Widom considered.

violence. Overall, 40% of the variance in delinquent violence was accounted for by the presence of paranoid symptoms and minor neurological deficits. It should be noted that the results of this study are of limited generalizability since the subjects were incarcerated and there was no matched nonincarcerated control group.

In another study Lewis, Pincus, Lovely, Spitzer, and Moy (1987) compared 31 delinquents with a matched sample of 31 nondelinquent subjects. Overall, the delinquents were much more likely to have been abused (77% vs. 13%) and to have witnessed family violence (61% vs. 23%). In addition, for the delinquents, either witnessing or being the victim of violence increased the violence of their delinquent acts. Similar, but weaker, results were found for the control sample. Physical abuse was also significantly related to violence, suggesting a transmission of violence effect in nondelinquent as well as delinquent youth.

In another investigation using a matched cohort design, Widom (1989b) found that 15.8% of a sample of 76 children who were physically abused prior to 11 years of age were arrested—but not necessarily convicted—as juveniles or adults on suspicion of committing a violent crime; this compared to 7.9% of 667 control subjects. Neglect was also related to arrests for violent crimes: 12.5% of 609 neglected children were accused of violent offenses. Interestingly, only 7.1% of the 70 children who were both abused and neglected were arrested. Ecological theory (Belsky, 1980; Starr, 1988) and research results (Dietrich et al., 1983) suggest that the presence of multiple forms of maltreatment, for example, both abuse and neglect, are indicative of greater disturbance in family functioning. However, only 7.1% of Widom's abused *and* neglected children were arrested—less than the results for her control group. While it is hard to interpret this latter finding, Widom discusses a number of factors that need to be considered. These include the reliance on official records, low-income reporting bias, the effects on family functioning of being labeled "maltreating," and the likelihood of concealed maltreatment in the control group. The overall effect of these factors cannot be determined.

Few studies have examined whether sexually abused children become sex offenders. Because of gender differences in the commission of sex crimes, this research has focused on male victims of childhood sexual abuse. Groth (1979) analyzed case histories of 348 men convicted of sex offenses. Thirty-one percent of his sample provided self-reports of childhood sexual trauma. Subjects were divided into groups of rapists and child molesters. Overall, 32% of child molesters and 29% of rapists reported childhood sexual trauma. The trauma for the rapists was typically an event involving pressure to have sex or some other sexually stressful situation (56%). Child molesters more frequently experienced a forcible sexual assault (70%). Other differences in the type of childhood assault for the two groups included the following: (1) assault by a family member was more common for the rapists (70% vs. 27%), (2) assaults by acquaintances were more common for the child molesters (48% vs. 16%), (3) rapists were more frequently assaulted by females (62% vs. 23%), and (4) child molesters were more frequently assaulted by a male (68% vs. 32%). Groth states that the offenses committed by the child molesters "often appear to duplicate" their childhood victimization but does not provide data concerning the frequency with which subjects committed repetitive acts.

Findings of a second study indicate that the experience of childhood sexual abuse is more common for child molesters than for rapists (Seghorn et al., 1987). The researchers report that 57% of a sample of incarcerated child molesters were victims of childhood sexual assaults, significantly greater than the proportion in a contrast sample of convicted rapists (23%). In agreement with Groth (1979), they report that the child molesters were more likely than the rapists to have been abused by a non-family member (33% vs. 7%) whereas intrafamilial sexual abuse occurred at a similar rate for both the molesters (7%) and the rapists (9%). An additional important finding is that the families of the molesters were much more likely to have some other form of sexual deviation that did not involve the molester (33% vs. 12%). The families of the child molesters who had such additional sexual problems were also more likely to have another child who was also sexually assaulted, regardless of the perpetrator.

However, data from other studies suggest that the relationship between child sexual abuse and the commission of adolescent and adult sex offenses is less strong. Becker (1988) reported that only 19% of adolescent sexual offenders seen in a treatment program reported sexual abuse during childhood. Almost 40% of these had been abused by a family member. Interestingly, more than 40% of the offenders were female, with few of these being relatives.

Discussion

Research evidence suggests that physically abused children are at a higher risk of growing up to commit criminal offenses and that children subjected to greater violence in their families tend to commit more violent offenses. At first glance it may seem that the relationship between abuse and delinquency is stronger than it is. Lewis et al. (1989) conclude that fewer than 20% of abused children grow up to become delinquent. However, we often focus on the flip side of this coin, that is, the recognition that a much higher percentage of delinquents—or abusers in the case of studies of intergenerational transmission—will report having been abused.

The picture for sexually abused children is less clear, owing in part to a lack of research and in part to the fact that physical abuse refers to violence within a family whereas sexual abuse includes both intrafamilial and extrafamilial maltreatment.

The results of many of these studies are difficult to interpret owing to the frequency with which multiple forms of maltreatment have occurred for a given subject. Neglect often accompanies physical or sexual abuse and, indeed, may play a primary role in delinquency. Thus, Widom (1989b) found that neglected children were only slightly less likely than abused children to be arrested for a violent offense. Interestingly, while 7.9% of her control group were delinquent, only 5.6% of her sample of 125 sexually abused youths were delinquent. Alfaro (1981), in a study concerned mainly with neglect, concludes that maltreatment in general is a more important determinant of delinquency than the particular type of abuse or neglect involved.

While the connection between physical abuse and violence makes logical sense, we need to ask about the factors that underlie the relationship between neglect and violence. One way to conceptualize this question is in terms of the ecology of the family. For example, Garbarino (1981) notes that abuse (and, by implication, neglect) deprives children of a chance to experience social relationships that are "normal." Both abused and neglected adolescents are seen as isolated from systems of prosocial support, with the result that they are often overly influenced by peer pressure to engage in delinquent acts. A second conceptualization is that the effect of neglect may be due to poverty and the chronicity of the deprivation neglected children experience. Abuse is generally an acute problem.

The link between neglect and delinquency may be characterized as follows. Neglect occurs with greater frequency in impoverished families. Poverty is related to aggression in two ways. The first is by the frustration of living under deprived conditions. Neglecting parents report less satisfaction with their relationships with others (Crittenden, 1983) and, by implication, are more frustrated. The second link between poverty and violence is that poorer families are more violent (Straus et al., 1980). There is, however, a common link between these two hypotheses; both of them involve a lack of or dissatisfaction with social support. In addition, research on physical abuse indicates that a lack of such support is an important correlate of abuse (Starr, 1988).

Child Maltreatment in Context

As the preceding discussion indicates, emotional maltreatment is an important component of physical abuse, neglect, and familial sexual abuse (Finkelhor, 1983; Garbarino, Guttman, & Seeley, 1986; Wolfe, 1987).

Regardless of how we define emotional maltreatment, it involves a failure to meet the emotional needs of the developing child. Thus, the psychological consequences for a child of an injury inflicted by an angry parent are likely to be considerably different from those following an accidental injury in which the parent also had a part. Psychological maltreatment includes rejecting, isolating, terrorizing, ignoring, and corrupting—acts that are part of all other forms of abuse and neglect. Most of the consequences of maltreatment are due more to the psychological component of the maltreatment than to such other aspects as injury or physical deprivation (Garbarino et al., 1986; Wolfe, 1987). Maltreated children commonly display disturbances in child–caregiver attachment and in cognitive, moral, social, and emotional development (see Cicchetti & Carlson, 1989; Cicchetti, Carlson, Braunwald, & Aber, 1987; Conte & Berliner, 1988; Haugaard & Reppucci, 1988). Investigators have conceptualized the mechanisms underlying these disturbances in different ways. Thus, Finkelhor (1983) compares abuse to brainwashing that leads victims to blame themselves for the maltreatment and to develop defective self-concepts. Peterson and Seligman (1983) conclude that emotional numbing and pathological passivity are common consequences of victimization and analyze these sequelae in terms of Seligman's learned helplessness model. Alternatively, others have conceptualized the sequelae of trauma in terms of posttraumatic stress disorder (Figley, 1985).

The long-term psychological consequences of maltreatment are relevant to life-span theory. More studies have been done on victims of childhood sexual abuse than on the long-term consequences of physical abuse or neglect. Sexual abuse has been related to many different disturbances in adult functioning for both men and women (see Browne & Finkelhor, 1986; Finkelhor & Browne, 1988; Haugaard & Reppucci, 1988; Wyatt & Powell, 1988). One summary of this literature (Finkelhor & Browne, 1988) concluded that only one of eight investigations that used nonclinical samples failed to find lasting effects of sexual abuse (Tsai, Feldman-Summers, & Edgar, 1979). Multivariate analyses of data were conducted in four of these studies (Bagley & Ramsay, 1985/1986; Finkelhor, 1984; Fromuth, 1984; Peters, 1988). Results for all except the Fromuth study indicate that sexual abuse has a major influence on psychological functioning even when the effects of other variables are controlled. However, Fromuth (1986) suggests that family variables play a significant role in mediating the effects of sexual abuse.

Disturbances that have been reported in nonclinical samples of adult victims of childhood sexual abuse include the following:

1. high levels of stress (Bagley & Ramsay, 1985/1986)
2. emotional problems (Sedney & Brooks, 1984)

3. depression (Bagley & Ramsay, 1985/1986; Briere, Evans, Runtz, & Wall, 1988; Briere & Runtz, 1988; Peters, 1988; Sedney & Brooks, 1984; Stein, Golding, Siegel, Burnam, & Sorenson, 1988)
4. suicidal ideation or acts (Briere et al., 1988; Sedney & Brooks, 1984)
5. affective disorder (Stein et al., 1988)
6. poor self-esteem (Bagley & Ramsay 1985/1986), particularly, concerning sexual relationships (Finkelhor, 1984)
7. psychosis (Bagley & Ramsay, 1985/1986)
8. anxiety disorders (Bagley & Ramsay, 1985/1986; Briere et al., 1988; Briere & Runtz, 1988; Fromuth, 1986)
9. dissociation (Briere et al., 1988; Briere & Runtz, 1988)
10. somatization (Briere & Runtz, 1988)
11. sleep disturbance (Briere et al., 1988; Sedney & Brooks, 1984)
12. homosexuality (Finkelhor, 1984)
13. sexual problems (Fromuth, 1986)
14. adult sexual victimization (Fromuth, 1986)
15. alcohol or substance abuse (Peters, 1988; Stein et al., 1988)

In spite of the vast array of symptoms that appear with greater frequency in adults who were sexually abused during childhood than in those who were not, these symptoms are not universally present in abuse survivors. The picture thus mirrors what we have described as the findings of studies of the intergenerational transmission of maltreatment and of violent behavior. Bagley and Ramsay, for example, found that 17% of abused and 9% of nonabused women were clinically depressed while 19% of abused and 5% of nonabused women had very poor self-esteem. On a more global level, Russell (1986) found that adult victims of incest reported more negative life experiences than did nonincest victims. Thus, 33% of incest victims had a positive outcome compared with 59% of Russell's control group. Sedney and Brooks (1984) found that 65% of women reporting childhood sexual experiences were depressed, 51% had trouble sleeping, 43% had emotional problems, and 39% thought of hurting themselves; comparable data for the control group were 43%, 29%, 22%, and 16%.

The only evidence available concerning the long-term sequelae of physical abuse comes from studies of clinical samples. Such studies have the disadvantage that the resulting data tend to overrepresent the frequency with which negative consequences result from maltreatment, but they have the advantage of providing more complete descriptions of symptoms (Haugaard & Reppucci, 1988). In one study of 188 psychiatric inpatients, 43% of the patients had been sexually and/or physically abused as children or adults (Carmen, Rieker, & Mills, 1984). The perpetrator was a family member in 90% of cases. About half of the maltreated patients had been physically abused, less than a third were both physically and sexually abused, and the remainder were sexually abused. Many patients had a history of chronic abuse as both children and adults. The abused patients were more likely than the nonabused ones to have attempted suicide (45% vs. 30%), to have been involved with the criminal justice system (15% vs. 5%), and to be abusive toward others (25% vs. 13%). On admission the only difference between the abused and contrast sample for nine symptom categories (e.g., suicidal, conduct disorder, depressive symptoms) was a decreased likelihood of organic symptoms in the abused sample. The only comparison of the effects of different types of maltreatment concerned the display of anger and aggression in the hospital (Rieker & Carmen, 1986); 30% of victims of both physical and sexual abuse displayed uncontrolled aggression directed toward themselves, compared to 20% of sexual abuse victims, 14% of physical abuse victims, and 10% of nonmaltreated patients. This last finding suggests that there may be differing sequelae for different forms of maltreatment. However, much more research needs to be done in this area before any conclusions can be reached.

Factors Protecting Children from the Effects of Maltreatment

The preceding review indicates that negative effects are far from universal consequences of childhood maltreatment. The key question is why different victims of similar abusive treatment show such different outcomes in adulthood. Indeed, this is the major challenge facing any investigator examining lifespan development. Research provides some suggestions concerning variables that protect maltreated children from psychological sequelae of maltreatment or buffer the effects of the maltreatment. This section of the chapter reviews this literature.

Studies note that parenting practices are multiply determined (Belsky & Vondra, 1989; Cicchetti & Rizley, 1981). Child maltreatment is similarly the result of a number of factors; single-cause explanations are simplistic. Thus, maltreatment is heterogeneous with regard to the presence of different forms of maltreatment, different etiological factors, and differential responses to the maltreatment (Cicchetti & Rizley, 1981).

As the preceding literature review indicates, it is difficult to trace the relative influence of factors that mediate and exacerbate maltreatment. Indeed, many of the negative behaviors that characterize maltreated children may be due to ecological correlates of maltreatment rather than the maltreatment itself (Wolfe, 1987). The sequelae of maltreatment can thus best be understood within a framework of developmental psychopathology (see Cicchetti, 1989, for a review) in which maltreatment is seen as but one of many potential types of disturbance in the transactional system containing parents, children, and the environment. One example of the role of compensatory and buffering factors that serve to decrease the likelihood of the intergenerational transmission of maltreatment is provided by Wolfe's (1987) three-stage transitional model. In the first stage there is a reduced parental tolerance for stress and a disinhibition of aggression, traits that can be modified by social support from a spouse and other role models, economic stability, and the reinforcing effect of success at work or school. In the second stage there is poor ability to manage acute crises and the provocative behaviors of the child, an ineffectiveness that can be buffered by changes in the child's behavior, participation in parent education programs, and the availability of coping resources. Finally, in the third stage compensatory factors can operate to limit continued aggression within families. Thus, parents can become dissatisfied with the use of corporal punishment, the child may respond positively to noncoercive controls, and the community may actively constrain parental use of aggression toward the child.

Alternatively, Kaufman and Zigler (1989) examine compensatory factors in terms of Belsky's (1980) application of Bronfenbrenner's (1977) ecological theory to child abuse. This broader framework focuses on person–environment interactions (Garbarino, 1982). However, Kaufman and Zigler focus on characteristics that lead parents to be at risk for maltreating their children or that protect them from the risk, rather than the characteristics that lead an abused child to grow up to be an adult with or without significant problems. There is limited longitudinal lifespan research concerning the role of potential buffering factors. Thus, we have to turn to the literature summarized by Kaufman and Zigler as well as to other research to obtain clues about important buffering and compensatory factors.

A final model emphasizes the development of coercive cycles of family interaction as indicators of the inability of parents to competently raise their children and of a lack of parental social skills (Burgess & Youngblade, 1988). Thus, research on parent–child interaction in maltreating families indicates that there are significant disturbances in daily interactions (see Starr, 1988; Wolfe, 1985). Both family and peer relations play important roles in the development of social skills and in buffering the effects of maltreatment.

Studies

The research and clinical literature on child maltreatment provides information about important differences between what have been termed survivors and nonsurvivors of maltreatment (Zimrin, 1986). The results of these studies generally support the importance of the potential buffers discussed by Kaufman and Zigler (1989), Wolfe (1987), and others.

Clinical reports support the concept of the vital role of buffers (e.g., Mrazek & Mrazek, 1987; Steele, 1986). Steele suggests that a critical buffer is the presence of some nurturing person who can give love and affection to the maltreated child. However, even in these cases there are usually some detectable sequelae of maltreatment. He cites the case of Jean Jacques Rousseau, whose mother died during childbirth and who was raised primarily by a punitive aunt but experienced placement in other foster homes as well. As an adult Rousseau wrote extensively on the needs of children but was unable to care for his own progeny: all of them were voluntarily placed in foundling homes.

Mrazek and Mrazek (1987) note 12 features that can improve the developmental resilience of abused children. It is interesting to note that some of these might initially be seen negatively but can turn out to have a positive developmental influence. Their list of adaptive personal characteristics includes the following: (1) hypervigilance in order to respond rapidly to danger, (2) precocious maturity to enhance self-esteem and a sense of internal locus of control, (3) dissociation to avoid the effects of further trauma, (4) obtaining information about environmental hazards in order to better avoid them, (5) an ability to quickly form and use close relationships for support, (6) fantasizing about the future to gain control in the present, (7) taking decisive risks as a means of developing a sense of personal responsibility, (8) developing a belief that one is loved by someone, even God, (9) identifying with other, positive, aspects of the aggressor, (10) restructuring prior negative experiences in a positive way, (11) becoming altruistic and giving to others what the individual did not himself or herself receive, and, most importantly, (12) having optimism and hope concerning oneself and the future.

The research literature provides evidence supporting many of the aforementioned conclusions based on clinical work. In an interesting study that provides indirect evidence concerning the role of buffers, Zimrin (1986) followed up 28 abused children 14 years after the abuse. She described 9 of them as survivors who were well adjusted and 19 as nonsurvivors who exhibited significant pathology. The two groups differed in that the survivors were optimistic, felt in control of their lives, had high self-esteem, did not exhibit self-destructive behaviors, were higher in cognitive ability, had hopeful fantasies, tended to be belligerent, and had a supportive adult in their life or were responsible for caring for someone else. No differences were found for aggression and the presence of difficulties in expressing feelings and forming relationships. The key variables leading to successful adaptation to abuse were good coping skills and a relative excess of resources, such as having a supportive adult available, over stressors. These findings are interpreted as supporting Lazarus's (Benner, Roskies, & Lazarus, 1980) model of coping under stress.

In another interesting study of adolescents in group homes, abused boys who saw their parents as rejecting or neglecting had more negative perceptions of their parents than did abused boys who saw the abuse as occurring as a result of factors that were not controllable by their parents (Herzberger, Potts, & Dillon, 1981). The latter group appeared to have greater resiliency. Thus, the way children perceive their own abuse may play an important role in determining the long-term impact of the maltreatment (see Wolfe & McGee, Chapter 11, this volume).

Other research supports the notion that the emotional response of the child to maltreatment is a critical variable. Tsai et al. (1979), in their comparison of sexually abused women who were and were not receiving psychotherapy, found that the groups differed in the degree to which they reported negative feelings about the molestation at the time it occurred. The women seeking psychotherapy were under greater pressure to participate in a sexual act, experienced more pain, felt more guilt, had a greater dislike for the abuser, and were more upset. However, these effects may be due to the greater severity of the molestation in the clinical sample. The child's emotional reactions to abuse represent a likely variable of importance in determining the long term effects of maltreatment.

Perceived and actual social support represent a second class of variables that mediate the effects of maltreatment. Fromuth (1986) found that psychological adjustment in women who were sexually abused as children was more closely related to the women's perceptions of the support provided them by their parents than to the sexual abuse per se. Women who described more parental support felt less emotionally neglected during childhood, saw their parents' marriage as happier, and were less likely to report both sexual and physical abuse. Wyatt and Mickey (1988) similarly found the presence of social support to children at the time of sexual victimization to be an important variable in determining attitudes toward males in adult women.

Another study demonstrated the importance of the way in which the abusive event is perceived by the victim (Harter, Alexander, & Neimeyer, 1988). This study compared nonabused and sexually abused college women on a variety of measures. While adult social adjustment was significantly lower in the abused subjects, this difference disappeared when analyses controlled for cognitive and family characteristics. Instead, the key determinants of adult social adjustment were background family adaptability and perceived social isolation. When cases of more severe paternal incest were examined, however, they were found to be related to later social adjustment. The finding of background family adaptability is probably similar to McCord's (1983) finding that having a self-confident mother was an important long-term buffer against the effects of abuse and neglect. Finally, Egeland, Jacobvitz, and Sroufe (1988) reported that mothers who are able to break the abusive cycle are more likely to have had a supportive nonabusive adult present during childhood, to have had extensive psychotherapy, and to have a satisfying, supportive relationship with their mate. Mothers who perpetuated the abusive cycle experienced more stress and were depressed, anxious, and immature.

The presence of and ability to use social support was only one of a number of factors found to buffer the intergenerational transmission of abuse in 40 families studied by Hunter and Kilstrom (1979). Thus, parents breaking the cycle had greater social resources; they were more likely to have supportive friends, to participate in community social groups, and to utilize agency services than were those who did not break the cycle of abuse. This networking provided not only support but also alleviated stress by aiding with child care and providing financial and other resources needed in times of crisis. The nonrepeating mothers were also more emotionally in touch with the maltreatment they suffered from during childhood, expressed more doubts about their parenting ability, and appeared to be better able to relive and discuss their childhood experiences.

Discussion

The research literature reviewed in this section suggests that many factors serve to buffer the effects of maltreatment, thus limiting the intergenerational continuity of abuse and neglect. However, the relative lack of research in this area, the reliance on retrospective analyses, the use of relatively small samples, and the paucity of studies explicitly designed to look at buffering factors make it difficult to fully understand those factors that determine adult outcomes of child maltreatment.

Perhaps it is best to consider maltreatment as but one of many marker variables that are indicative of a problem family. As Rutter (1983, 1989) indicates, psychosocial disabilities and parenting problems frequently accompany each other. The problems commonly seen as the result of maltreatment are similar to those seen in other persons whose parents had such significant difficulties as drug addiction and psychopathology. Conducting appropriate prospective longitudinal studies will not be easy. But it is the only way in which we can more completely understand the life course in relation to the consequences of maltreatment.

A LIFE-SPAN DEVELOPMENTAL
APPROACH TO MALTREATMENT

As the preceding review indicates, there are significant limitations in the existing research on adult sequelae of child maltreatment. Across several areas, similar methodological difficulties emerge, and many of the most important questions can only be answered by well-designed longitudinal studies. A key recognition in creating such designs is that simple main-effects models are unlikely to successfully disentangle the deep interconnections that characterize these phenomena. The connections between childhood experiences of maltreatment and later developmental outcomes are the result of multiple factors that interact dynamically with each other. Indeed, research models that do not permit analyses of these complex relationships may provide unclear and sometimes misleading results.

On the other hand, the best available evidence does suggest that there are significant adult sequelae of child maltreatment. Understanding these life course continuities is of major practical and theoretical importance. We contend that in order to explore these connections it will be necessary to employ a conceptual model that recognizes the organizational properties of the self-system (Cicchetti, 1989; Keating & MacLean, 1988; Rutter, 1989), the social organization of the ecological setting (Belsky & Vondra, 1989; Rutter, 1989; Starr, 1988), and the critical nature of developmental timing as key features.

In the remainder of this chapter, we highlight three themes to bear in mind in pursuing this research agenda: the use of developmentally sensitive constructs for assessing outcomes, the social organization of potentiating and compensatory risk factors, and the role of developmental timing in efforts for prevention and intervention. We focus especially on the possibilities and difficulties involved in applying this conceptual model to a life-span time frame.

Developmentally Sensitive Outcome Measures

As we have seen in the review of research, many studies of adult outcomes have quite naturally focused on relatively straightforward and discrete behaviors, such as maltreating as parents, criminal records, especially violent acts, sex offenses, and so on. We suspect that such a main-effects approach may underestimate the serious consequences of child maltreatment for at least two reasons. First, the reporting rate of these discrete behaviors may vary with many other factors, such as social class, cultural background, and so on. Second, many personality and psychosocial burdens that may exist as real outcomes of child maltreatment may not manifest themselves in behaviors that can be identified in such measures but that may nonetheless be serious enough to engender significant personal and family dysfunction.

Moving beyond an assessment of specific behavioral outcomes as the sole criteria is most productive if it is theoretically guided (Cicchetti, 1989). Central to this conception is the recognition that the self-system undergoes substantial structural reorganization throughout development. Thus, measures that are sensitive to these organizational issues are most likely to yield meaningful information on outcomes. Cicchetti (1989), for example, describes development as "consisting of a number of important age and stage-appropriate tasks which, upon emergence, remain critical to the child's continual adaptation, although decreasing somewhat in salience relative to other newly emerging tasks" (p. 385). Here we would only add that this remains true throughout adolescence and adulthood. Identifying and assessing these crucial developmental indicators is an important part of the research agenda, a point to which we return later.

The use of such a model for childhood outcomes has been explored by Aber et al. (1989). They studied three groups of children: maltreated children, who were also in poor families as indexed by receipt of AFDC (Aid to Families with Dependent Children); an economically matched (i.e., also receiving AFDC) sample of nonmaltreated children; and a middle-class control group of nonmaltreated children. The researchers constructed several measures designed to tap developmentally sensitive issues for preschoolers and early school-age children. These were combined into two constructs: secure readiness to learn and outer-directedness. In addition, they looked at behavioral symptomatology, which has of course been the key dependent measure for most previous outcome studies. Of particular interest here is that the results for the socioemotional outcomes revealed a somewhat different pattern than did those for behavioral symptomatology. Clear group differences were observed for the former, but behavioral differences were significant only for school-age children, not for preschoolers. Moreover, the patterns of relationships between the measures of developmental organization and the behavioral symptoms were different for the various samples of preschoolers. Secure readiness to learn was predictive of behavioral symptomatology for the maltreated sample, whereas outer-directedness was predictive for the economically matched nonmaltreated sample. Although there are several possible interpretations of the pattern of results (which are too complex to describe here), we suggest that the inclusion of developmentally sensitive, theoretically guided assessments offers an opportunity for understanding that is unavailable through consideration of behavioral symptomatology alone.

Drawing on such an approach to examine life-span developmental outcomes is no doubt challenging, but it is necessary. As noted earlier, Rutter (1989) identifies adult personality outcomes as more clearly discernible by research instruments than the transmission of specific behaviors. Constructing appropriate assessments of developmental organization for adolescents and adults requires consideration of the major developmental tasks of each period as well as of which of these may be most sensitive for detecting sequelae of maltreatment.

At adolescence, for example, the issues of separation and individuation within the family, as well as the accompanying cognitive differentiation and reintegration, appear to be crucial (Keating, 1990). Such issues may well be especially sensitive for adolescents who have been maltreated in that they echo and revive critical developmental conflicts of early childhood (e.g., Aber et al., 1989). Similarly sensitive issues at adolescence, young adulthood, and beyond may be fruitfully identified and explored from a life-span developmental perspective.

In employing such an approach, the notion of developmental organization needs to remain at the forefront. There are myriad complex features of any developmental level; systems, however, are self-organizing. Discovering the principles behind the organization at any specific level is an enterprise that can productively join developmental theory and developmental psychopathology (Cicchetti, 1989; Keating & Rosen, 1990). One such organizing principle is likely to be the cognitive structures that allow individuals to interpret the experiences of their socialization history (Keating & MacLean, 1988). Indeed, as some of the evidence reviewed earlier suggests, the individual's interpretation of the experience of maltreatment plays a significant role in the overall level of functioning. This further implies that a potentially important compensatory factor may be the cognitive reorganization of experienced events, whether it occurs naturally or with therapeutic assistance. The more we learn about the life-span developmental outcomes of maltreatment, the more likely we are to make deliberate intervention of this sort effective.

One further topic merits comment within this theme. Relatively few studies of the interactions between parents and children have taken into account the developmental organization of each individual. Two speculative examples suffice to illustrate the importance of this approach. Consider the parent of an adolescent who may be at risk for maltreating behavior, whether or not this has occurred previously. The entry of one's own child into adolescence raises a number of stressful issues, not the least of which are the separation and individuation conflicts noted earlier, which are in turn related to identity seeking. This added family stressor occurs for many parents at the point in their own development when similar identity issues are being revived in the guise of concerns about generativity. The co-occurrence of these developmental issues may increase negative risk factors, leading to the renewal of or newly initiated maltreating behaviors, or they may provide an opportunity for more positive resolutions of earlier dysfunctional relations. Such matches or mismatches of parent and child developmental organization and crises may yield a cycling of maltreatment and reconciliation, leading to diverse patterns of adult outcomes.

A second example highlights the potential effects of interpersonal relationships in later development for individuals with a history of maltreatment. There has been considerable interest in the developmental effects for the child of a secure versus an insecure attachment relationship. But note that the quality of this relationship also has an effect on the mother (or primary caretaker). For a parent with a history of having been maltreated, the socioemotional effects of a positive or stressful relationship with one's own child may be powerful. Rutter (1989, p. 340) notes that risk tends to be cumulative, so that poor parenting (and thus, presumably, a lower quality attachment relationship) increases in likelihood with a sequence of negative developmental outcomes, as described earlier. On the other hand, compensatory factors, such as a less discordant home and a more positive marital relationship, improve the chances of better parenting. In this framework, a secure attachment may work not only to break the cycle of maltreatment for the child but may have significant adult developmental consequences of a positive nature for the parent.

Social Organization of the Ecological Setting

We noted previously Rutter's (1989) description of research findings that suggest that events that tend to potentiate maltreatment do not operate independently in the social setting. Both the ecological system and the self-system are organized. A number of the potentiating risk factors for child maltreatment (Belsky & Vondra, 1989; Cicchetti, 1989; Rutter, 1989), whether of enduring or transient nature, arise from systemic features of the social ecology. Factors such as poverty, economic marginalization, unemployment, marital discord, and chaotic neighborhoods are often related in the real world. Thus, *nonmaltreated* children from AFDC families exhibit many substantial developmental effects that resemble but are less severe than those found for maltreated children from AFDC families (Aber et al., 1989). It is, of course, incorrect to suggest that child maltreatment always occurs in families with the burden of such stressors, or that it does not occur in families immune to such burdens. But when we examine the range of risk factors for maltreatment, it is important to recognize that a parent's history of having been maltreated is only one specific factor enmeshed in an intricate network of other factors. For research focusing on the sequelae of maltreatment, it is necessary to disentangle the specific effects of maltreatment from these potentially confounding associated factors. For research focusing on the etiology of maltreatment, it is important to recognize that the accumulation of negative risk factors may well be adequate to trigger these behaviors, even in the absence of a parental history of maltreatment. And for research on prevention, it is crucial to realize that these broad social system factors increase family burdens dramatically, such that the incidence of maltreatment is likely to increase under their weight, with or without a previous history of maltreatment. Breaking a cycle of maltreatment requires a dual focus on the development of the individual parent who may engage in it and on the social risk factors that potentiate it.

Prevention and Intervention from a Developmental Perspective

Most of the issues relevant to the prevention and intervention of maltreatment of children have been discussed; here we focus on key factors from a developmental perspective.

It is helpful to consider prevention both in terms of the self-system and the social system. We have already noted that many social risk factors do not occur independently, that they are themselves organizationally related. One implication of this is that by construing development as not just an individual history but as a transaction of the individual and the social environment, we can identify more clearly the critical features of that ecology. Although we need more systematic research from this perspective, the main outlines are reasonably clear. The burdens on families arising from major social dislocations constitute significant potentiating risk factors for child maltreatment. Even in the absence of maltreatment, the developmental sequelae of such dislocations are significant (Aber et al., 1989). From this perspective, it may be useful to conceive of maltreatment in the traditional sense as the special case of intrafamilial maltreatment. In a larger sense, this is a subset of a system of general child maltreatment, another subset of which may be termed social maltreatment. The latter is an important aspect of contemporary childrearing in the United States, when one considers the large and increasing proportion of the child population growing up in officially defined poverty. Prevention of child maltreatment in terms of social systems could productively address these broad risk factors, which are highlighted by an explicitly developmental perspective.

At the individual level, several aspects of a developmental model are crucial for both prevention and intervention. First, it is important to generate a broader research base for the understanding of issues that reflect the appropriate level of developmental organization and, within that, to focus on those that are especially sensitive to long-term effects of maltreatment. In other words, the identification and deliberate enhancement of compensatory factors depends crucially on a better understanding of the individual's level of developmental organization. Second, dynamic models of development recognize not only that there are multiple determinants that interact in a complex system but also that the cause-effect relationship is often nonlinear. Events that appear small in magnitude may have major effects on subsequent outcomes, depending on the timing of those events. Similarly, a self-system that has settled into a stable but dysfunctional organization may be resistant to seemingly major efforts at intervention. Discovering critical developmental periods during which plasticity is highest, for example, would be of great value for providing positive intervention as well as for targeting periods of highest risk in order to guide efforts at prevention.

From our review of the literature on maltreatment and its developmental sequelae, it strikes us rather forcibly that the field has embarked on a new phase in its own development. The research agenda arising from the application of explicitly developmental models such as those described here is challenging, but it also offers the hope of achieving a much deeper theoretical understanding and far more effective methods of prevention, intervention, and therapy.

REFERENCES

Aber, J. L., Allen, J. P., Carlson, V., & Cicchetti, D. (1989). The effects of maltreatment on development during early childhood: Recent studies and their theoretical, clinical, and policy implications. In D. Cicchetti & V. Carlson (Eds.), *Child maltreatment: Theory and research on the causes and consequences of child abuse and neglect* (pp. 579–619). New York: Cambridge University Press.

Alfaro, J. D. (1981). Report on the relationship between child abuse and neglect and later socially deviant behavior. In R. J. Hunner & Y. E. Walker (Eds.), *Exploring the relationship between child abuse and delinquency* (pp. 175–219). Montclair, NJ: Allanheld, Osmun.

American Association for Protecting Children. (1988). *Highlights of official child neglect and abuse reporting 1986.* Denver: American Humane Association.

Bagley, C., & Ramsay, R. (1985/1986). Sexual abuse in childhood: Psychosocial outcomes and implications for social work practice. *Journal of Social Work and Human Sexuality, 4,* 33–47.

Baltes, P. B. (1987). Theoretical propositions of life–span developmental psychology: On the dynamics between growth and decline. *Developmental Psychology, 23,* 611–626.

Becker, J. V. (1988). The effects of child sexual abuse on adolescent sexual offenders. In G. E. Wyatt & G. J. Powell (Eds.), *Lasting effects of child sexual abuse* (pp. 193–207). Newbury Park, CA: Sage.

Belsky, J. (1980). Child maltreatment: An ecological integration. *American Psychologist, 35,* 320–355.

Belsky, J., & Vondra, J. (1989). Lessons from child abuse: The determinants of parenting. In D. Cicchetti & V. Carlson (Eds.), *Child maltreatment: Theory and research on the causes and consequences of child abuse and neglect* (pp. 153–202). New York: Cambridge University Press.

Benner, P., Roskies, E., & Lazarus, R. S. (1980). Stress and coping under extreme conditions. In J. F. Dimsdale (Ed.), *Survivors, victims, and perpetrators* (pp. 219–258). New York: Hemisphere.

Bersani, C. A., & Chen, H-T. (1988). Sociological perspectives in family violence. In V. B. Van Hasselt, R. L. Morrison, A. S. Bellack, & M. Hersen (Eds.), *Handbook of family violence* (pp. 57–88). New York: Plenum.

Blumberg, M. L. (1974). Psychopathology of the abusing parent. *American Journal of Psychotherapy, 28,* 21–29.

Briere, J., Evans, D., Runtz, M., & Wall, T. (1988). Symptomatology in men who were molested as children: A comparison study. *American Journal of Orthopsychiatry, 58,* 457–461.

Briere, J., & Runtz, M. (1988). Symptomatology associated with childhood sexual victimization in a nonclinical adult sample. *Child Abuse & Neglect, 12,* 51–59.

Bronfenbrenner, U. (1977). Toward an experimental ecology of human development. *American Psychologist, 32,* 513–531.

Browne, A., & Finkelhor, D. (1986). Impact of child sexual abuse: A review of the research. *Psychological Bulletin, 99,* 66–77.

Burgess, R. L., & Youngblade, L. M. (1988). Social incompetence and the intergenerational transmission of abusive parental practices. In G. T. Hotaling, D. Finkelhor, J. T. Kirkpatrick, & M. A. Straus (Eds.), *Family abuse and its consequences: New directions in research* (pp. 38–60). Newbury Park, CA: Sage.

Carmen, E. H., Rieker, P. P., & Mills, T. (1984). Victims of violence and psychiatric illness. *American Journal of Psychiatry, 141,* 378–383.

Cicchetti, D. (1989). How research on child maltreatment has informed the study of child development: Perspectives from developmental psychopathology. In D. Cicchetti & V. Carlson (Eds.), *Child maltreatment: Theory and research on the causes and consequences of child abuse and neglect* (pp. 377–431). New York: Cambridge University Press.

Cicchetti, D., & Carlson, V. (Eds.). (1989). *Child maltreatment: Theory and research on the causes and consequences of child abuse and neglect.* New York: Cambridge University Press.

Cicchetti, D., Carlson, V., Braunwald, K., & Aber, J. L. (1987). The sequelae of child maltreatment. In R. J. Gelles & J. B. Lancaster (Eds.), *Child abuse and neglect: Biosocial connections* (pp. 277–298). Hawthorne, NY: Aldine.

Cicchetti, D., & Rizley, R. (1981). Developmental perspectives on the etiology, intergenerational transmission, and sequelae of child maltreatment. *New Directions for Child Development, 11,* 31–55.

Conte, J. R., & Berliner, L. (1988). The impact of sexual abuse on children: Empirical findings. In L. E. A. Walker (Ed.), *Handbook on sexual abuse of children: Assessment and treatment issues* (pp. 72–93). New York: Springer.

Crittenden, P. (1983, November). *The relationship of quality of network support to quality of child-rearing and child development.* Paper presented at the Forum for Developmental Research, Richmond, VA.

DeYoung, M. (1982). *Sexual victimization of children.* Jefferson, NC: McFarland.

Dietrich, K. N., Starr, R. H., Jr., & Weisfeld, G. E. (1983). Infant maltreatment:

Caretaker–infant interaction and developmental consequences at different levels of parenting failure. *Pediatrics, 72,* 532–540.

Egeland, B., Jacobvitz, D., & Papatola, K. (1984, May). *Intergenerational continuity of abuse.* Paper presented at the Social Science Research Council Committee on Biosocial Perspectives on Parent Behavior and Offspring Development Conference on Child Abuse and Neglect, York, ME.

Egeland, B., Jacobvitz, D., & Sroufe, L. A. (1988). Breaking the cycle of child abuse. *Child Development, 59,* 1080–1088.

Figley, C. R. (1985). From victim to survivor: Social responsibility in the wake of catastrophe. In C. R. Figley (Ed.), *Trauma and its wake: The study and treatment of post-traumatic stress disorder* (pp. 398–415). New York: Brunner/Mazel.

Finkelhor, D. (1983). Common features of family abuse. In D. Finkelhor, R. J. Gelles, G. T. Hotaling, & M. A. Straus (Eds.), *The dark side of families: Current family violence research* (pp. 17–28). Beverly Hills, CA: Sage.

Finkelhor, D. (1984). *Child sexual abuse: New theory and research.* New York: Free Press.

Finkelhor, D., & Browne, A. (1988). Assessing the long-term impact of child sexual abuse: A review and conceptualization. In G. T. Hotaling, D. Finkelhor, J. T. Kirkpatrick, & M. A. Straus (Eds.), *Family abuse and its consequences: New directions in research* (pp. 270–284). Newbury Park, CA: Sage.

Fromuth, M. E. (1986). The relationship of childhood sexual abuse with later psychological and sexual adjustment in a sample of college women. *Child Abuse & Neglect, 10,* 5–15.

Garbarino, J. (1981). Child abuse and juvenile delinquency: The developmental impact of social isolation. In R. J. Hunner & Y. E. Walker (Eds.), *Exploring the relationship between child abuse and delinquency* (pp. 115–127). Montclair, NJ: Allanheld, Osmun.

Garbarino, J. (1982). *Children and families in the social environment.* New York: Aldine.

Garbarino, J., Guttman, E., & Seeley, J. W. (1986). *The psychologically battered child.* San Francisco: Jossey-Bass.

Giovannoni, J. M., & Billingsley, A. (1970). Child neglect among the poor: A study of parental adequacy in families of three ethnic groups. *Child Welfare, 49,* 196–204.

Goodwin, J., McCarthy, T., & DiVasto, P. (1981). Prior incest in mothers of abused children. *Child Abuse & Neglect, 5,* 87–95.

Gray, E. (1988). The link between child abuse and juvenile delinquency: What we know and recommendations for policy and research. In G. T. Hotaling, D. Finkelhor, J. T. Kirkpatrick, & M. A. Straus (Eds.), *Family abuse and its consequences: New directions in research* (pp. 109–123). Newbury Park, CA: Sage.

Groth, A. N. (1979). Sexual trauma in the life histories of rapists and child molesters. *Victimology: An International Journal, 4,* 10–16.

Harter, S., Alexander, P. C., & Neimeyer, R. A. (1988). Long-term effects of incestuous child abuse in college women: Social adjustment, social cognition, and family characteristics. *Journal of Consulting and Clinical Psychology, 56,* 5–8.

Hastdorf, A. H., Richardson, S. A., & Dornbusch, S. M. (1958). The problem of relevance in the study of person perception. In R. Tagiuri & L. Petrullo (Eds.), *Person perception and interpersonal behavior* (pp. 54–62). Stanford, CA: Stanford University Press.

Haugaard, J. J., & Reppucci, N. D. (1988). *The sexual abuse of children.* San Francisco: Jossey-Bass.

Herrenkohl, E. C., Herrenkohl, R. C., & Toedter, L. J. (1983). Perspectives on the intergenerational transmission of abuse. In D. Finkelhor, R. J. Gelles, G. T. Hotaling, & M. A. Straus (Eds.), *The dark side of families: Current family violence research* (pp. 305–316). Beverly Hills, CA: Sage.

Herzberger, S. D., Potts, D. A., & Dillon, M. (1981). Abusive and nonabusive parental treatment from the child's perspective. Journal of Consulting and Clinical Psychology, 49, 81–90.

Hunner, R. J., & Walker, Y. E. (1981). *Exploring the relationship between child abuse and delinquency.* Montclair, N.J.: Allanheld, Osmun.

Hunter, R. S., & Kilstrom, N. (1979). Breaking the cycle in abusive families. *American Journal of Psychiatry, 136,* 1320–1322.

Kaufman, J., & Zigler, E. (1987). Do abused children become abusive parents? *American Journal of Orthopsychiatry, 57,* 186–192.

Kaufman, J., & Zigler, E. (1989). The intergenerational transmission of child abuse. In D. Cicchetti & V. Carlson (Eds.), *Child maltreatment: Theory and research on the causes and consequences of child abuse and neglect* (pp. 129–150). New York: Cambridge University Press.

Keating, D. P. (1990). Adolescent thinking. In S. Feldman & G. Elliott (Eds.), *At the threshold: The developing adolescent* (pp.54–89). Cambridge, MA: Harvard University Press.

Keating, D. P., & MacLean, D. J. (1988). Reconstruction in cognitive development: A post-structuralist agenda. In P. B. Baltes, D. L. Featherman, & R. M. Lerner (Eds.), *Life-span development and behavior* (Vol. 8, pp 283–317). Hillsdale, NJ: Erlbaum.

Keating, D. P., & Rosen, H. (Eds.). (1990). *Constructivist perspectives on atypical development.* Hillsdale, NJ: Erlbaum.

Lewis, D. O., Mallouh, C., & Webb, V. (1989). Child abuse, delinquency, and violent criminality. In D. Cicchetti & V. Carlson (Eds.), *Child maltreatment: Theory and research on the causes and consequences of child abuse and neglect* (pp. 707–721). New York: Cambridge University Press.

Lewis, D. O., Pincus, J. H., Lovely, R., Spitzer, E., & Moy, E. (1987). Biopsychosocial characteristics of matched samples of delinquents and nondelinquents. *Journal of the American Academy of Child and Adolescent Psychiatry, 26,* 744–752.

Lewis, D. O., Shanok, S. S., Pincus, J. H., & Glaser, G. H. (1979). Violent juvenile offenders: Psychiatric, neurological, psychological, and abuse factors. *Journal of the American Academy of Child Psychiatry, 18,* 307–319.

Mash, E. J., & Wolfe, D. A. (1991). Methodological issues in research on physical child abuse. *Criminal Justice and Behavior, 18,* 8–30.

McCord, J. (1983). A forty year perspective on effects of child abuse and neglect. *Child Abuse & Neglect, 7*, 265–270.

McCord, J. (1988). Parental aggressiveness and physical punishment in long-term perspective. In G. T. Hotaling, D. Finkelhor, J. T. Kirkpatrick, & M. A. Straus (Eds.), *Family abuse and its consequences: New directions in research* (pp. 91–98). Newbury Park, CA: Sage.

Monahan, J. (1981). *Predicting violent behavior: An assessment of clinical techniques.* Beverly Hills, CA: Sage.

Mrazek, P. J., & Mrazek, D. A. (1987). Resilience in child maltreatment victims: A conceptual exploration. *Child Abuse & Neglect, 11*, 357–366.

National Committee for the Prevention of Child Abuse and Neglect. (1978, November). Public service announcement shown at the conference *Child Abuse: Cultural Roots and Policy Options,* Philadelphia.

Peters, S. D. (1988). Child sexual abuse and later psychological problems. In G. E. Wyatt & G. J. Powell (Eds.), *Lasting effects of child sexual abuse* (pp. 101–117). Newbury Park, CA: Sage.

Peterson, C., & Seligman, M. E. P. (1983). Learned helplessness and victimization. *Journal of Social Issues, 39*, 103–116.

Pianta, R., Egeland, B., & Erickson, M. F. (1989). The antecedents of maltreatment: Results of the Mother-Child Interaction Research Project. In D. Cicchetti & V. Carlson (Eds.), *Child maltreatment: Theory and research on the causes and consequences of child abuse and neglect* (pp. 203–253). New York: Cambridge University Press.

Polansky, N. A. (1976). Analysis of research on child neglect: The social work viewpoint. In Herner & Co., *Four perspectives on the status of child abuse and neglect research.* Washington, DC: National Center on Child Abuse and Neglect. (NTIS No. PB-250 852).

Polansky, N. A., Chalmers, M. A., Buttenwieser, E., & William, D. P. (1981). *Damaged parents.* Chicago: University of Chicago.

Rieker, P. P., & Carmen, E. H. (1986). The victim-to-patient process: The disconfirmation and transformation of abuse. *American Journal of Orthopsychiatry, 56*, 360–370.

Rosenfeld, A. A. (1977). Sexual misuse and the family. *Victimology, 2*, 226–235.

Russell, D. E. H. (1986). *The secret trauma: Incest in the lives of girls and women.* New York: Basic Books.

Rutter, M. (1983). Stress, coping, and development: Some issues and some questions. In N. Garmezy & M. Rutter (Eds.), *Stress, coping, and development in children* (pp. 1–41). New York: McGraw-Hill.

Rutter, M. (1989). Intergenerational continuities and discontinuities in serious parenting difficulties. In D. Cicchetti & V. Carlson (Eds.), *Child maltreatment: Theory and research on the causes and consequences of child abuse and neglect* (pp. 317–348). New York: Cambridge University Press.

Sandberg, D. N. (1989). *The child abuse—delinquency connection.* Lexington, MA: Lexington Books.

Sedney, M. A., & Brooks, B. (1984). Factors associated with a history of childhood sexual experience in a nonclinical female population. *Journal of the American Academy of Child Psychiatry, 23,* 215–218.

Seghorn, T. K., Prentky, R. A., & Boucher, R. J. (1987). Childhood sexual abuse in the lives of sexually aggressive offenders. *Journal of the American Academy of Child and Adolescent Psychiatry, 26,* 262–267.

Spinetta, J. J., & Rigler, D. (1972). The child-abusing parent: A psychological review. *Psychological Bulletin, 77,* 296–304.

Starr, R. H., Jr. (1978). The controlled study of the ecology of child abuse and drug abuse. *Child Abuse & Neglect, 2,* 19–28.

Starr, R. H., Jr. (1988). Physical abuse of children. In V. B. Van Hasselt, A. S. Bellack, R. L. Morrisson, & M. Hersen (Eds.), *Handbook of family violence* (119–155). New York: Plenum.

Steele, B. F. (1986). Notes on the lasting effects of early child abuse throughout the life cycle. *Child Abuse & Neglect, 10,* 283–291.

Stein, J. A., Golding, J. M., Siegel, J. M., Burnam, M. A., & Sorenson, S. B. (1988). Long-term psychological sequelae of child sexual abuse: The Los Angeles epidemiologic catchment area study. In G. E. Wyatt & G. J. Powell (Eds.), *Lasting effects of child sexual abuse* (pp. 135–154). Newbury Park, CA: Sage.

Straus, M. A. (1979). Family patterns and child abuse in a nationally representative American sample. *Child Abuse & Neglect, 3,* 213–225.

Straus, M. A. (1983). Ordinary violence, child abuse, and wife-beating: What do they have in common? In D.Finkelhor, R. J. Gelles, G. T. Hotaling, & M. A. Straus (Eds.), *The dark side of families: Current family violence research* (pp.-213–234). Beverly Hills, CA: Sage Publications.

Straus, M. A., Gelles, R. J., & Steinmetz, S. K. (1980). *Behind closed doors: Violence in the American family.* New York: Anchor Press.

Tsai, M., Feldman-Summers, S., & Edgar, M. (1979). Childhood molestation: Variables related to differential impacts on psychosexual functioning in adult women. *Journal of Abnormal Psychology, 88,* 407–417.

Widom, C. S. (1988). Sampling biases and implications for child abuse research. *American Journal of Orthopsychiatry, 58,* 260–270.

Widom, C. S. (1989a). Does violence beget violence? A critical examination of the literature. *Psychological Bulletin, 106,* 3–28.

Widom, C. S. (1989b). The cycle of violence. *Science, 244,* 160–166.

Widom, C. S. (1989c). Child abuse, neglect, and adult behavior: Findings on criminality, violence, and child abuse. *American Journal of Orthopsychiatry, 59,* 355–367.

Will, D. (1983). Approaching the incestuous and sexually abusive family. *Journal of Adolescence, 6,* 229–246.

Wilson, J. W. (1987). *The ghetto underclass, poverty, and social dislocations.* Chicago: University of Chicago.

Wolfe, D. A. (1985). Child-abusive parents: An empirical review and analysis. *Psychological Bulletin, 97,* 462–482.

Wolfe, D. A. (1987). *Child abuse: Implications for child development and psychopathology.* Newbury Park, CA: Sage.

Wolock, I., & Horowitz, B. (1984). Child maltreatment as a social problem: The neglect of neglect. *American Journal of Orthopsychiatry, 54,* 530–543.

Wyatt, G. E., & Mickey, M. R. (1988). The support by parents and others as it mediates the effects of child sexual abuse: An exploratory study. In G. E. Wyatt & G. J. Powell (Eds.), *Lasting effects of child sexual abuse* (pp. 211–226). Newbury Park, CA: Sage.

Wyatt, G. E., & Powell, G. J. (Eds.). (1988). *Lasting effects of child sexual abuse.* Newbury Park, CA: Sage.

Zimrin, H. (1986). A profile of survival. *Child Abuse & Neglect, 10,* 339–349.

2

A Longitudinal Study of High-Risk Families: Issues and Findings

BYRON EGELAND
University of Minnesota

In 1975 my colleagues and I began a prospective longitudinal study of a sample of 267 high-risk infants and their families. The purpose was to determine the antecedents of good and poor parenting for individuals at risk for abusing their children. Over the years we have attempted to determine the causes and the consequences of various forms of maltreatment. In addition, we are interested in tracing the developmental pathways of good and poor child developmental outcomes and in identifying factors that influence those outcomes. The sample consisted of primiparous women who were enrolled during their last trimester of pregnancy and who were patients at the Minneapolis Public Health Clinics. The children currently range in age from 13 years 8 months to 15 years 4 months.

Our sample of mothers and children was selected to ensure a greater than average incidence of poor quality caretaking and developmental problems and disorders. The mothers were at risk for a variety of reasons, including age. Mean age at parturition was 20.5, with a range of 12 to 37 years; 62% were single; only 13% of the biological fathers were in the home 18 months after the child's birth; 86% of the pregnancies were unplanned; and 40% had not completed high school. These were multi-problem families from lower socioeconomic backgrounds living in chaotic and disruptive environments. For example, 80% of the sample moved in the first two years of the child's life and the mean number of moves was four. The risk status of the sample has been confirmed in a variety of ways. For example, 45% of the infants were classified as anxiously attached at 12 months of age. Over 50% of the children in each grade were referred for special education services. Many of the mothers had been physically abused and, as we have reported in earlier publications, approximately 15% of the children were physically and sexually abused and/or physically or emotionally neglected (Egeland, & Brunnquell, 1979; Egeland & Sroufe, 1981; Egeland, Sroufe, & Erickson, 1983; Egeland & Erickson, 1987; Pianta, Egeland, & Erickson, 1989).

Detailed and comprehensive assessments of each family began during the last trimester of pregnancy and have continued at regularly scheduled intervals through the sixth grade. Extensive data have also been collected on characteristics of the child (e.g., temperament), parents, child–parent interaction, and the environment, which includes life circumstances and stress. Data on child adaptation, the family, and environment were obtained using multiple data-gathering procedures and multiple sources of information. These comprehensive and wide-ranging assessments have allowed us to account for quality of caretaking as well as developmental outcomes of the child. We have examined the course of the development of competence/incompetence through the sixth grade, and have identified factors that account for deflections in development. At each developmental period we have a detailed picture of the adaptation of these children, and we have identified some of the factors and interactions of factors that account for good as well as poor developmental outcomes. Even though a central focus of this investigation is the study of the development of these high-risk children, this chapter will focus on child maltreatment, particularly the consequences of different patterns of maltreatment through the early school years. In the sections that follow, general issues and problems involved in the prospective study of high-risk families and their children are discussed, the findings on the consequences of maltreatment are summarized, and relevant methodological issues are identified.

DESIGN: THE AT-RISK APPROACH

In recent years the prospective longitudinal study of children and families at risk for poor outcomes has become a popular approach to the study of pathology. This recent interest is a result of the data coming from long-term follow-up studies of disturbed children (e.g., Robbins, 1978). A major question emerging from this longitudinal research is, Why do some behavior-problem children adjust and cope adequately as adults while others are maladjusted? At-risk research is also a response to the questionable conclusions that frequently result from retrospective research. Comparing deviant populations with normal or other clinical groups generally results in group differences, but these differences tell us little about what factors were important in the development of the pathology (Egeland & Brunnquell, 1979).

Distinguishing cause from consequence has always been a problem in retrospective research. In comparing abusers with nonabusers it is impossible to determine whether differences between groups lead to or result from abuse. Retrospective studies suffer from what Garmezy (1974) refers to as "etiological error": looking backward in time always provides a "cause," but the inferred relationship is misleading. Causes and effects established from retrospective approaches oftentimes are not confirmed using a prospective longitudinal design. An at-risk prospective approach provides a framework for studying the complex interaction of factors that must be considered in the etiology of maltreatment. Comparisons of abusers and nonabusers often result in simple linear explanations of the cause of maltreatment. The causes and consequences of maltreatment are complex and cannot be understood using a simple linear framework.

One strategy for learning more about complex etiologies is to examine the exceptions to predicted outcomes. For example, even though there is a strong link between abuse across generations, the results from prospective studies indicate that the relationship is not perfect (cf. Starr, MacLean, & Keating, Chapter 1, this volume). There are a number of exceptions to this predicted outcome: many individuals who were abused as children do not abuse their children. It is important that we account for why some parents were able to break the cycle of abuse and others were not. Examining the exceptions to intergenerational continuity of child abuse has provided important knowledge for understanding the antecedents of abuse (Egeland, Jacobvitz, & Sroufe, 1988; Egeland, 1988). No single theory or simple causal model will explain the complex phenomena of child abuse. However, by using high-risk subjects and attempting to identify the precipitating factors that differentiate high-risk families that abuse their children from similar families that provide adequate care, we can come closer to understanding the etiologies of abuse.

Much retrospective research is plagued by the problem of finding an adequate control group. This is basically not a problem for prospective studies, since the controls come from the same risk sample. The at-risk methodology is "probabilistic" in its approach to pathology. It is based on the assumption that a group can be identified in which a certain problem will occur with a frequency great enough to warrant extensive study of a large sample of individuals. The first step in risk research is the selection of this high-risk sample to be followed. Within this group a large percentage of the sample will not develop the target problem. This basically healthy group provides an excellent group for comparison of the effects of the various factors that put the child at risk, for it is only in contrast to good outcomes within the same sample that the major influences in the poor outcomes can be identified (Egeland & Brunnquell, 1979).

GENERAL ISSUES IN MEASUREMENT SELECTION

In planning our assessments of child adaptation we were guided by an organizational view of development (Sroufe, 1979; Sroufe, in press). Within an organizational perspective, development is viewed in terms of changing organization and patterns of behavior. In short, a holistic picture of behavior and development is sought in which the changing integration and organization of capacities are investigated rather than emphasizing the measurement of specific capacities in isolation. Adaptation is defined in terms of the salient developmental issues of a particular age. Behavior, then, is reorganized around a series of developmental tasks. In our own work we have been guided by Bowlby (1969), Erikson (1963), Sroufe (1983), and others.

The development of a secure emotional attachment between parent and infant is an example of a salient developmental issue during the infancy period, and it provides an excellent illustration of assessing adaptation and demonstrating coherence of development. Attachment is a construct that is reflected in the organization of behavior (quality of attachment) rather than the frequency of specific behaviors. Through the use of Ainsworth's Strange Situation (Ainsworth, Blehar, Waters, & Wall, 1978), individual differences in the organization (pattern) of attachment behavior have been shown to be stable over time (Egeland & Farber, 1984; Waters, 1978) whereas various discrete attachment behaviors are not stable across situations or time. In fact, most attachment behaviors change dramatically over time. For example, dependency/proximity seeking is pronounced during the infancy period, but during the toddler period, where issues of autonomy are important, proximity seeking changes dramatically. One problem with many longitudinal studies is that they have focused on examining the stability of static traits over time. As we and others have shown, specific behaviors such as proximity seeking are not stable over time. What is needed in order to predict behavior over time is a more dynamic developmental perspective, one in which *lawful transformations* of behavior over time, rather than complete stability, are sought. This approach has yielded much more powerful relationships. Developmental relationships are lawful but complex. A number of recent studies have demonstrated this coherence of individual child development over time (e.g., Bates, Maslin, & Frankel, 1985; Block & Block, 1980; Sroufe, 1983).

One example of coherence of adaptation from our own work involves children with histories of avoidant attachment patterns in infancy. These infants showed high levels of physical aggression and hostility toward peers starting in preschool (Erickson, Sroufe, & Egeland, 1985) and in the early school years (Renken, Egeland, Marvinney, Mangelsdorf, & Sroufe, 1989). An anxious avoidant pattern of attachment is characterized by a failure to seek contact with the caregiver following distress. We predicted that these infants later would be aggressive with their peers in preschool and early elementary school. Such a prediction does not follow in a simple way from the behavior shown in Ainsworth's Strange Situation; yet from developmental considerations the intense contactseeking and neediness exhibited by these children toward supportive preschool teachers was expectable (Sroufe, 1983). Parental rejection led to the avoidant pattern (Cassidy & Kobak, 1988; Egeland & Farber, 1984) but also left the child unresourceful and in need of nurturance. The intense neediness, the frustration resulting from parental rejection and unavailability, and the child's lack of adequate resources to cope resulted in anger.

The coherence of development was revealed by different manifest behavior. No explicit aggression or anger is shown in the infant attachment assessment, and, indeed, these assessments are done too early to capture meaningful differences in aggression at that time. But, again, from the inference that avoidant attachment reflects chronic rejection or caregiver unavailability, the later pattern of hostility and aggression toward peers was predicted and confirmed (Erickson et al., 1985; Renken et al., 1989).

Our longitudinal research has been guided by "process" rather than linear causality. Linear causality involves predicting later outcomes from earlier outcomes or events, and assumes that this direct relationship is causal in nature. A process approach involves the study of the effects of moderator variables on developmental adaptation. The failure to examine moderator variables is a shortcoming of much of the research on the consequences of child maltreatment. In order to account for the range of outcomes found among abused children, child characteristics such as IQ, temperament, and past developmental history must be considered along with parent characteristics, the parent–child relationship, and the families' life circumstances, including life stress and social support. Certainly, child maltreatment has been shown to adversely affect the child's development; however, the severity and pattern of outcomes vary. Some leaders in abuse research have acknowledged the need to move beyond prediction of outcomes to more process-oriented research (Aber & Allen, 1987); unfortunately, too few investigations of outcome employ such an approach.

In the original conceptualization of our longitudinal study and in the selection of measures of child adaptation, parenting, and moderator variables, we were guided by Sameroff and Chandler's transactional model (1975). This model presents the environment and the child as mutually influencing; the continued manifestation of maladaptation or adaptation depends on the environmental response, and the child characteristics, in part, determine the nature of the environment. This model goes beyond the linear model, which demands simple one-to-one causal relationships, to a formulation of developmental continuity that can embrace both change and stability. Disordered behavior results from a complex set of mutually influencing interactive factors, an ongoing adaptation between child and parent and between environment and family.

Many investigations of the outcomes of child abuse can be criticized for focusing on single outcomes. For example, focusing on academic achievement as a consequence of abuse may lead to the conclusion that abuse does not adversely affect all children. Some abused children will not show academic deficits, but this does not mean they are competent in all areas of functioning. Using an assessment of only one area of competence and adaptation provides an incomplete picture of the effects of abuse. Bergman (1988) and Magnusson and Bergman (1990) talk about this as variable-oriented research, which consists of the study of the stability of single aspects of functioning. They, along with Cairns (1986), note that variable-oriented research needs to be complemented with person-oriented research, in which the person is the main unit of interest. This view is consistent with our approach to adaptation as defined by the salient developmental issues of a particular age. A related problem exists in using the same measure of a specific behavior across a wide age range. For example, measures of acting-out behaviors, such as noncompliance, have very different meanings for children of different ages. A 2-year-old who is noncompliant is displaying normal behavior for this developmental period whereas the same behavior observed in an 8-year-old indicates a problem. This behavior has very different meanings across these two developmental periods. From the perspective of a transactional model, it is clear that heterotypic continuity (continuity of patterns of behavioral organization) is to be sought rather than what Kagan (1971) calls complete continuity or stability of the frequency of discrete behaviors from Time 1 to Time 2. Since environment and child are viewed as mutually influencing, it follows that behavior at Time 2 reflects not only quality of adaptation at Time 1 but also the intervening environmental inputs and supports.

The importance of comprehensive measures of child adaptation and the need to examine development from a transactional process orientation has guided our decisions regarding particular measures and testing schedules. We were also guided by a number of practical considerations, including issues of statistical power and subject-to-variable ratio. Our emphasis has been on broad-based comprehensive measures. The actual number of measures included in a particular assessment battery must be within acceptable limits, depending on the number of subjects and the type of statistical analyses to be conducted.

There are many other practical considerations. For example, we have moved away from paper and pencil tests of parenting attitudes and skills. Some of our parents read below the third-grade level, and in general, paper and pencil tests of parenting are poor predictors of actual parenting behavior. For example, parents' ratings of their child's behavior on the Child Behavior Checklist (Achenbach & Edelbrock, 1980) did not significantly relate to teacher ratings or our observation of the child.

Many measures were not suited for use with a poverty sample. At the time the study began, there were no available stressful life event inventories appropriate for this group. We developed our own measure of life stress that included a qualitative scoring of the degree of disruptiveness of each event (Egeland, Breitenbucher, & Rosenberg, 1984). Even asking straightforward questions in an interview format often resulted in inaccurate information. Drug and alcohol use, discipline practices, mother's relationship history, and even sample questions about friends and social support often resulted in misleading information. Mothers told us that they had many friends, but when asked specifics, they did not know addresses or phone numbers and had not seen the individuals for months.

Classifying and categorizing information from interviews is often not as simple as it appears on the surface. For example, we have always been interested in family relationship status. Even the basic categories of "single parent" or "intact family" are not straightforward. Men move in and out of the household and relationships change frequently. Over the years we have developed an increasing number of qualitative scoring and coding systems for interview data having to do with parenting, satisfaction with spouse, emotional support, and so forth. Even though there are problems in accurately "rating" qualitative data, we have found that often it is more valid than quantitative approaches. Obviously, the success of qualitative ratings depends on the skills of the interviewer and coder. We have gone to great lengths to select the most qualified interviewers and coders and we spend considerable time training them.

We have also used qualitative approaches in the coding of parent–child interaction. There are many highly sophisticated procedures for counting specific interaction behaviors. We have tried these approaches, but invariably we end up using more global qualitative ratings. Gottman (1983), Patterson (1980), Bakeman and Brown (1980), and others have developed highly sophisticated sequential analytic techniques. While such techniques have been found to be useful, they are time consuming and there is some evidence to suggest that they are not as valid as the more global qualitative approaches.

One final consideration in making decisions about measures has to do with the psychometric properties of the measure. Researchers and practitioners often take for granted that most measures, particularly those with a long history, are valid and reliable. In considering the psychometric propensities of a measure, reliability and validity cannot be considered separately. A high level of reliability is essential, but high reliability is useless if the measure does not measure the desired construct. Many important constructs studied in the behavioral sciences cannot be measured with great accuracy. There must be a balance between reliability and validity.

In summary, we have attempted to assess child adaptation as defined by the salient developmental issues of a particular period. Selecting the best measures was balanced by economic reality and practical considerations. Measures were also selected because they were noninvasive of the children's privacy. We have used multiple measures and multiple sources of information. For example, our peer relations/social competence data gathered in the sixth grade come from school records and teacher interviews, ratings, and ranking of the children in the class on social competence. In addition, for a subsample of children ($n = 100$) we observed the child in the classroom on at least two occasions and completed ratings on a 7-point scale and a Q-sort. Finally, we conducted a summer camp for 48 children (16 each summer for three summers), during which time we videotaped and did detailed and intensive observations of the children.

ISSUES IN SUBJECT SELECTION

This section discusses some of the broader issues and experiences in the recruitment and retention of subjects. Sample characteristics of the 267 high-risk families enrolled in the Mother–Child Project will not be described, since they were briefly discussed in earlier sections of this chapter and in prior project publications (Egeland & Brunnquell, 1979; Egeland, Kalkoske, Gottesman, & Erickson, 1990; Sroufe, Egeland, & Kreutzer, in press).

From September 1975 to May 1977 we recruited 267 pregnant women from the Minneapolis Public Health Clinics. Every attempt was made to enroll fathers, but without much success. Altogether, 87 fathers agreed to participate, but this number decreased dramatically after they completed the three-month assessment. We decided to not include fathers in future assessments since most refused to cooperate and many threatened to also withdraw their wives and infants from the study. We regret not having father participation; however, excluding the father was necessary in order to keep the mother and child involved in the study. We are currently conducting family assessments and have invited the man in the house (approximately 70% of the mothers currently are living with a man) to participate in the assessment. About one-third of the men have agreed to participate. Not including fathers leaves major gaps in knowledge about the study of child abuse and parenting in general (cf. Biller & Solomon, 1986).

Originally 414 mothers were contacted, of whom 147 were unable to participate. In 19 cases, the husband or boyfriend refused to let the mother participate, 31 were moving, 22 delivered before the prenatal testing, 5 babies were placed for adoption, 3 babies were born with physical problems, and 2 babies died during delivery. The remainder declined to participate for a variety of reasons, such as language problems, lack of time, and refusal to be observed during feeding of infant. A comparison of the clinic records of the families who participated versus those who declined did not reveal any differences between the groups in terms of age, education, occupation, clinic staff judgment of risk, and other variables recorded in the files.

Despite not finding differences on broad demographic variables, I would imagine that there were important differences between those who agreed to participate and those who declined. Were those who declined more or less at risk for caretaking problems? Unfortunately, the answer is not known, but I have a hunch that those who declined make up a bimodal distribution on the risk continuum. Some came from highly dysfunctional multiproblem families, and others met the poverty criteria but could not be considered high-risk. This low-risk group consisted of women who were college students who qualified for free medical care, who had husbands who were college students, or who had held good jobs but were currently out of work. Paikin et al. (1974) examined the characteristics of a group of individuals who refused participation in a longitudinal study of adoption. Because of the particular nature of the data base from which these investigators identified their subject pool (the population registers uniformly maintained on Danish citizens), it was possible to conduct statistical tabulations of characteristics of "refusers." Demographic characteristics that differentiated participants and refusers included the following: marital status (more unmarried refused), parental status (nonparents refused more often), and social class (significantly more male refusals were categorized as being in the lower social classes). In addition to studying characteristics of refusers, these researchers also studied the tenacity of the refusals in the face of repeated attempts at persuasion to participate. These repeated attempts were conducted over a period of several years. Neither financial incentives nor the personal touch was successful in convincing refusers to participate.

For any research there exists the question of the representativeness of the sample and the generalizability of the results. This is particularly crucial in research with abusing families. Abusing families recruited from child protective services (CPS) files will likely be different from families recruited from Parents Anonymous. Within each population there are probably differences between those who agree to participate and those who decline. Very few investigations in the abuse area report the number of subjects contacted and the proportion that agree to participate. In a classic follow-up study, Elmer (1977) began with a large subject pool of all abused hospitalized children and control groups who were also hospitalized for reasons other than abuse. She was able to recruit 40% for her four-year follow-up and less than 20% for her eight-year follow-up. Is this small fraction of the total population representative of the total population? Perhaps the reason she basically found no difference between the abused and control groups is that she was unable to find or recruit those children who were most severely abused. The most severely abused are likely to come from the most dysfunctional families, which are the most difficult to find and recruit.

Dropout is a major problem in longitudinal research. Attrition is not a randomly distributed event since certain types of individuals are more likely to refuse continual participation. Disadvantaged, single-parent, multiproblem families are generally more difficult to locate (Harway, 1984). Generalizing from a cohort where attrition is high is likely to result in errors of interpretations. Such errors are particularly problematic in pursuing research questions in the abuse area; those at greatest risk are those most likely to drop out.

At the time of our 18-month assessment we had 212 mother–infant pairs. The reasons for losing 55 mothers were the following: 20 moved out of the city, 4 babies died, 1 baby had a serious medical problem, 10 we could not find, and 20 gave no specific reason for refusing further participation in the study (the majority in this group had boyfriends who did not want them participating). At the time of the 42-month assessment we had a total of 194 subjects; this declined to 190 at first grade, 186 at second grade, and 186 at third grade. Our rate of attrition was highest for the first few years of the study. Because of the excellent rapport and trust we have with the mothers, we have had very little attrition since preschool. We have learned many lessons.

The fact that we lost only approximately 25% of our sample is quite good considering the mobility and nature of the sample. Initially we lost a number of families because we could not find them. We have since developed a number of procedures for keeping track of the families. Our testers have excellent rapport with the families (one of them has been with the project for 14 years and knows most of the families well). Mothers are given postcards addressed to the Mother–Child Project and they are asked to inform us of any change in address. This procedure works, but we have found that more personalized approaches are more effective. Over the years we have gotten to know the mothers' families and friends. We keep track of their addresses and phone numbers and, if necessary, contact them if we are having difficulty finding the mother.

Preventing dropout and keeping track of where the families live are major tasks of longitudinal research. Our relative success in this area is most likely due to a number of factors, including paying mothers (and now the child) in cash to participate, providing selective feedback to families, and at times presenting small gifts. For example, we did not gather data at 36 months. In order to keep in contact with the family we delivered "project T-shirts" to the children on their third birthday. Probably the most important reason for the low dropout rate is the previously mentioned excellent rapport and trust we have established with the families. Some families are in hiding (because of problems with welfare agencies, for example) and cannot be found and tested unless they trust the tester and are confident that the data will remain confidential.

The importance of having interviewers and testers who are sensitive and understanding of the problems experienced by many poverty families cannot be overemphasized. It is important that the tester be persistent and flexible in searching out families; much of our testing has been done at odd hours and on weekends. We stress to mothers that we will do the testing at a time that is convenient for them. We have found that it is important to keep mothers informed about what we are doing and to let them know how much we need their help. The mothers and their children are treated as people, not as "research subjects." Two final reasons for the low dropout rate of our study is that we have had an excellent working relationship with the various city and county social agencies, who have been helpful in various ways, and Dr. Amos Deinard, a coinvestigator for the first six years of the project, served as the pediatrician at the Maternal and Infant Care Clinics for most of the children.

ETHICAL ISSUES

In the United States and Canada we have come to value highly the freedom of scientific inquiry. We also have a strong respect for each individual's right of privacy. The behavioral scientist is often faced with the need to reconcile these two contradictory values. Because of the frequency with which subjects are observed and tested, longitudinal research presents a greater threat to the individual's right of privacy than most investigations employing a cross-sectional design. However, the issue of invasion of privacy is minimized if the subjects are fully informed and their consent to participate is obtained without coercion.

No doubt there are many instances of subtle pressure on individuals to participate in research. Patients recruited from medical centers or social service agencies are bound to feel some pressure to participate. The patients may feel that their treatment and quality of care are threatened if they do not cooperate with the research. Abusing parents may feel that if they do not participate they may lose their child, end up in jail, receive other forms of punishment, or not receive help. We were careful to indicate to our pregnant women that they were free to choose whether or not to participate and that if they chose not to participate (or if they decided to drop out) their medical care through Maternal and Infant Care Clinics would not be affected. It is important that the recruitment of subjects for longitudinal research be done face-to-face and that the recruiter be sensitive to possible subtle pressures to participate. This is particularly crucial for potential subjects (such as abusing parents) who may feel vulnerable to issues of reduced treatment (or termination of child rights).

Legislation was enacted in 1974 requiring all federally funded research projects to obtain written informed consent from all research subjects. With uneducated individuals, like many of those in the Mother–Child Project, obtaining informed consent may be difficult. Most do not understand the research procedures or the reasons for assessing a variety of complex variables. We have taken great care to write our consent letters in simple language (written consent is obtained at the beginning of each funding period). The testing schedule is explained, along with a description of measurement procedures and information about where the assessments will take place. We also point out that we hope to keep following the sample beyond the five-year grant period, but that this depends on future funding. The consent letters are delivered in person and explained to the mother (and now the child). We have found that a personal explanation by a staff member whom the mother knows is important.

In the consent letter we did not say we were interested in studying child abuse or poor developmental outcomes in the children. We told the mothers that we were interested in looking at the range of caretaking and developmental outcomes. Perhaps this is misleading, but we would not have been able to conduct the research if we informed parents that we were looking for child abuse. Certain research questions cannot be answered without concealing the true nature of the research (Harway, 1984). Fully revealing the nature of a measure may invite bias or may cause the individual to feel inadequate. There are no simple guidelines on how to write a consent letter, other than making every effort to uphold and maintain the individual's dignity. Researchers must give careful consideration to the importance of the study and the extent of potential harm to the dignity of the participant in developing their research procedures.

During the first year of the child's life we did 10 assessments of the mothers and babies, most of which were conducted in the mothers' homes. We got to know the families very well, and as a result we discovered instances of abuse, violence, serious drug and alcohol use, and many other serious family problems. Ethically and legally, we were obligated to see that the family received help. We used a number of different procedures. If we suspected abuse we generally reported it to the public health nurse, who investigated and reported it to CPS. If the family did not have a public health nurse or the abuse was discovered after the child was too old for one, we met with the family and asked if they would like help, including help through CPS. We have never had an instance of a family refusing help. The families trusted us and were willing to get help as long as they knew that we were their advocates. We have a good relationship with CPS and other social agencies that have been responsive to the needs of our families. I have learned over the years that abusing and troubled families are willing to get help if they receive proper guidance and support and, most importantly, if they trust the professional. We have never had to turn in a family to CPS, but if an abusing family declined help we would have no choice but to report them.

Every researcher must balance the importance of the study and the potential risk to the subject. For longitudinal research such as ours there is some degree of psychological risk. Certain interview and test questions (such as, How were you cared for as a child?) may stimulate memories of painful past experiences. We are using Main and Goldwyn's Adult Attachment Interview (1985) as part of the follow-up measure for mothers in our intervention project. Many mothers have become very upset while completing this interview. The interviewer must be sensitive to such psychological effects. If the mother shows signs of distress, she must be given the opportunity to get psychological help. Any research project dealing with potentially upsetting material must be sensitive to the psychological risk and make available psychological help.

Another crucial ethical issue for longitudinal researchers is maintaining confidentiality of the data. At any one time we have approximately 25 students and staff working on the project; our staff is constantly reminded of the importance of maintaining confidentiality. We have given a number of local speeches that include case descriptions, we are quoted in the newspapers, and we have presented the data (including case descriptions) in a number of books and journals. Test scores and other qualitative data are stored on a computer by an identification number, and we save all the raw data. All of this, plus the length of time we have studied the families, makes us conscientious about maintaining the individual's confidentiality. There are many procedures for maintaining confidentiality (such as storing data in a secure space, allowing only the statistician access to data, etc.); however, the most important safeguard is to have a mature and professional staff. It is the researcher's—and the entire staff's—responsibility to make sure data remain confidential. For reasons of confidentiality we have not given our data to a centralized data bank or other investigators for secondary analyses.

The amount of space devoted here to these ethical issues does not signify their importance. There are many difficult issues for which there are no simple answers or guidelines. All research must start with a basic respect for the dignity of the participant. Each research staff member, regardless of position, must perform his or her duties in a highly professional fashion.

THE MOTHER–CHILD PROJECT: ISSUES AND FINDINGS

This section summarizes the findings on the consequences of child maltreatment and discusses some of the methodological concerns involved in the study of the effects of child maltreatment.

The methodological issues involving risk research, measures, subject selection, and attrition discussed earlier certainly apply to the study of the effects of maltreatment. Much research in the area fails to look at moderator variables that may exacerbate the affects of abuse or serve as a protective factor. Many studies suffer from the lack of adequate control groups, poor definitions of abuse, and a failure to examine subtypes of maltreatment (e.g., comparing abused and neglected children). Those researchers who have compared physically abused children with neglected children have found differences: abused children tend to be more aggressive, and neglected children are more withdrawn, helpless, and developmentally delayed (Crittenden, 1985; Hoffman-Plotkin & Twentyman, 1984). Failure to separate groups may obscure important differences between maltreated and nonmaltreated children. The difficulty in identifying subgroups of maltreatment is the lack of clear-cut criteria. As Aber and Cicchetti (1984) discussed in their review of maltreatment research, there is no hard, clear line separating subtypes of maltreatment. It has certainly been our experience that subtype groups overlap—a fact researchers should not deny by attempting to force cases into one group or another. Research also might address the question of whether different combinations of types of maltreatment lead to different consequences for children.

One major advantage in using a high-risk sample and longitudinal format in the study of the consequences of abuse is that the nonabused children from the high-risk sample serve as an excellent control group. An important question in the study of the consequences of abuse is, To what extent are the child's problems due to maltreatment per se or to other aspects of the environment in which the child is reared? We have found that maltreatment does have consequences above and beyond the effects of poverty and its correlates. Comparing maltreated children with non-maltreated children, we have found maltreated children to function more poorly in a number of areas (Egeland & Erickson, 1987; Egeland, Jacobvitz, & Sroufe, 1988; Egeland & Sroufe, 1981; Erickson, Egeland, & Pianta, 1989). We are confident that the differences we found are due to maltreatment and not to poverty, life stress, poor quality schools, or a variety of other factors that are often associated with maltreatment.

Consequences of Different Patterns of Maltreatment

Defining abuse groups in a consistent fashion is a major problem among researchers in the area. There are no objective criteria or operational definitions of maltreatment, particularly regarding neglect and emotional maltreatment. As Aber and Zigler (1981) and others have noted, definitional issues account for a great deal of the variance in the results of empirical studies of child maltreatment.

Our conceptualization of maltreatment has been based upon what we consider to be the parameters of caretaking that enhance optimal development of the child. It has been a consistent finding in the parenting literature that available, sensitive, and responsive caretaking within an organized home environment enhances the development of the child (Maccoby & Martin, 1983). In addition to sexual abuse, physical abuse, and neglect, the forms of maltreatment we have identified using this framework are hostile/rejecting and psychologically unavailable parenting. Thus, our definition of maltreatment was based on developmentally appropriate caretaking parameters and not solely upon cases identified by CPS.

A wide variety of data, including interviews with mothers and observation in home and laboratory, were used to make judgments about the quality of care provided to the child. Using all available data, a team of project staff members discussed and classified subjects into one or more maltreatment groups. Despite the subjective nature of identifying maltreating mothers, there was nearly perfect agreement among staff members.

This process identified four groups of women who were maltreating their 2-year-old children: physically abusive ($n = 24$), hostile/verbally abusive ($n = 19$), psychologically unavailable ($n = 19$), and neglectful ($n = 24$). As is often the case in maltreatment classifications using specific categories, there were some women who fit more than one classification (Cicchetti & Rizley, 1981; Gersten, Coster, Schneider-Rosen, Carlson, & Cicchetti, 1986). Altogether there were 44 women who fit at least one category of maltreatment (cf. Pianta, et al., 1989). It is unfortunate—from a classification perspective—that behavioral patterns that compose a function as complex as caretaking do not group themselves into neat, nonoverlapping categories. However, it is apparent from our observations of these mothers that it is not unusual for children to experience more than one subtype of maltreatment at a given point in time (Pianta et al., 1989).

Behaviors of the mothers in the physically abusive group ranged from frequent and intense spanking in disciplining their children to unprovoked angry outbursts resulting in severe injuries such as cigarette burns. In all cases the abuse was seen as physically damaging to the child. All of the women in this group were involved with CPS, as reported by the mothers and cross-checked with county files.

Mothers in the hostile/verbally abusive group chronically found fault with their children and criticized them in an extremely harsh fashion. This form of maltreatment involved constant berating and harassment of the child. The findings from this group will not be summarized, since they are similar to those of the physically abusing group.

The mothers in the psychologically unavailable group were unresponsive to their children and, in many cases, passively rejected them. These mothers appeared detached and uninvolved with their children, interacting with them only when it appeared necessary. For example, in the problem-solving situation at 24 months, these mothers would ignore their child's cues for help and assistance, offer no encouragement to the child even if the child was failing to perform the task, and would appear comfortable even when the child was highly frustrated. In general, these mothers were withdrawn, displayed flat affect, and seemed depressed. There was no indication that they derived any pleasure or satisfaction from their relationship with their children.

Mothers in the neglect group were irresponsible or incompetent in managing the day-to-day activities and care of their children. Interviews and observation indicated that they did not provide adequate physical or health care and did little to protect the children from dangers in the home. In several cases, the children were observed to have extremely poor hygiene and appeared malnourished.

Finally, we identified a group of good caretakers to use as a control group (n = 85). These mothers were identified by agreement among staff members using the criterion that they could not have been considered candidates for classification in any of the maltreatment groups. That is, they represent an *average* sample within the high-risk group, not a sample of excellent caretakers. Generally, mothers in this group were characterized by responsive, sensitive caretaking; they managed to see to it that their children's needs for emotional and physical nurturance were met on a regular basis, and there was no evidence whatsoever that any of their children suffered from any form of maltreatment. These good caretaking controls were selected from the same high-risk sample as the maltreatment groups and did not differ from them on the demographic characteristics of age or income level. Our definition of maltreatment yields a base rate of approximately 16%; that is in excess of the 5% cited nationwide (Gil, 1970) and confirms the risk status of our sample. This increased prevalence of maltreatment within our sample may be explained by three possibilities. First, the sample was selected in order to increase the probability of maltreatment and therefore was expected to include a greater than base rate prevalence of maltreating mothers. Second, conceptualizing maltreatment in terms of the broad parameters of good parenting mentioned earlier increases the prevalence of identified maltreatment victims beyond the prevalence based on overt physical or sexual insult, the common basis of identification. This procedure may have resulted in a less stringent definition of maltreatment than the legal definition. However, it should be noted that comparison of CPS cases from within our maltreatment group with the non-CPS cases from our maltreatment group did not result in any differences on child outcome measures. Both maltreatment groups were functioning poorly. Finally, our close association with these families over the years has enabled us to obtain information on quality of care that it would not be possible to obtain in cross-sectional or retrospective studies. Our findings on prevalence of child maltreatment suggest that it is a more prevalent phenomenon than statistics indicate and is consistent with estimates of Garbarino (1982) and Straus, Gelles, and Steinmetz (1988).

Each maltreatment group was compared to the control group on the measures of adaptation given at 12, 18, 24, 42, and 54 months, and at the end of first, second, and third grade in school. Since physical abuse often accompanies other forms of maltreatment, two sets of analyses were performed: one in which each maltreatment group was compared to the control group, and one in which physically abused children were subtracted from each maltreatment group. These findings, which have been reported in detail elsewhere (Egeland & Sroufe, 1981; Egeland, Sroufe, & Erickson, 1983; Erickson, Egeland, & Pianta, 1989), are summarized here. (Again, findings from the hostile/verbally abusive group are not reported here since they are similar to those of the physical abuse group.)

Consequences of Physical Abuse

At 18 months significantly more physically abused children were classified as anxiously attached; at 24 months they were more angry, frustrated with their mother, and noncompliant, and they exhibited less enthusiasm for a problem-solving situation than did the control group. In preschool they were observed to be more hyperactive and distractible, to lack self-control, and to express more negative affect. They had lower self-esteem ratings, and when observed with mother the physically abused children were more noncompliant, negativistic, and avoidant of her. In preschool they continued to be noncompliant and angry and to express a great deal of negative affect.

The anger, defiance, and negative affect characterized the physically abused children's behavior in preschool and the early school years. These children scored lower on the Wechsler Preschool and Primary Scale of Intelligence (WPPSI) and on most achievement subtests than did those in the control group. On the Child Behavior Checklist (Achenbach & Edelbrock, 1980) they were rated by their teachers as inattentive, unpopular, aggressive, self-destructive, and obsessive-compulsive. These children lacked self-control, which made it very difficult for them to be successful in school. All but one physically abused child were referred for special education services.

There were a number of differences between boys and girls who were physically abused. Abused girls were not significantly lower on the Peabody Individual Achievement Test (Dunn & Markwardt, 1970) compared to control girls, but had more internalizing behavior problems compared to the abused boys.

Consequences of Neglect

During the infancy period significantly more neglected children were anxiously attached, compared to the control group. There were no differences on the Bayley Scales of Infant Development at 9 months, but the neglected children showed a significant decline in Bayley scores between 9 and 24 months. In the problem-solving task at 24 months the neglected children lacked enthusiasm and were angry, frustrated, and noncompliant. In the Barrier Box at 42 months they showed poor impulse control and were inflexible and uncreative in their approach to the problem. They had low self-esteem, and they often withdrew from the problem. In the Teaching Task with their mothers at 42 months, they were incompetent on all measures. They had difficulty coping and they were rated high on dependency and anger.

Neglected children continued to show a decline in functioning in the early school years. They were significantly lower on all achievement subtests, and by second grade all of the neglected children were referred for special education services. In general, these children had difficulty coping with the demands of school. They were lower on both the internalizing and externalizing scales of the Child Behavior Checklist (CBC) and on the

WPPSI and the Wechsler Intelligence Scale for Children (WISC). On the Devereux rating scale (Spivack & Swift, 1967) they were rated as extremely inattentive, uninvolved, reliant, and lacking creative initiative. In general, the neglected children were doing poorly in school in almost every area assessed. They have poor work habits and are dependent and isolated.

Consequences of Psychological Unavailability

The most striking characteristic of children whose mothers are psychologically unavailable is the severe decline in functioning in the early years. Children in the psychologically unavailable group actually looked more robust than children in the control group shortly after birth and at 3 months. There were no differences on the 9-month Bayley or 12-month assessments of attachment. By 18 months all but two were anxiously attached, and by 24 months children in the psychologically unavailable group showed a 40-point decline on the Bayley. In both observation tasks with mother at 24 and 42 months, these children were angry, noncompliant, and extremely frustrated. At 42 months they were extremely avoidant of their mothers. They showed many pathological signs in preschool and were extremely dependent and lacking in self-control.

As these children entered school they showed a fairly consistent pattern of aggression and classroom disturbance, although they were not as low in achievement as the other maltreatment groups. The severe decline in social and emotional functioning seemed to level off as the children entered school. They appeared depressed and highly dependent, and of the 55% who were referred for special education services all but one was referred for social and behavioral problems.

CONCLUSIONS

The findings indicate that children who are maltreated experience significant problems. Controlling for the effects of poverty and other aversive environmental conditions associated with maltreatment, the maltreated children showed maladaptation at each period of assessment. The range of outcomes varied, but each child showed some negative effect of maltreatment. No one was immune or invulnerable to the effects of maltreatment (Farber & Egeland, 1987).

There were both similarity of behavioral consequences and specific patterns of adaptation associated with particular patterns of maltreatment. Some of the differences included poor achievement in the children of neglectful mothers. These children had a history of environmental deprivation and lack of stimulation. They were observed to lack persistence, to have difficulty dealing with frustration, and to have poor coping skills. The deprivation, poor coping skills, and dependency do not provide the child with a good foundation for coping with the demands of school. Whereas the neglected children were socially isolated in school, the physically abused children were highly unpopular and rejected. The children of psychologically unavailable mothers were also unpopular, but they differed from the other two groups in that they were more withdrawn; like their mothers, they were emotionally unresponsive and unavailable. Thus, it appeared that the children of neglectful mothers lacked social skills, the abused children were unpopular because of their aggression, and the children of psychologically unavailable mothers were unpopular because of their social withdrawal. As observed by Bowlby, deprived children have superficial relationships, lack a capacity to care for others, and are emotionally inaccessible. Within the theory of attachment it can be said that they have developed an inner working model of not having their emotional needs met. Based on their past history of maltreatment they expect abuse, rejection, and emotional unresponsiveness from others. The influence of these expectations on social behavior and relationship patterns is clear. Our maltreated children were experiencing major social problems in the preschool and elementary school years. For those maltreated children who are not provided with an alternative model of a loving caregiver, it is likely that they will enter into abusive and unsatisfying relationships as adolescents and young adults. Unfortunately, some of these individuals will abuse their own children.

Acknowledgment. This research was supported by grants from the National Center on Child Abuse and Neglect, Administration for Children, Youth and Families (DHEW 90-C-424); the Maternal and Child Health Service of the Department of Health, Education and Welfare (MC-R-270416-01-0); the Office of Special Education, Department of Education (G008300029); the Wm. T. Grant Foundation, New York, NY; and the National Institute of Mental Health (MH 40864 01).

REFERENCES

Aber, J. L., & Allen, J. P. (1987). The effects of maltreatment on young children's socioemotional development: An attachment theory perspective. *Developmental Psychology, 23*, 406–414.

Aber, J. L., & Cicchetti, D. (1984). The socio-emotional development of maltreated children: An empirical and theoretical analysis. In H. Fitzgerald, B. Lester, & M. Yogman (Eds.), *Theory and research in behavioral pediatrics* (Vol. 2, pp. 147–205). New York: Plenum.

Aber, J. L., & Zigler, E. (1981). Developmental considerations in the definition of child maltreatment. In R. Rizley & D. Cicchetti (Eds.), *New directions in child development: Developmental perspectives in child maltreatment* (pp. 1–29). San Francisco: Jossey-Bass.

Achenbach, T., & Edelbrock, C. (1980). *Child Behavior Checklist - teacher report form.* University of Vermont: Child Psychiatry Associates.

Ainsworth, M. D. S., Blehar, M., Waters, E., & Wall, W. (1978). *Patterns of attachment.* Hillsdale, NJ: Erlbaum.

Bakeman, R., & Brown, J. V. (1980). Early interaction: Consequences for social and mental development at three years. *Child Development, 51*(2), 437–447.

Bates, J. E., Maslin, A., & Frankel, K. A. (1985). Attachment security, mother–child interaction, and temperament as predictors of behavior-problem ratings at age three years. In I. Bretherton & E. Waters (Eds.), Growing points of attachment theory and research. *Monographs of the Society for Research in Child Development, 50,* 167–193.

Bergman, L. R. (1988). Modelling reality: Some comments. In M. Rutter (Ed.), *Studies of psychosocial risk: The power of longitudinal data* (pp. 354–366). Cambridge: Cambridge University Press.

Biller, H. B., & Solomon, R. S. (1986). *Child maltreatment and paternal deprivation: A manifesto for research, prevention, and treatment.* Lexington, MA: Heath.

Block, J. H., & Block, J. (1980). The role of ego control and ego resiliency in the organization of behavior. In W. A. Collins (Ed.), *Minnesota Symposium in Child Psychology, 13,* 39–101.

Bowlby, J. (1969). *Attachment and loss: Vol. 1. Attachment.* New York: Basic Books.

Cairns, R. B. (1986). Phenomena lost: Issues in the study of development. In J. Valsinger (Ed.), *The individual subject and scientific psychology.* New York: Plenum.

Cassidy, J., & Kobak, R. R. (1988). Avoidance and its relation to other defensive process. In J. Belsky & T. Nezworski (Eds.), *Clinical implications of attachment* (pp. 300–322). Hillsdale, NJ: Erlbaum.

Cicchetti, D., & Rizley, R. (1981). Developmental perspectives on the etiology, intergenerational transmission, and sequelae of child maltreatment. In R. Rizley & D. Cicchetti (Eds.), *Developmental perspectives on child maltreatment* (pp. 31–55). San Francisco, CA: Jossey-Bass.

Crittenden, P. M. (1985). Maltreated infants: Vulnerability and resilience. *Journal of Child Psychology and Psychiatry, 26,* 85–96.

Dunn, L. M., & Markwardt, F. C., Jr. (1970). *Peabody Individual Achievement Test.* Circle Pines, MN: American Guidance Service.

Egeland, B. (1988). Breaking the cycle of abuse: Implications for prediction and intervention. In K. D. Browne, C. Davies, & P. Stratton (Eds.), *Early prediction and prevention of child abuse* (pp. 87–99). New York: Wiley.

Egeland, B., Breitenbucher, M., & Rosenberg, D. (1984). Prospective study of the significance of life stress in the etiology of child abuse. *Journal of Consulting and Clinical Psychology, 48*(2), 195–205.

Egeland, B., & Brunnquell, D. (1979). An at-risk approach to the study of child abuse: Some preliminary findings. *Journal of the American Academy of Child Psychiatry, 18*, 219–235.

Egeland, B., & Erickson, M. F. (1987). Psychologically unavailable caregiving: The effects on development of young children and the implications for intervention. In M. Brassard, B. Germain, & S. Hart (Eds.), *Psychological maltreatment of children and youth* (pp. 110–120). New York: Pergamon Press.

Egeland, B., & Farber, E. A. (1984). Infant–mother attachment: Factors related to its development and changes over time. *Child Development, 55*(3), 753-771.

Egeland, B., Jacobvitz, D., & Sroufe, L. A. (1988). Breaking the cycle of abuse. *Child Development, 59*(4), 1080–1088.

Egeland, B., Kalkoske, M., Gottesman, N., & Erickson, M. F. (1990). Preschool behavior problems: Stability and factors accounting for change. *Journal of Child Psychology and Psychiatry. 31*(6), 891–909.

Egeland, B., & Sroufe, L. A. (1981). Developmental sequelae of maltreatment in infancy. In R. Rizley & D. Cicchetti (Eds.), *New directions for child development: Developmental perspectives in child maltreatment* (pp. 77–92). San Francisco, CA: Jossey Bass.

Egeland, B., Sroufe, L. A., & Erickson, M. F. (1983). Developmental consequences of different patterns of maltreatment. *Child Abuse & Neglect, 7*, 459–469.

Elmer, E. (1977). A follow-up study of traumatized children. *Pediatrics, 59*, 273–279.

Erickson, M. F., Egeland, B., & Pianta, R. (1989). The effects of maltreatment on the development of young children. In D. Cicchetti & V. Carlson (Eds.), *Child maltreatment: Theory and research on the causes and consequences of child abuse and neglect* (pp. 647–684). New York: Cambridge University Press.

Erickson, M. F., Sroufe, L. A., & Egeland, B. (1985). The relationship between quality of attachment and behavior problems in preschool in a high-risk sample. In I. Bretherton & E. Waters (Eds.), *Monographs of the Society for Research in Child Development, 50*(1–2), 147–166.

Erikson, E. (1963). *Childhood and society* (2nd ed.). New York: Norton.

Farber, E. A., & Egeland, B. (1987). Invulnerability among abused and neglected children. In E. J. Anthony & B. Cohler (Eds.), *The invulnerable child* (p. 253–288). New York: Guilford Press.

Garbarino, J. (1982). *Children and families in the social environment.* New York: Aldine.

Garmezy, N. (1974). Children at risk: The search for the antecedents of schizophrenia: Part 1. Conceptual models and research methods. *Schizophrenia Bulletin*, No. 8, 14–90.

Gersten, M., Coster, W., Schneider-Rosen, K., Carlson, V., & Cicchetti, D. (1986). The socio-emotional bases of communicative development and early maltreatment. In M. E. Lamb, A. L. Brown, & R. Rogoff (Eds.), *Advances in developmental psychology* (Vol. 4, pp. 105–151). Hillsdale, NJ: Erlbaum.

Gil, D. G. (1970). *Violence against children: Physical child abuse in the United States.* Cambridge: Harvard University Press.

Gottman, J. (1983). How children become friends. *Monographs of the Society for Research in Child Development, 48* (whole No. 201).

Harway, M. (1984). Some practical suggestions for minimizing subject attrition. In S.A. Mednick, M. Harway, & K.M. Finello (Eds.), *Handbook of longitudinal research: Volume #1. Birth and Childhood Cohorts* (pp. 133–137). New York: Praeger.

Hoffman-Plotkin, D., & Twentyman, C. T. (1984). A multimodal assessment of behavioral and cognitive deficits in abused and neglected preschoolers. *Child Development, 55,* 794–802.

Kagan, J. (1971). *Change and continuity in infancy.* New York: Wiley.

Maccoby, E., & Martin, J. (1983). Socialization in the context of the family: parent–child interaction. In E. M. Hetherington (Ed.), *Handbook of child psychology; Vol. 4, Socialization, personality and social development* (pp. 1–101). New York: Wiley.

Magnusson, D., & Bergman, L. R. (1990). A pattern approach to the study of pathways from childhood to adulthood. In L. Robins & M. Rutter (Eds.), *Straight and devious pathways from childhood to adulthood* (pp. 101–115). New York: Cambridge University Press.

Main, M., & Goldwyn, R. (1985). An adult classification and rating system. Unpublished manuscript, University of California at Berkeley.

Paikin, H., Jacobsen, B., Schulsinger, F., Godtfredsen, K., Rosenthal, D., Wender, P., & Kety, S. S. (1974). Characteristics of people who refuse to participate in a social and psychopathological study. In S. A. Mednick, F. Schulsinger, J. Higgins, & B. Bell (Eds.), *Genetics, environment, and psychopathology.* Amsterdam: North-Holland.

Patterson, G. R. (1980). Mothers: The unacknowledged victims. *Monographs of the Society for Research in Child Development, 45* (Whole No. 186).

Pianta, R., Egeland, B., & Erickson, M. F. (1989). The antecedents of maltreatment: Results of the mother–child interaction research project. In D. Cicchetti & V. Carlson (Eds.), *Child maltreatment: Theory and research on the causes and consequences of child abuse and neglect* (pp. 203–253). New York: Cambridge University Press.

Renken, B., Egeland, B., Marvinney, D., Mangelsdorf, S., & Sroufe, L. A. (1989). Early childhood antecedents of aggression and passive-withdrawal in early elementary school. *Journal of Personality. 57*(2), 257–282.

Robbins, L. N. (1978). Sturdy childhood predictors of adult antisocial behavior: Replication from longitudinal studies. *Psychological Medicine, 8,* 611–622.

Sameroff, A. J., & Chandler, M. J. (1975). Reproductive risk and the continuum of caretaking casualty. In F. D. Horowitz (Ed.), *Review of child development research* (Vol. 4, pp. 187–244). Chicago: University of Chicago Press.

Spivack, G., & Swift, M. (1967). *Devereux Elementary School Behavior Rating Scale.* Devon, PA: The Devereux Foundation.

Sroufe, L. A. (1979). The coherence of individual development. *American Psychologist, 34,* 834–841.

Sroufe, L. A. (1983). Patterns of individual adaptation from infancy to preschool. In M. Perlmutter (Ed.), *Minnesota Symposium in Child Psychology, 16,* 41–91.

Sroufe, L. A. (1990). An organizational perspective on the self. In D. Cicchetti & M. Beeghly (Eds.), *The self in transition: Infancy to childhood* (pp. 281–307). Chicago: University of Chicago Press.

Sroufe, L. A., Egeland, B., & Kreutzer, T. (1990). The fate of early experience following developmental change: Longitudinal approaches to individual adaptation in childhood. *Child Development.* *61*(5): 1363–1373.

Straus, M. A., Gelles, R. J., & Steinmetz, S. K. (1988). *Behind closed doors: Violence in the American family* (2nd ed.). Beverly Hills, CA: Sage.

Waters, E. (1978). The reliability and stability of individual differences in infant–mother attachment. *Child Development, 49,* 483–494.

3

The Developmental Consequences of Child Abuse: The Lehigh Longitudinal Study

ROY C. HERRENKOHL
ELLEN C. HERRENKOHL
BRENDA P. EGOLF
PING WU
Lehigh University

BACKGROUND AND OBJECTIVES

The Lehigh Longitudinal Study began in 1974 as the evaluation component of a state-funded child abuse prevention and treatment demonstration program in two counties of northeastern Pennsylvania. Several federal grants were subsequently obtained. The first, from the National Center on Child Abuse and Neglect (NCCAN), was to conduct a follow-up of all families cited for abuse in the two county area during the period 1967–1976. The objective of the study was to determine the frequency with which abuse recurred. A second project, funded by the National Institute of Mental Health (NIMH) in 1975, concerned coping styles and family functioning in abusing and nonabusing families. Families in this study were from the abuse and the protective service units of two county child welfare agencies, from Head Start, and from day care programs. In this study each family had at least one preschool child between the ages of 18 months and 6 years. In 1980–1982 with funding from NCCAN a lon-

ped by reassessing families and children from
unded studies. At that time an additional mid-
is included. In the 1980–1982 assessment all
d school and most were in the 3rd to 5th

ork (1986–1989), funded by NIMH, involved
is of data from the preschool-age and school-age stud-
us was the consequences of preschool-age maltreatment for
ol-age children's cognitive, educational, emotional, social, and physical development. The analyses were in two parts: one focused on the
causal link between maltreatment and developmental status, and the other
sought to identify individual and family characteristics that differentiate
more competent from less competent children.

Hypotheses in the initial study focused on coping behaviors in abusive families. Abuse was seen as a distorted, destructive way of coping
with the stress of parenting. In this study considerable attention was given
to identifying the antecedents and consequences of abuse (R. C. Herrenkohl & E. C. Herrenkohl, 1981; R. C. Herrenkohl, E. C. Herrenkohl, &
Egolf, 1983).

Hypotheses about the school-age children focused on the longer-term
developmental consequences of abuse. Specifically, we predicted that children who were abused as preschoolers would manifest not simply the
short-term physical and emotional trauma often associated with physical
and emotional abuse but also longer term developmental consequences to
cognitive, educational, emotional, and social functioning—what we have
come to refer to as social competence (Zigler & Trickett, 1978).

In the 1985–1988 reanalyses of the preschool- and school-age data
sets we continued to examine the impact of maltreatment on children's
social competence. We wanted to examine more carefully the validity of
the relationship between maltreatment and social competence by identifying and then seeking to rule out plausible rival hypotheses (Cook &
Campbell, 1979) to the hypothesized causal link between maltreatment
and development.

As a subfocus of the causal analysis study we sought to identify
abused children who did not manifest the developmental dysfunction that
was characteristic of many abused children. It was hypothesized that the
family and community environments of such children would in some way
provide social supports that were not present in the families of nonre-
silient abused children.

In the paragraphs that follow, the overall methodology of the study is
described. This is followed by a discussion of methodological problems
and findings for each of the studies undertaken.

METHODOLOGY

Research Design

The research design was developed in 1976 for the preschool assessment. The experimental group contained families served by child welfare agencies who were identified as abusive. There were four comparison groups, each focused on a distinctive aspect of maltreatment or socioeconomic status (SES): child welfare neglectful, Head Start, day care, and middle income. The number of children in each group was as follows: child welfare abuse, 144; child welfare neglectful, 105; Head Start, 70; day care, 64; and middle income, 74—for a total of 457.

Subject Sample

Selection of the sample of abusive and neglectful child welfare families was accomplished by the two county child welfare agencies' referring to the study, over a two-year period, all new and some ongoing cases in which there was in the home at least one abused or neglected child 18 months to 6 years of age. The referred families were informed of the study by the agency and were approached by a member of the study staff to request their participation. In addition to the previously mentioned criteria we wished to have a preschool classroom or group setting in which to observe children's behavior outside the home. The child welfare children participated in one of several different types of group settings (e.g., day care family and classroom settings and Head Start classrooms) where observers could assess the child's functioning. Comparison group children were obtained directly through child care programs. Program staff described the study to all of their participating families. Study staff then approached families to obtain their agreement to participate. The programs, geographically spread throughout the two counties, included 13 Head Start centers, 12 day care programs, 2 programs for handicapped children, 3 Home Start workers, and 8 nursery school programs.

Of the children in the study 248 (54.3%) are male and 209 (45.7%) are female. While the preschool assessment focused on children 18 months to 6 years of age, we included a few older siblings. The income level of 63% of the children's families at the first (1976–1977) assessment was below $700 per month. The remainder ranged to over $3,000 per month. The numbers of children assessed in each of the 297 families are as follows: 155 (52.2%) families in which one child was assessed, 128 (43.1%) in which two children were assessed, and 14 (4.7%) in which three or four children were assessed. The demographic characteristics of the families were as follows: 83% were white, 12% had Spanish surnames, and 5% were Black; 62% were Protestant, 24% were Catholic, and less than 1% were Jewish; 86% had both a male and female head, although not necessarily married; and 34% of the female heads and 31% of the male heads had at least a high school education.

How representative of abusive families generally is our sample? The best available information is from a 1987 incidence/prevalence study of abuse (USDHHS, 1988) which provides information on three relevant issues. First, to what extent is the income level in our sample comparable to that of abusive families in the national survey? In the present study, 71% of abusive families had incomes below $15,000; national data indicate that, in 1976–1977, 99% and in 1980–1982, 72% of families labeled "abusive" were below that figure. A second issue is whether there are differences depending on geographic location. The national survey found that whether the county was major urban, urban, or rural "had no reliable impact on the incidence of maltreatment according to any measure of type or severity" (p. 5–39). This is evidence that a study done in our two-county area has relevance to other geographic areas. A further question concerns differences in severity of injuries due to abuse. The national survey found that "moderate injuries predominated, occurring in 72% of the countable cases" (p. xxi). This is quite similar to our finding of 75% moderate injuries (R.C. Herrenkohl & E. C. Herrenkohl, 1981). While our sample is not a probability sample of abused families, these comparisons point to the comparability of our sample to the larger national population of abusive families. But that universe is itself rapidly changing as the proportion of abused children reported to authorities increases. We regard it as a major strength of our initial sample that we have located many more cases of severe and abusive parenting through our in-depth interviews on disciplinary practices of supposedly normal (control) cases. For such cases, however, there is no identified universe. The previously unidentified instances in our study were indicated to have occurred "prior to the last three months," and where needed, referrals for services were made.

In the school-age assessment 83 participants (18.1%) assessed in the preschool assessment were not reexamined. This raises the possibility that participants lost to attrition were different from those who remained in the study. Several analyses were done to examine this issue. First, we tested the equality of attrition across groups. The percentage lost from each group was reasonably similar: abuse (19.4%), neglect (15.2%), Head Start (21.4%), day care (15.6%), and middle income (20.3%). We then examined differences on a number of independent and dependent variables. There were no statistically significant differences for SES variables, for sex of child, for the parent interaction variables, for all but one discipline practices variable (fathers in families lost were *less* severe than fathers in those remaining) or for children's cognitive ability scores. There was, however, a difference in children's age. The average age (in 1988) of children in the school age assessment was 15.9 years, and the average age of those lost to the school age assessment was 15.0 years. Thus, out of a rather large number of variables tested, only two were statistically significant.

Measurement Procedures

In each of two assessments a large amount of data was collected. Interviews with the mother and/or father and observations of the quality of the parent–child interactions in the home were done in both assessments. These included both observations of specific behaviors and more global ratings (E.C. Herrenkohl, R.C. Herrenkohl, Toedter, & Yanushefski, 1984). Cognitive testing of the children was done in both assessments using the McCarthy Scale in the preschool study and the Wechsler Intelligence Scale for Children—Revised (WISC-R) in the school-age study. Observations of the child in the preschool classroom were made in the preschool assessment. Observations of the (preschool-age) child's behavior were done with a rating scale that was completed by the parent–child interaction observer, by both classroom observers, and by the cognitive testing administrator. A modified form of the Achenbach Scale (Achenbach, 1978; Achenbach & Edelbrock, 1979) was completed in the school age assessment by the child's mother, father, and teacher. The child's hospital birth record was analyzed in the preschool assessment. The child's school records were analyzed in the school-age assessment. A locus of control measure (Nowicki & Strickland, 1975) was administered to the child at school age. In the school-age assessment the Rosenzweig Picture Frustration Test (Rosenzweig, 1978) was administered in the appropriate version to the parents and to the child. A case record analysis of the child welfare records of all families being served by the child welfare agencies was done in the preschool assessment and updated in the school-age assessment.

Data Analysis and Testing of Models

The research designs used in our own and others' studies of maltreatment are quasi-experimental, that is, research using such designs must cope with rival hypotheses (see Cook & Campbell, 1979) such as selection bias. In addition, difficulties arise due to lower than desirable reliability and validity of some measurement procedures. The nonequivalent control group design (Cook & Campbell, 1979; Judd & Kenny, 1981), the design on which this project is based, requires an adjustment for selection bias. The selection bias of particular concern is social status. At the correlational level the occurrence of abuse is clearly associated with various social class indicators. In exploring the causal impact of maltreatment, those few studies that have tried to control for social class have uniformly used matching or regression adjustment procedures almost certain to *under adjust* and to leave open the possibility that the findings represent residual "underadjusted selection biases" (Cook & Campbell, 1979; R. C. Herrenkohl & Wu, 1991).

The analytic strategy we have used is a progressive one. Initially, descriptive statistics and graphic methods were used to examine the distributions of variables. Correlations provided preliminary evidence of relationships between variables. Data reduction using factor analysis was done for variables presumed to measure the same construct. Descriptive statistics and reliabilities were obtained for the variables that resulted from the data reduction. Next, relationships between the variables were examined, beginning with graphic methods to identify unusual qualities of distributions; after this, simple correlational analyses were done. Multiple regression was used when appropriate. The next step was to test models proposed as explaining variation in child outcomes, beginning with the impact of maltreatment and then proceeding to more complex models. In our study of resilience in children, one-way analysis of variance and discriminant analysis were used to examine the degree to which different constructs differentiate between children characterized by high, medium, and low levels of social competence.

Testing the models was done in several steps. Since LISREL (Joreskog & Sorbom, 1984) requires at least two measures of the same construct, selecting the best operational representations of the construct is important. In most instances potential measures for a construct were selected for face validity; then, using confirmatory factor analysis, their relationship to a single construct was examined. Finally, the best representatives of a construct were tested in a two construct LISREL analysis. If this test showed that the measurement model for the construct was reasonably robust, it was continued in use; if not, additional measures were sought (Rindskopf, 1978, discusses the use of multiple measurement methods for convergent validation).

RESULTS

Preschool-Age Study

Analysis of data from the preschool study had two goals: one, construct definition, involved extensive analyses to identify empirically those vari-

ables that reflected a construct of interest and ther
provide a reliable index of that construct; the second
relationships between variables or constructs. In the
cross-sectional data were available, and analyses ten
tifying features of abusive parenting and then seekin
antecedents. Some consideration was also given to po:

Definition of Variables

Our abuse (experimental) group was defined by the service category into
which the agency had placed the family. A part of the preschool study was
an extensive content analysis of child welfare case records of families in
the experimental abuse group. We were particularly interested in differentiating between children in the abuse group by type and frequency of
abuse. The content analyses provided this information, as well as information about any other domestic violence reported in the case record.

Analyses of the case records showed that the number of *formal*
charges of physical, emotional, and sexual abuse and gross neglect often
greatly underestimated the amount of abuse indicated in a family's record.
Among families with valid formal charges 75% had one charge, 20% had
two, and the remainder had no more than five. Among these same families
33% had only one incident recorded in the case record, 28% had two,
25% had three to five incidents, and 14% had from 6 to over 15 incidents
(R. C. Herrenkohl, E. C. Herrenkohl, Egolf, & Seech, 1979).

The case record also provided information on the separations, particularly foster care, experienced by children served by child welfare. We
found that 62% of abused and neglected children experienced a living situation outside the home (i.e., either formal placement or informal
arrangements to live outside the home). We also found that 62% of the
children who were placed experienced two or more moves from one living
situation to another while outside the home and that of those returned
home 44% were reabused (see E. C. Herrenkohl & R. C. Herrenkohl,
1979). The separations and unstable living arrangements are clearly both
a consequence of abuse and an added source of stress.

Information on 39 discipline practices was obtained from the parent
interviews. Both parents were asked about the frequency with which each
practice was used, both in the last three months and prior to the last three
months, by all disciplinarians of each study child in the family. Practices
ranged from mild discipline to very severe/abusive discipline. Responses
were factor analyzed and the following categories were identified: burning, hitting so as to bruise, shaking/slapping, oral discipline (e.g., pepper
in the mouth), positive discipline, isolating or restricting, depriving of
meals, extreme threats, and frequently used practices such as spanking or

ting child to chair or room. This information was available for all
ildren and provided an alternative approach to identifying abuse only
by means of the case records.

Observations of parent–child interactions provided information on the
ongoing quality of the relationship in contrast to the episodic quality of the
discipline practices. Initially, these involved individual observation categories and ratings of specific behaviors. Later, factor analyses were done
that identified groups of related variables. The five groupings of the
observed parent behaviors were the following: negative/controlling, task
supportive, miscellaneous talking, agreeing/disagreeing, and positive affect.
The six groupings of the children's observed behavior were the following:
task involvement, negative behaviors, visual focus on parent, talking to
observer, positive affect, and child helps parent. The three groupings of
observer ratings—nervousness, warmth, and hostility—were the same for
parents and children (see E. C. Herrenkohl et al., 1984).

Examination of Relationships

In a series of analyses we learned several things. First, our original view
that the presence and extent of maltreatment was defined by the "abuse"
group designation was too simple. Within that group there were variations in type, severity, and duration of abuse that needed to be considered.
We had also begun to suspect, based on cursory case record analyses, that
there was abuse in the child welfare, "protective service" group. Second,
while bizarre instances of maltreatment were identified, abuse more frequently occurred as a part of everyday child-rearing activities, not in
response to unusual or exceptional events (R. C. Herrenkohl et al., 1983).
Abuse thus reflected inadequate strategies of coping with childrearing and
could be placed on a continuum of quality of parenting (Belsky, 1984).
Third, while we found few objective differences in abused and nonabused
children at birth, we did find that parents perceived the abused children as
more difficult (R. C. Herrenkohl & E. C. Herrenkohl, 1981). Fourth, parents who used harsh discipline techniques were more negative in interacting with their children, and those who were both neglecting and harshly
disciplining were more negative and hostile and exhibited less task-sup-
portive behavior (E. C. Herrenkohl et al., 1984). Fifth, abused children
were found to be more negative, less warm and less task involved in interaction with their parents (E. C. Herrenkohl et al., 1984). In non-family
settings they were more aggressive than non-abused children (R. C. Herrenkohl & E. C. Herrenkohl, 1981). Finally, while a statistically significant relationship was found between parents' childhood experiences of
harsh discipline and their own harsh discipline techniques, roughly half of
those abused as children did *not* abuse their children. We concluded that

experiencing abuse as a child increases the risk of one's being abusive but that other factors are influential in enhancing or diminishing that risk (E. C. Herrenkohl, R. C. Herrenkohl, & Toedter, 1983).

School-Age Study

The school-age study, conducted four years later, allowed us to determine what longer-term consequences resulted from the experience of abuse. To accomplish this, an extensive reassessment of the children and their families was done. This included parent interviews, cognitive testing of the children, observations of parent–child interactions, analysis of school records, completion by parent and teacher of a behavior inventory (Achenbach, 1978), and an analysis of the case records of all families served by child welfare. Data analyses utilized multiple regression to examine the relationship between preschool-age factors—age, sex, income level, and maltreatment indicators—and indicators of the child's developmental status at school age.

Further Definition of Maltreatment

At the outset we sought to clarify the extent of maltreatment in the non-abusive control groups. Content analyses of the case records of the protective service group of families revealed that 89.5% of these families had maltreatment incidents comparable to those for which there were formal charges of abuse in the experimental "abuse" group; 46% of the protective service children were found to have been physically abused. We also examined parents' reports of the discipline practices they used, one of which was "hit the child so as to bruise." When the frequency of use of this dimension, reported by the mother, was examined across the groups, the results were as follows: abuse, 81%; protective service, 57%; Head Start, 82%; day care, 65%; and middle-income, 40%. These results indicate that a subgroup in each of the control groups had used physical discipline that could be labeled very harsh or abusive.

Correlates of Developmental Status

The school-age study report (R. C. Herrenkohl, E. C. Herrenkohl, Egolf, & Sibley, 1984) focused on the child's developmental status as defined by school age cognitive test scores, by the Achenbach (1978) Scale, by the child's school record, and by the mother's report of the child's health at school age. Independent variables were the self-reported discipline methods at preschool age, the quality of the parent's interaction with the child at preschool age and the child's physical status at birth. Analyses were done by multiple regression with the child's age and sex and family income level controlled.

Generally, positive discipline methods were associated with higher IQs and with academic achievement as rated by the child's teacher whereas more negative methods were associated with poorer performance in school, although no single method stood out as particularly helpful or devastating. Mothers who used severe emotional discipline had children who exhibited poorer emotional adjustment. Discipline practices had little relationship to the child's health. In the parent–child interactions, negative behavior on the part of the mother was associated with lower IQ in the child whereas affectionate contact, greater overall involvement, and positive affect were associated with higher IQ. Negative interaction behavior predicted to total illnesses experienced by the child. Higher income level was positively related to IQ and to academic success, while lower income level was associated with failure to behave in a socially acceptable manner. Mothers with higher income levels were also likely to view their children in a favorable light and less likely to see their children as problematic.

A general picture emerged in which parental involvement and support, as well as mild discipline, of a preschooler was associated with higher achievement and healthier social, emotional, and physical status as a school-age child. In addition, the notable impact of income level on developmental status indicators raised the question of the role that SES plays in the overall process. A shortcoming that became apparent was that little attention was given in the analyses to neglect as distinct from physical and emotional discipline. Generally, a more comprehensive approach to defining maltreatment was needed.

Structural Equation Modeling Study

In an effort to obtain greater clarity we proceeded to reanalyze the longitudinal data using structural equation (LISREL) modeling (Joreskog & Sorbom, 1984). This method of analysis offered several conceptual and methodological improvements. It provided a strategy for taking a more comprehensive approach to measurement by focusing on constructs (e.g., emotional health, social functioning) and their relationships rather than individual variables (e.g., "friendly"). LISREL was also capable of handling a number of problems in our data such as selection bias (Cook & Campbell, 1979). Selection bias was present because the abusive families were of lower SES than were families in two of the comparison groups. LISREL could also deal with underadjustment of confounding influences that resulted from measurement error. LISREL had a further advantage in providing a basis for exploring a causal interpretation of the relationship between early maltreatment and later developmental status by allowing the evaluation of alternative hypotheses.

The use of LISREL required the development of models of the relationships to be studied. The model involved in much of the published work on the consequences of abuse is simply a two-construct model in which abuse, or some feature of abuse, is considered to influence developmental status or some feature of developmental status. A three-construct model was required to incorporate SES into the relationship between abuse and developmental status.

To implement LISREL models it was also necessary to reexamine the measurement procedures. LISREL measurement models require parallel measures to define a construct and to provide a basis for calculating reliability coefficients. Development of measurement models—that is, operational definitions of multiple measures—required to assess a construct (cf. Campbell & Fiske, 1959), even for single hypothesis testing, proved to be a sizable task.

Definition of Developmental Status Constructs

Consideration was given to developmental status as defined by the Achenbach (1978) measure. This scale examines a broad range of developmental characteristics and has reasonably good psychometric properties. Originally, a scoring procedure was developed from factor analytic results. After reconsideration, it was decided to develop a different scoring procedure more clearly oriented to social competence (Zigler & Trickett, 1978) and involving four subsets of items: *physical* well-being, *emotional* functioning, *cognitive/educational* functioning, and *social* functioning. Each item on the Achenbach scale was categorized in one of these four groups. The physical and cognitive item sets had high reliabilities as groups and were treated as single scales. The emotional and social item groups were large but, as groups, did not have high reliabilities. Each group was factor analyzed separately, and three emotional subscales and two social subscales were identified, each with acceptably high (internal consistency) reliabilities. The seven resulting dimensions and reliability coefficients were the following: physical difficulties (r_{xx} = .82), academic excellence (r_{xx} = .90), angry/negative (r_{xx} = .93), self-respecting/happy (r_{xx} = .87), withdrawn/anxious (r_{xx} = .85), acting out/destructive (r_{xx} = .93), and affectionate/friendly (r_{xx} = .87). Parallel forms of each dimension were developed by dividing the items on each dimension into two scales.

Definition of Constructs Hypothesized to Influence Development

The responses on the 39 discipline practices were scored for severity. This was accomplished by using the responses of 24 child development/ child welfare professionals who had rated each of the 39 discipline practices for severity, depending on the age of the child and the frequency of use. Mean severity ratings were used as severity weights and were assigned to each practice for each child. The practices were divided into physical practices and emotional practices. After several scoring procedures were tested and their psychometric properties considered, the physical and the emotional severity ratings were summed separately, giving a single physical discipline score (r_{xx} = .68) and a single emotional discipline score (r_{xx} = .50) for each parent's discipline of each child. The two measures of discipline (i.e., during the last three months and prior to the last three months) were available. Although analyses also indicated that mothers' and fathers' physical discipline could be used to define a single construct, ultimately only mothers' discipline methods were used, so that single parent families could be included.

Neglect was assessed using several ratings of the child done by the two parent–child interaction observers. These focused directly on the child's condition and on the parent's treatment of the child. The items were the following: evidence of emotional neglect, evidence of physical neglect, and observable injuries. Our current judgment is that these dimensions reflect the degree of neglect.

The measures of severity of physical discipline, severity of emotional discipline, and degree of neglect were available for children in both experimental and control groups. This we considered a major accomplishment. First, severity of discipline was continuous rather than categorical. Second, analyses were no longer based on the labels that child welfare agencies assigned. Comparisons of children in and out of the child welfare system could be made on the same dimensions. Third, we were also in a position to examine relationships between the maltreatment variables and other variables that might influence or be influenced by them.

Two groupings were among the parent interaction dimensions, one reflecting a positive quality and one reflecting a negative quality of parent interaction. These included both frequency counts of observed behaviors and global ratings of parental behavior. Interobserver reliability was 96% agreement (cf. E. C. Herrenkohl et al., 1984). These data were used in the LISREL analyses to indicate quality of interaction. Analyses also indicated that mothers' and fathers' interactions comprised separate constructs.

On the basis of factor analysis, several indicators of SES were selected: level of education completed by mother and by father, occupational status of mother and of father, level of family income, and number of rooms in the family dwelling (Wu, 1988). LISREL analyses indicated that analyses using the mother's occupational status and educational level led to results that paralleled those obtained when the same variables for the fathers were used. This was important for including single parent families in the analyses.

We also moved from separate indicators of the child's condition at birth to a single index based on the child's hospital birth record and the parents' interview information about the child's physical status at birth. From this information an index was developed that provided an indication of the child's status at birth. The development of this index followed a procedure suggested by Sameroff (Sameroff, Seifer, & Zax, 1982).

Children's gender differences have not as yet been examined. They will be a part of the process of examining alternative hypotheses about influences on developmental status.

Testing of Hypotheses

The strategy selected was to test two-construct models and then proceed to three-construct models. D. Campbell (personal communication, 1985) prepared a working paper for the project in which he proposed the single hypothesis approach on the grounds of parsimony and the need to avoid problems with degrees of freedom when several variables or constructs were examined simultaneously. This approach provided a baseline set of results for comparison with other studies that, for the most part, had used two-construct models, that is, maltreatment and development.

Tests of Two-Construct Models

The primary hypothesis is that maltreatment results in impaired social competence. There is no control for SES. This hypothesis was tested by examining the relationship between each of the nine abuse/interaction indicators and the seven Achenbach competence indicators. Results (LIS-REL gammas) indicated several statistically significant relationships. There was a significant relationship between emotional abuse and two social competence dimensions, academic excellence and self-respecting/ happy. Significant relationships were found between neglect and all but one (friendly) of the social competence variables. Similarly, the mother's positive and negative interactions were significantly related to all seven of the social competence variables. The father's positive interactions were related to none of the social competence indicators. The father's negative interactions were, however, related to four of the social competence variables. These were academic excellence, angry/negative, self-respecting/ happy, and acting out/destructive.

Two additional two-construct hypotheses, both involving SES, were examined. The first is that the higher the SES, the greater the social competence. This hypothesis was tested by examining the relationship between SES and the seven social competence dimensions. Results indicated a strong statistically significant relationship between SES and each social competence dimension in the predicted direction.

The second hypothesis is that SES influences maltreatment such that the lower the SES, the more severe the maltreatment. This hypothesis was tested by examining the relationship between the SES construct and each of the maltreatment indicators. Results indicated a statistically significant relationship in the predicted direction between SES and each of the maltreatment indicators except emotional discipline. The results for the maltreatment indicators are in general agreement with those of Straus, Gelles, and Steinmetz (1980).

The findings clearly indicated the potential for SES to confound the relationship between maltreatment and social competence. The strong relationship between SES and the social competence indicators and the weaker but still impressive relationship between SES and the maltreatment/interaction measures meant that the two-construct relationship between the maltreatment/interaction indicators and the social competence indicators to some degree reflected the influence of SES. To account for the effect of SES required a three-construct model in which the relationships between SES and maltreatment/interaction and between SES and social competence were considered.

Test of Three-Construct Model

The three-construct model tests the relationship between maltreatment and social competence as well as the relationship between SES and each of those two constructs (R. C. Herrenkohl, Wu, & E. C. Herrenkohl, 1988; R. C. Herrenkohl & Wu, 1991). This model adjusts for the influence of SES on maltreatment and social competence. With SES controlled in this way tests of the relationship between each maltreatment indicator and each developmental status indicator revealed only three statistically significant maltreatment/social competence relationships based on LISREL analyses. Two were between emotional maltreatment and social competence (self-respecting/happy and affectionate/friendly) and one was between father's negative interaction and the child's being angry/negative. The relationships between SES and the developmental status dimensions remained strong, however.

There were several possible explanations for these results. The effect of maltreatment could be sufficiently small that the effect of SES overpowers it (cf. Elmer, 1977; Werner, 1987). Another possibility was that the most damaging effects of maltreatment will not appear until later in the child's life (Lazar & Darlington, 1982). It is also possible that the maltreatment indicators, which were considered one at a time, were not sufficiently comprehensive to reveal their effect.

A Comprehensive Definition of Maltreatment

The explanation that a more comprehensive maltreatment construct was needed was examined. Rather than treating each type of maltreatment and parent interaction as separate constructs, we considered them jointly. Interrelationships among the different types of maltreatment were examined in an effort to determine the latent variable structure underlying them. Results indicated two possible structures. One was a single parenting construct defined by positive and negative parental interaction, parental neglect, and parental physical discipline. Results indicated that parental interactions and neglect were more central in defining the construct, with loadings in the .70s, while the two physical discipline indicators had much lower loadings. Emotional discipline did not load on this construct and, as measured, does not appear to constitute a construct of its own.

The second possible structure involved two parenting constructs. One was defined by negative and positive parental interaction and neglect, with loadings for each indicator in the expected direction in the .70s. The second construct was defined by the physical discipline indicators, with loadings ranging from the .80s to the .50s. Again, emotional discipline failed to load on this construct. Some preliminary results, described in the following section, point to the greater explanatory value of the two-construct definition of parenting.

Reexamining Maltreatment and Developmental Status

The next step was to reexamine the relationship between the maltreatment construct(s) and the social competence constructs. Initially, the measurement model for the cognitive/educational construct was reconsidered. Originally, parallel measures of the teacher's ratings of the child's cognitive/educational ability were used as indicators of the construct. The teacher's ratings and the mother's ratings were then used together. These correlated at the $r = .60$ level. Confirmatory factor analysis indicated a reasonably well defined construct; that is, factor loadings for these variables ranged from .74 to .84. These results suggested that the mother's view and the teacher's view of the child's cognitive/educational status were in reasonable accord. They agreed with the child's cognitive test score as well, which correlated with both mother's and teacher's ratings at about the same level, $r = .59$. Thus, all three were used to define a single cognitive/educational ability construct.

This definition of the cognitive/educational construct was then used to test a model that involved the SES, parenting, and the cognitive/educational constructs. First, parenting defined as a single construct was tested. Results indicated a significant relationship between parenting and cognitive status (LISREL beta = .19). With the dual-construct model of parenting there was a significant relationship between the interaction/neglect construct and the cognitive/educational construct (LISREL beta = .17), but the relationship between the discipline construct and the cognitive/educational construct was not significant (LISREL beta = .10). These results suggest that there is a significant relationship between parenting and cognitive/educational competence of the child, even while controlling for SES, and that the dominant influence is the interaction/neglect aspect of parenting.

A next step was to examine the relationship between SES, parenting, and the three emotional dimensions of competence. Again, the indicators of the emotional construct were reconsidered to determine if the mother's and teacher's ratings of the child's emotional well-being could be used to define a single construct, as was done with the cognitive/educational construct. The correlations between the teacher's and mother's ratings of the three emotional dimensions were low (r = .41, .33, .20). When factor analyses were done the loadings for the mother's ratings were lower (.28 – .55) than the teacher's ratings (.70 – .75). This led us to judge that for the child's emotional status there were two constructs, one for the mother and one for the teacher, and that the mother and teacher view the child's emotional status somewhat differently.

Analyses were done using the two-construct definition of parenting and the teacher's rating of the child's emotional status. Separate analyses were done with the mother's rating of emotional status. The results were striking. The relationship between SES and the parent interaction/neglect construct and between SES and the discipline construct were roughly equivalent in the two analyses. The relationship between SES and the emotional status construct was considerably higher in the analysis using the teacher's ratings than in the analysis using the mother's ratings, although both were statistically significant. In the analysis with the teacher's ratings of emotional status, the relationship between the parent interaction/neglect construct and the emotional construct was modest but significant (LISREL beta = .19), but the relationship between discipline and the emotional construct was low and not significant. In the analysis with the mother's ratings of the child's emotional status, the reverse was found. The relationship between interaction/neglect and the emotional construct approached zero whereas the relationship between the physical discipline construct and the emotional construct was statistically significant and strong (LISREL beta = .54). The relationship between the quality of the parent's interaction and the child's emotional status as indicated by the teacher's ratings accords with our previous findings (related to cognitive/educational ability) that parent interaction is a statistically significant influence whereas discipline is not. The finding that the reverse occurs with the mother's ratings, that discipline has a strong relationship to emotional status as rated by the mother, suggests that mothers perceive the children they discipline harshly as having emotional difficulties and probably as more difficult children. Perhaps this perception serves as a rationalization for harsh discipline.

To date, we have operationalized the SES construct, the abusive parenting (discipline and interaction/neglect) constructs, the social competence (cognitive/educational, emotional and social) constructs and the birth status construct. We have also shown that negative, uninvolved, neglecting parenting at preschool age has an impact on social competence at school age even when SES is controlled. Furthermore, we have found that for the academic excellence dimension of social competence, teachers' ratings, mothers' ratings, and cognitive test scores are in reasonable agreement concerning the child's level of capability and that the latter, in turn, is significantly influenced by the parent interaction/neglect dimension. In contrast, the teacher and mother are less in agreement on the child's emotional functioning. The severity of parental discipline was found to be strongly related to the mother's ratings of emotional functioning while negative interaction/neglect is related to the teacher's ratings. We have not yet analyzed mother's and teacher's ratings of the child's social behavior.

Study of Resilient Children

The study of resilient children began by determining which were resilient and which were damaged children. Resilient children were defined as those abused children who, on our scoring of the Achenbach measure, were in the top 40% on the cognitive/educational, social, and emotional dimensions. Eleven of the 144 children in the original abuse group were found to be at or above this level of functioning. Case studies were prepared on each child. A review of these suggested that a higher IQ, more positive parenting, and parental modeling of resilience might buffer the child against the negative consequences of abuse. Using these suggestions as a guide, the parent–child interactions of the high, medium, and low competence groups were compared on specific variables. Results showed that both parental behavior and child's IQ varied with the level of competence of the child. Mothers of more competent children were found to be more involved, more affectionate, more supportive, and less hostile, and their appearance reflected that they took more pride in themselves. The children in both the resilient abuse group and the larger group of more competent children drawn from the entire study population were found to be brighter at both preschool-age and school-age testings. This study also led to questions about the significance of other risk factors and buffering factors and to speculation about the individual characteristics contributing to a shield for high risk children. Analysis of data relevant to these factors is in progress; results to date are given in E. C. Herrenkohl and R. C. Herrenkohl (1987).

CURRENT STATUS AND FUTURE ACTIVITIES

Hypotheses Currently Being Tested

To date we have tested three broad hypotheses and are currently testing two more.

Abusive Parenting at Preschool Age Negatively Influences
School-Age Social Competence

This hypothesis has been tested in our current research, and abused children have generally been found to have significantly lower social competence than nonabused children. The child's level of cognitive/educational functioning as seen by the child's teacher and mother and as reflected by cognitive test scores are comparable. The interaction/neglect construct is influential on this cognitive dimension whereas the discipline dimension is not. Other research has not discriminated between the effects of abusive discipline and the effects of the negative quality of the interaction. For example, as a group, maltreated children have been considered to perform poorly on formal intelligence measures and exhibit learning problems (Elmer, 1977; Elmer & Gregg, 1967; Martin, Beezley, Conway, & Kempe, 1974; Morse, Sahler, & Friedman, 1970; Sandgrund, Gaines & Green, 1975). This poor performance has been at least implicitly attributed to the effect of harsh discipline. The quality of the parent–child interaction has, however, not been disentangled in these studies.

The relationship between maltreatment and emotional/personality development is more complex. The child's mother and teacher are not in close accord about the status of the child's emotional functioning. When these perspectives are distinguished, different factors are found to be at work. The severity of discipline strongly influences the mother's assessment of the child. That is to say, the mother's perception of the child's level of emotional functioning is strongly related to the severity of discipline reported by the mother. By contrast, the quality of the parent's interaction is strongly related to the teacher's perception of the child's level of emotional functioning. The child's emotional functioning as the teacher sees it is also influenced by SES. This raises questions about the findings of others, for example, Martin et al. (1974), who list distinctive personality characteristics of abused children, such as an impaired capacity to enjoy life, hyperactivity, low self-esteem, and withdrawal (Garbarino & Vondra, 1987; Gaensbauer & Sands, 1979). These observations may reflect the influence of the parent–child interaction or of SES more than they reflect harsh discipline.

A third dimension of social competence, physical development, has not been found in analyses to date to be influenced by discipline, neglect, or quality of interaction. This is in general agreement with the findings of Sherrod, O'Connor, Vietze, and Altemeier (1984).

The fourth dimension, social functioning, has not yet been examined. We expect that the effect of maltreatment on social behavior will prove to be as complex as the effect on emotional behavior. We have found effects in earlier analyses (R. C. Herrenkohl & E. C. Herrenkohl, 1981) and expect to find a relationship between some aspect of abusive parenting and social behavior. Abused children generally have been found to have poor peer relationships (Perry, Doran, & Wells, 1983; Mash, Johnston, & Kovitz, 1983), including heightened aggression to peers (George & Main, 1979; Reidy, 1977).

The remaining two hypotheses involve SES.

Preschool SES Influences Parenting

Specifically, this hypothesis is that the higher the SES, the more adequate the parenting. Our research to date has demonstrated the presence of this relationship. A major concern has been to remove the confounding influence of SES on analyses of the relationship between maltreatment and competence in children. One dimension of this confounding effect is the influence SES has on severity of discipline. Wandersman's (1973) review concludes that coercive and physically assertive techniques are more frequently used by lower class mothers (Bee, Van Egeren, Streissguth, Nyman, & Leckie, 1969; Hess & Shipman, 1965). Our own data revealed a significant correlation between SES and severity of discipline. We have also found SES to be related to the presence of neglect and to the quality of the parent–child interaction (R. C. Herrenkohl & Wu, 1991). What is not clear is what specifically about SES leads to these results.

Preschool SES Influences School-Age Social Competence

We hypothesized that the higher the SES, the greater the social competence. Our research has also demonstrated this relationship. Elmer (1977) found few overall developmental differences between abused children and accident victims in her study and suggested that this is due to their common poverty. Relationships between SES and developmental status have also been found, for example, in the areas of personality and emotional development (Sewell & Haller, 1956), intelligence and learning (Hess, 1970; Sontag, Baker, & Nelson, 1958), social skills (Reiss, 1959; Sears, Maccoby, & Levin, 1957; Sewell & Haller, 1956), and language ability (Bernstein, 1970). Again, the question is, What is it about SES that gives rise to these results?

The two preceding hypotheses involving SES underscore what has become a major theme of our research: disentangling the influence of SES from the influence of abusive parenting. From a methodological perspective the identified relationships between SES and abusive parenting and between SES and indicators of social competence suggest that the relationship between abusive parenting and developmental status is confounded by SES.

From a conceptual perspective it is important to explore how SES exerts its influence in the relationship between abuse and development. For example, are parental educational inadequacies at the root of SES's effect on parenting or are other facets of SES the source of the influence?

Two as yet untested hypotheses round out the small set to be examined as part of these relatively simple conceptual models.

Preschool Parenting Influences School-Age Parenting

Over time inadequate, abusive parenting will continue and, as the child becomes more independent, will become worse. Exploratory analyses indicate that angry, rejecting behavior by the parent during parent–child interactions is positively correlated with angry, rejecting behavior by the child (E. C. Herrenkohl et al., 1984). The mutually rejecting behavior is likely to reinforce both parent's and child's negative responses to the other. Over time this process is likely to result in alienation of the child.

School-Age Parenting Influences School-Age Social Competence

This hypothesis extends the prediction that abusive, inadequate parenting at preschool age will result in the child's manifesting lowered social competence at school age. Our prediction is that this will continue to be true as the child grows older. Data analysis on this issue is currently under way.

Hypotheses Proposed for Testing

The models tested to date provide a baseline against which other models can be compared. For example, the status of the child at birth (that is, whether the child is premature, has birth defects, etc.) can be added as a construct and examined in relationship with abusive parenting, social competence, and SES. The measurement model for the birth status construct has already been developed.

Similarly, other constructs—such as marital conflict, amount of overall stress in the family, or degree of social isolation, all available in our existing data—can each be tested as part of a larger model. The objective would be not only to determine the nature of their relationships to the other variables but also to determine if the overall adequacy of the model, an issue in LISREL modeling, is improved by the inclusion of the additional construct(s).

The adequacy of the structural equation model has not been placed at the forefront of our efforts. Rather, we have seen this issue as a later stage. The first concern was to develop adequate measurement models of each of the constructs to be examined. The second concern was to test simple two-construct models not only to establish a baseline against which to compare later stages of the work but also to provide comparison with other research because many, possibly most, of the tests of relationships between indicators of abusive parenting and developmental status have involved two constructs or variables. The third concern is to proceed to develop more adequate—in the sense of "fit"—models.

The Future of the Lehigh Longitudinal Study

Were we to proceed further with data collection, it would involve a third assessment of the children, who are now adolescents. Broadly, our view is that abusive preschool-age parenting that continues into the school-age years will result in lowered social competence during the school-age years and during adolescence. We anticipate that children whose social competence is low will grow into adolescents with equally low or even poorer levels of social competence. Inadequate, abusive parenting in the school-age years will result in weakened parent–child bonds. This will in turn result in the absence of parental support when the child becomes an adolescent. This weakened support will result in further lessening of motivation for the adolescent to behave competently. This poor social competence is expected to lead to deviant behavior and to the selection of adolescent peers who support the deviant behavior. Such behaviors include assault, theft, robbery, vandalism, drug use, drug sales, and prostitution (teenage pregnancy can also be included even though it is neither delinquency nor a status offense).

In addition, we would like to test several hypotheses about the resilient survivors of maltreatment. We expect to find that resilience in maltreated adolescents is associated with several conditions: (1) A parent or parent surrogate who has provided a sense of caring and concern in the adolescent's life is one possibility. Exploratory analyses of preschool-age and school-age data suggest that resilient school-age children have such an anchor in their lives. (2) In the resilient adolescent's early life history there will be at least a minimum of stability in the home situation. We anticipate either no foster placements or one stable placement outside the home during the first five years of life. It is predicted that trust in others and developmental competence are negatively affected by frequent changes of caretaking figures and associated disruptions of attachment. (3) Higher levels of intellectual capability, as measured by the Wechsler Adult Intelligence Scale, will be found. Exploratory analyses to date have revealed significant differences between average IQ levels of high- and low-functioning children from maltreating homes. (4) An ability to mobilize anger at the injustices they have experienced in an effort to protect themselves from further victimization will be present. (5) We expect to find an ability to envision an improved existence and a determination to achieve a better life than they have experienced as children. Clinical experience has suggested that those persons who have achieved high levels of functioning despite serious abuse in their past have been able to say, in some fashion, "never again" and aim their vision at a dream for the future, thus avoiding the sense of hopelessness and helplessness that tends to characterize lower functioning victims of abuse. (6) A support network of other high-functioning peers is predicted. While delinquent youth have frequently been found to have associations with deviant peers who reinforce each other's antisocial behavior, the same reinforcing value, in the opposite direction, of high-functioning peers is expected to be found for resilient adolescents.

Acknowledgments. Preparation of this paper was funded in part by Grant No. MH41109 from the National Institute of Mental Health. The authors express their gratitude to Donald Campbell and to David Rindskopf for their helpful suggestions.

REFERENCES

Achenbach, T. M. (1978). The child behavior profile: I. Boys aged 6–11. *Journal of Consulting and Clinical Psychology, 46*(3), 378–488.

Achenbach, T. M., & Edelbrock, C. S. (1979). The child behavior profile: II. Boys aged 12–16 and girls aged 6–11 and 12–16. *Journal of Clinical and Consulting Psychology, 47*(2), 223–333.

Bee, H. L., Van Egeren, L. F., Streissguth, A. P., Nyman, B. A., & Leckie, M. (1969). Social class differences in maternal teaching strategies and speech patterns. *Developmental Psychology, 1*, 726–734.

Belsky, J. (1984). The determinants of parenting: A process model. *Child Development, 55*, 83–96.

Bernstein, B. (1970). A sociolinguistic approach to socialization. In F. Williams (Ed.), *Language and Poverty* (pp. 25–61). Chicago: Markham.

Campbell, D. T., & Fiske, D. W. (1959). Convergent and discriminant validation by the multitrait–multimethod matrix. *Psychological Bulletin, 56*, 81–105.

Cook, T. D., & Campbell, D. T. (1979). *Quasi-experimentation: Design and analysis issues for field settings.* Boston: Houghton-Mifflin.

Elmer, E. (1977). *Fragile families, troubled children.* Pittsburgh: University of Pittsburgh Press.

Elmer, E., & Gregg, G. S. (1967). Developmental characteristics of abused children. *Pediatrics, 40*, 327–330.

Gaensbauer, T. J., & Sands, K. (1979). Distorted affective communications in abused/neglected infants and their potential impact on caretakers. *Journal of the American Academy of Child Psychiatry, 18(2)*, 236–251.

Garbarino, J., & Vondra, J. (1987). Psychological maltreatment: Issues and perspectives. In M. R. Brassard, R. Germain & S. N. Hart (Eds.), *Psychological maltreatment of children and youth* (pp. 25–44). New York: Pergamon Press.

George, C., & Main, M. (1979). Social interactions of young abused children: Approach, avoidance and aggression. *Child Development, 50*, 306–318.

Herrenkohl, E. C., & Herrenkohl, R. C. (1979, October). *Foster care of abused children: What happens after placement?* Paper presented at the National Conference on Child Abuse and Neglect, Los Angeles.

Herrenkohl, E. C., & Herrenkohl, R. C. (1987, July). *Resilience in the socioemotional development of abused children.* Paper Presented to Third National Family Violence Conference for Researchers, Durham, NH.

Herrenkohl, E. C., Herrenkohl, R. C., & Toedter, L. J. (1983). Perspectives on the intergenerational transmission of abuse. In D. Finkelhor, R. J. Gelles, G. T. Hotaling & M. A. Straus (Eds.), *The dark side of families: Current family violence research* (pp. 305–316). Beverly Hills: Sage.

Herrenkohl, E. C., Herrenkohl, R. C., Toedter, L., & Yanushefski, A. M. (1984). Parent–child interactions in abusive and non-abusive families. *Journal of the American Academy of Child Psychiatry, 23*, 641–648.

Herrenkohl, R. C., & Herrenkohl, E. C. (1981). Some antecedents and developmental consequences of child maltreatment. In R. Rizley & D. Cicchetti (Eds.), *Developmental perspectives on child maltreatment* (pp. 57–76). San Francisco: Jossey-Bass.

Herrenkohl, R. C., Herrenkohl, E. C., & Egolf, B. P.(1983). Circumstances surrounding the occurrence of child maltreatment. *Journal of Consulting and Clinical Psychology, 51*(3), 424–431.

Herrenkohl, R. C., Herrenkohl, E. C., Egolf, B. P., & Seech, M. (1979). The repetition of child abuse: How frequently does it occur? *Child Abuse & Neglect, 3*, 67–72.

Herrenkohl, R. C., Herrenkohl, E. C., Egolf, B. P., & Sibley, M. (1984). *Child abuse and the development of social competence* (Final report of the project A Longitudinal Study of the Consequence of Child Abuse). Bethlehem, PA: Lehigh University, Center for Social Research.

Herrenkohl, R. C., & Wu, P. (1991). *The validity of the relationship between abusive parenting and children's developmental status.* Unpublished manuscript.

Herrenkohl, R. C., Wu, P., & Herrenkohl, E. C. (1988, October). *The effect of SES and maltreatment on children's developmental status.* Paper presented at the meeting of the Society for Applied Sociology, Chicago.

Hess, R. D. (1970). The transmission of cognitive strategies in poor families: The socialization of apathy and under-achievement. In V. L. Allen (Ed.), *Psychological factors in poverty* (pp. 73–92). Chicago: Markham.

Hess, R. D., & Shipman, V. C. (1965). Early experiences and socialization of cognitive modes in children. *Child Development, 36*, 869–886.

Joreskog, K., & Sorbom, D. (1984). *LISREL VI user's guide.* Mooresville, IN: Scientific Software.

Judd, C. M., & Kenny, D. A. (1981). *Estimating the effects of social interventions.* Cambridge: Cambridge University Press.

Lazar, I., & Darlington, R. (1982). Lasting effects of early education: A report from the Consortium for Longitudinal Studies *Monographs of the Society for Research in Child Develolopment,* 47(2–3, Serial No. 195).

Martin, H. P., Beezley, P., Conway, E. F., & Kempe, C. H. (1974). The development of abused children. *Advances in Pediatrics,* 21, 25–73.

Mash, E. J., Johnston, C., & Kovitz, K. (1983). A comparison of mother–child interactions of physically abused and non-abused children during play and task situations. *Journal of Clinical Child Psychology,* 12, 337–346.

Morse, C. W., Sahler, O. J. Z., & Friedman, S. B. (1970). A three-year follow-up study of abused and neglected children. *American Journal of the Diseases of Children,* 120, 439–446.

Nowicki, S., & Strickland, B. L. (1975). A locus of control scale for children. *Journal of Consulting and Clinical Psychology,* 40(1), 148–154.

Perry, M. A., Doran, L. D., & Wells, E. A. (1983). Developmental and behavioral characteristics of physically abused children. *Journal of Clinical Child Psychology,* 12, 320–324.

Reidy, T. J. (1977). The aggressive characteristics of abused and neglected children. *Journal of Clinical Psychology,* 33(4), 1140–1145.

Reiss, A. J. (1959, Summer). Are educational norms and goals of conforming, truant and delinquent adolescents influenced by group position in American society? *Journal of Negro Education,* 28, 309–333.

Rindskopf, D. M. (1978). Secondary analysis: Using multiple analysis approaches with Head Start and Title I data. In R. Boruch (Ed.), *Secondary analysis: New directions for program evaluation* (pp. 75–88). San Francisco: Jossey-Bass.

Rosenzweig, S. (1978). *The Rosenzweig Picture-Frustration Study: Basic Manual.* St. Louis: Rana House.

Sameroff, A. J., Seifer, R., & Zax, M. (1982). Early development of children at risk for emotional disorder. *Monographs of the Society for Research in Child Development,* 47(7, Serial No. 199).

Sandgrund, A., Gaines, R. W., & Green, A. W. (1975). Child abuse and mental retardation: A problem of cause and effect. *American Journal on Mental Deficiency,* 3, 327–330.

Sears, R., Maccoby, E., & Levin, H. (1957). *Patterns of child-rearing,* Evanston, IL: Row-Peterson.

Sewell, W. H., & Haller, A. O. (1956). Social status and the personality adjustment of the child. *Sociometry,* 19, 114–125.

Sherrod, K. B., O'Connor, S., Vietze, P. M., & Altemeier, W. A. (1984). Child health and maltreatment. *Child Development,* 55, 1174–1183.

Sontag, L. W., Baker, C. T., & Nelson, V. L. (1958). Mental growth and personality development: A longitudinal study. *Monographs of the Society for Research in Child Develvlopment,* 23(2, Serial No. 68).

Straus, M., Gelles, R., & Steinmetz, S. (1980). *Behind closed doors: Violence in the American family.* Garden City, NY: Anchor.

USDHHS. (1988). *Study Findings: Study of national incidence and prevalence of child abuse and neglect: 1988 Office of Human Development Services.* Washington, DC: U.S. Department of Health and Human Services.

Wandersman, L. P. (1973). Stylistic differences in mother–child interaction: A review and re-evaluation of the social class and socialization research. *Cornell Journal of Social Relations, 8*(2), 197–218.

Werner, E. (1987). Vulnerability and resiliency in children at risk for delinquency: A longitudinal study from birth to young adulthood. In J. D. Burchard & S. N. Burchard (Eds.), *Prevention of delinquent behavior* (pp. 16–43). Beverly Hills, CA: Sage.

Wu, P. (1988). *The impact of family socio-economic status on child development.* Unpublished manuscript, Lehigh University, Center for Social Research, Bethlehem, PA.

Zigler, E., & Trickett, P. K. (1978). Social competence and evaluation of early childhood intervention studies. *American Psychologist, 33,* 780–798.

4

The Early Screening Project

PETER M. VIETZE
New York State Institute for Basic Research in Developmental Disabilities
SUSAN O'CONNOR
KATHRYN B. SHERROD
WILLIAM A. ALTEMEIER
Vanderbilt University and Nashville General Hospital

The Early Screening Project was conceived as an interdisciplinary research study to identify the antecedents of child maltreatment. We believed that if the predisposing factors that led a parent to physically abuse or neglect a child were known, effective preventive interventions could be developed. Several assumptions were made, based on our reading of the extant literature in 1974 when the project was designed. The first was that in a very large number of cases, child abuse and neglect begin early in the child's life. The second was that maltreatment persists until the family receives treatment of some sort. It was also assumed that child maltreatment was more prevalent among families living in impoverished homes either because of overreporting among these families and underreporting among families living in better circumstances or because of the negative effects of poorer socioeconomic conditions. Finally, there was an emerging view about the role of children in families which suggested that children influenced their parents in interactions and activities that affected them both. This view was crystallized by Sameroff and Chandler (1975) in their presentation of the "transactional" perspective of early development. The Early Screening Project was conceptualized around these assumptions.

SOME HISTORICAL ROOTS

Earlier in this century concern for the continuing health and welfare of children during infancy became focused on occasions when infants were separated from their mothers either permanently or for long periods of time. Investigations of infants raised in institutions without their biological mothers suggested that absence of the mother was the cause of the infants' depressed motor, social, emotional, and intellectual development (Bowlby, 1969). These findings suggested that if maternal deprivation led to such dire consequences for the infant, then maternal presence must provide an infant with the necessary ingredients to ensure healthy development. This early perspective that the mother herself was the exclusive agent of social stimulation for the young infant came under attack from a variety of sources.

Casler (1963), Yarrow (1963), and others have suggested that the importance of the infant's mother for adequate development resides in the caregiving activities in which she is engaged with her infant. Bakwin (1949) noted that infants hospitalized for long periods of time showed depressed behavior similar to that shown by the infants observed by Spitz (1945). He further noted that extra stimulation experiences in the hospital, such as those provided by mothers, led to improvement among these hospitalized infants. Interest in the effects of maternal deprivation as a mediator of general stimulus deprivation in infancy has had broad consequences for research and practice. Its effects on research have been seen in the vast number of studies of mother–infant separation as well as in the formulation of theories of infant attachment (Ainsworth, 1973; Bowlby, 1969). This increased awareness of the importance of environmental ingredients for healthy infant development has spread to a variety of settings and populations: day care settings, hospital wards, and programs for children with handicaps. Nevertheless, much of this emphasis is based on interpretations of unidirectional models of caregiver–infant influence.

Recent attempts to identify precursors of parental childrearing practices have emerged in part as a result of shifts in the understanding of parental influences on child development. Early ideas about behavioral development understood infants as being shaped by their parents, making little or no contribution to their own socialization and development. Forty years ago a bidirectional view of parent–child interaction and socialization was proposed by Sears (1951), but it was not recognized widely in the research or child welfare literature until more recently. It is now accepted that the infant's behavior and characteristics can have powerful effects on the caregiver's behavior in interaction with the baby (Lewis & Rosenblum, 1974). These changing views concerning mother–infant interaction make it possible to consider interactional disorders, like child abuse and neglect, in families where parents and infants are not physically separated.

Explanations of the early origins and social context of variations in child development including developmental retardation, behavior disorders, and infant mortality and morbidity have incorporated bidirectional parent–infant influences. Child development researchers construe child outcomes as having multiple historical and causal determinants rather than single-factor causes. Sameroff and Chandler (1975) proposed a model that views the multiple transactions between environmental forces, caregiver characteristics, and infant attributes as continuing, reciprocal contributions to the events and outcomes of child development. This transactional view suggests that to understand a child's development in terms of those factors that influence it, single events cannot have the salient effects once thought to exist. Instead, environmental responses to particular infant characteristics must be considered dynamically. Continuing interactions of the infant with the environment, as well as the characteristics of both infant and context, must be examined. Sameroff and Chandler (1975) proposed that the caregiving environment exists as a continuum that influences how particular child characteristics are expressed. The transactional–developmental perspective can explain child maltreatment as a disorder of parent–child interaction rather than as a result largely of parental psychopathology.

When the Early Screening Project was conceived, existing research on child maltreatment suffered from methodological weaknesses. Either the studies were retrospective analyses in which evaluations of the children and families were done with knowledge of the presenting symptoms, or there were no adequate comparison groups evaluated in a similar manner. Thus, associations made between child maltreatment and family background and history may have been spurious or exaggerated. There are many ways in which parents, especially mothers, are labeled as having character defects that result in child maltreatment, with none of these factors being justified scientifically. Labeling prior to assessment seriously confounds the results and interpretations of these earlier studies.

The diagnosis of child maltreatment has significant consequences for both mother and child. After a diagnosis has occurred, for example, in the case of nonorganic failure to thrive (NFT), an attempt is made to help the mother to increase the weight gain of the infant. If the symptoms are severe and intervention attempts fail, children are frequently hospitalized and treated under more controlled conditions. Hospitalization usually results in a rapid weight gain to normative levels. The transactional approach suggests that negative behavioral patterns are established early in life between mother and child and that these may have contributed to the growth retardation. Such patterns may serve as later obstacles to normal development.

In our study, the transactional approach suggested by Sameroff and Chandler (1975) was applied to identify factors that might be useful in predicting child maltreatment. In using a prospective longitudinal approach, several assumptions were made based on the research literature and on clinical practice at Nashville General Hospital. First, it was assumed that child maltreatment has its roots early in the child's life. This suggests that there might be evidence of a disturbance in the early parent–child relationship. This could only be assumed from the retrospective studies that had been reported to date. Secondly, although there is reason to question the "sick or defective parent" notion regarding the parent who maltreats a child, we do recognize that there may be factors in the parent's background that conspire with contemporaneous events to produce child maltreatment. Indeed, we expected to find patterns of parental history that would be good predictors of parenting practice when combined with characteristics of the child and the interaction between child and parent. Finally, we assumed that environmental factors that produce stress for the families would also contribute to formulating a multivariate transactional view of child maltreatment (Altemeier et al., 1979).

Our prospective approach makes it possible to prenatally identify families at risk for maltreatment, so that preventive interventions might be implemented. Since part of the group studied in the Early Screening Project was selected randomly, it was possible to observe the complete range of parenting styles that existed in this low income population. This allowed for the identification of optimal, as well as detrimental, parent–child combinations.

A TRANSACTIONAL MODEL FOR UNDERSTANDING CHILD MALTREATMENT

In order to explore the transactional approach as it applied to child maltreatment, a hypothetical model was proposed (see Figure 4.1). This model considers the interplay of parental, child, and parent–child interactional influences as determinants of the continuum of parenting practices, one extreme of which is child maltreatment. There are many possible influences. Thus, potential influencing factors we examined in evaluating the transactional model included (1) environmental factors that have indirect effects on children—socioeconomic status, level of stressful events, social support; (2) parental history and background variables that might have a more direct influence on childrearing practices—experiences as a child, current childrearing attitudes, and knowledge and information about child development; and (3) the parents' ability to cope with stress and discomfort—temperamental factors that probably affect parenting

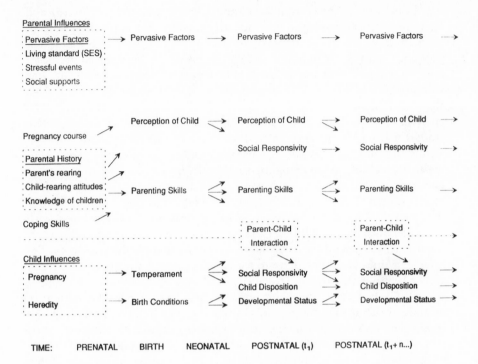

FIGURE 4.1. A transactional model of early child development for understanding child maltreatment.

practices. All of these factors were measured prenatally; when combined with data concerning the actual course of the pregnancy, they constitute the background factors that could potentially influence later parent–child interaction patterns.

The influence of the child was also examined. While prenatal influences may exist, they are difficult to assess. Thus, we focused on such perinatal variables as the course of the pregnancy, infant temperament, and infant behavior while interacting with the parent. These variables, together with such pervasive factors as social class, interact to produce the climate in which the child is raised. The Early Screening Project was designed to identify which factors and what levels of these factors are important in predicting child maltreatment.

Methodological Issues

The Early Screening Project was conceived as a response to the limitations of earlier, largely retrospective studies. Since our aim was to identify precursors of child maltreatment, we took a prospective, longitudinal approach beginning prior to the birth of the child. This methodology allowed us to predict outcome in the real sense of prediction, not merely in the statistical sense. The longitudinal design was necessitated by our desire to understand the emerging aspects of child maltreatment. Our original proposal was to formulate two groups based on extreme responses to an interview in both directions: a high-risk group and a no-risk group. We were persuaded by the funding agency (which probably was persuaded by reviewers) to select a random sample as well as the high-risk group. This sampling strategy strengthened the study for a number of reasons. First, it permitted us to estimate risk in the general population. It also gave us the freedom to conduct several levels of analysis beyond the initial questions of concern. The sample and data are still quite fertile in terms of our being able to continue to ask interesting questions. The fact that we had selected a sufficiently large sample permitted us to observe families in which maltreatment had actually occurred. Thus, we were not observing risk factors or probabilities but actual cases of abuse and neglect both before and after they were identified. The fact that we were successful in identifying a high-risk group as well as a low-risk group meant that we could observe families in which conditions for maltreatment were present but maltreatment had not been identified. Hence, it may still be possible for us to find immunizing conditions in such families.

Sample size was also a limiting factor in our study. In order to conduct certain analyses we were limited by the relatively small number of affected children. This is in part due to the low prevalence rates for the phenomena we were studying. Since child maltreatment is a low-prevalence problem, despite the attention it receives in the mass media, an even larger sample is necessary to conduct any but the simplest analyses. Many of our analyses were simple due to the available sample size. In addition, the prevalence issue may have contributed to the attrition. It is easy to understand why stressed families might be less willing to continue in a study with little or no treatment benefits for them and time-consuming data collection requirements. Although we sought to follow these families until the infants were 18 months old, our attrition was so high that some analyses could not be performed because they would have contained more variables than subjects. This continues to be a problem for studies on "rare" phenomena.

Finally, the reliance on mothers as respondents presents a serious problem in that evidence shows men to be frequent perpetrators of child maltreatment (Starr, Dubowitz, & Bush, 1990). We chose to focus on mothers because they were more readily available. Were we to repeat this study now, we would make fathers as well as mothers the subject of our investigation.

Approach

As mentioned earlier, we sought to mitigate the problems engendered by a retrospective approach and hence adopted a prospective longitudinal approach. Since we assumed that child maltreatment occurs early in a child's life, we sought to begin as early as possible. We believed that if we wanted to identify the earliest evidence of how the child contributed to his or her well-being, we would need to begin antenatally. This timing would also permit us to measure the familial antecedent circumstances without interference from the index child. Thus, the first phase of the project consisted of an interview administered during the mother's initial prenatal clinic visit. The second phase, which began when the woman gave birth, included information concerning the perinatal period. The usual perinatal variables were recorded from each woman's medical chart and from her infant's record. In addition, Brazelton's (1973) Neonatal Behavioral Assessment Scales (NBAS) were administered. Finally, prior to discharge the infant and mother were observed during a feeding using a behavioral coding system which preserved the sequence and timing of interactional events (Anderson, Vietze, Faulstich, & Ashe, 1978). The third phase began at discharge with the collection of the follow-up data. Data included maternal perceptions of infant temperament, observations of interaction during feeding and play, a developmental assessment, child health information coded from medical records, and maltreatment information from child protective services. The information obtained from the protective services organization was combined with records of weight gain to form the outcome measures.

In summary, our approach was to interview all the women in the prenatal clinic, make a risk determination, and follow the 20% thought to be at greatest risk for child maltreatment. For comparison, we followed a random sample of 20% of the 1,400 women interviewed prenatally in order to estimate the incidence of maltreatment in our population as well to validate our prediction criteria.

The Prenatal Questionnaire

An initial pilot questionnaire was developed from the child maltreatment literature to allow identification of factors in the background of the prospective mother that might predispose her to maltreat her infant. Variables assessed included maternal feelings about her pregnancy, the availability of social support, maternal childhood history, current stressors, parenting skills, and personality characteristics.

This questionnaire initially was administered in interview format to 200 women who had come to Nashville General Hospital for their first antenatal visit. This open-ended interview was subsequently refined, and response weights were determined so that the interview could be easily administered and coded. In addition, data were collected using a life stress inventory, to document recent stressful life events, and a questionnaire about child development knowledge.

Observations of Mother–Child Interaction

In order to ascertain the quality of the interaction between mother and infant, observations were made during feeding while the mother and infant were in the hospital prior to discharge. In addition, similar observations were carried out at home using an observational coding system (Anderson et al., 1978). The codes for the mother and the infant each consisted of nine mutually exclusive and exhaustive combinations of four basic behavior categories and one code to represent none of the other coded behaviors (see Table 4.1). Satisfactory interobserver reliability was obtained throughout the duration of the project.

The system of continuous recording permitted the computation of the duration as well as frequency of occurrence of individual mother and

TABLE 4.1. Outline of Observational Categories

Infant behavior patterns	Caregiving
Vocalize	Feed
Look at mother	Bathe-diaper/dress
Look/smile	Put to sleep
Vocalize/look	No caregiving
Vocalize/look/smile	Infant state
Vocalize/smile	
Smile	Active-awake
Cry	Quiet-awake
Cry/look	Drowsy
No signaling behavior	Asleep
Maternal behavior	Maternal proximity
Vocalize to infant	Holds infant
Look at infant	Within 3 feet
Look/smile	Greater than 3 feet
Vocalize/look	Out of room
Vocalize/look/smile	
Vocalize/tactile play	
Vocalize/look/smile/tactile play	
Tactile play	
No behavior to infant	

infant behaviors and of dyadic behavior. Proportion of total session time
for each of the five maternal and five infant behavior categories (including
no response) were computed.

Measures of the nature of the dyadic interaction were also obtained
from the observational records. By using a strategy for reducing the observations to conditional probabilities (Bakeman & Brown, 1977), it was
possible to construct interactional variables that measured maternal initiation, maternal continuation, maternal stopping, maternal contingent join-
ing, and maternal contingent stopping.

Outcome Measures

To determine whether the study infants had been maltreated, files of all
reports of child abuse and neglect in Tennessee were reviewed. In addition, nonorganic failure to thrive (NFT) was monitored in the study
infants. Infants were weighed at each well- and sick-child medical ap-
pointment and during each home visit. NFT was defined as growth retardation that could not be attributed to an organic disorder and therefore
was apparently due to inadequate feeding. Failure to thrive was defined as
a continuing weight gain of less than two-thirds of the Harvard 50 percentile curve (Vaughan, McKay, & Nelson, 1975). All failure to thrive
charts were reviewed by a physician; those children without substantial
growth failure or who had an organic abnormality that could explain the
failure were excluded from the diagnosis.

The Sample

Between September 1975 and December 1976, all women who registered
for the prenatal clinic were asked to participate in the Early Screening Project. Of 1,500 women, 6.6% refused, leaving 1,400 women who agreed to
be interviewed. One-third of these women were black, and about 25%
were less than 18 years old. With regard to marital status, 700 women
were married and living with their husbands, 457 were single, and 243
were divorced or separated. Thus, half of the sample mothers had no live-
in partner. It should be noted that, since we were contacting these women
through a public city hospital, it is reasonable to assume that the number
of single women was overestimated. For example, if a woman was receiving welfare, she might not have been truthful about whether she had a
partner. Still, the number of women who were actually without a partner
was quite high. Further, since the hospital served mainly indigent patients,
it is safe to assume that a large proportion of the infants were born into
family settings that may have been stressed from the beginning. The proportion of unmarried black women was significantly higher than that of

unmarried white women. This clearly was not due to any difference in the number of women under 18 in the two groups, since the numbers of subjects in the under-18 subgroups were comparable. One other noteworthy aspect of the sample was that a large proportion of the women had grown up in single-parent homes themselves; this did not differ appreciably by race. (Further details about the sample can be found in Altemeier et al., 1979.)

The determination of high risk for maltreatment was based on the prenatal interview. Extreme response cutoffs had been established based on responses of the pilot sample. The criteria consisted of any one category falling above the 99th percentile, two categories above the 95th percentile, or an average above the 75th percentile for all eight categories of the interview. In addition, since we had trained the interviewers to be sensitive to signs that might predispose the woman to maltreat her child, we also asked them to note any woman who appeared to be answering the questions in a way that made her seem risk-prone (we did not tell the interviewers that we included these women—there were 50 of them—in the high-risk category). The distribution of how the women designated as high risk fulfilled the criteria is shown in Table 2. As indicated earlier, we followed two groups of women—those who were judged to be high risk and a random sample of 20% of the 1,400 women interviewed. Of course, this procedure meant that some of those in the random sample would be considered high risk: in fact, 55 of the women in the random sample were so designated. A low-risk sample of 225 subjects was then developed by removing the 55 women from the random sample. In examining attrition, we analyzed the high-risk and the low-risk groups to determine whether there was any systematic difference in subject loss. These results are shown in Table 4.3. The only noteworthy differences were in the rate of fetal or nursery death and the number of mothers who gave their child up. Both of these were higher in the high-risk groups.

We also examined the two groups with regard to several other noteworthy characteristics. These are presented in Table 4.4. As can be seen,

TABLE 4.2. Criteria Used to Select 273 High-Risk Mothers

	Only one criterion	One other	Two others	Three others
Subjective Identification	50	24	10	6
1 Category > 99th percentile	49	46	40	6
2 Categories > 99th percentile	33	55	42	6
3 Categories > 75th percentile	19	25	33	6

TABLE 4.3. Loss of Study Infants

	High risk		Low risk	
	N	%	N	%
Total receiving interview	273	100.00	225	100.00
Total born at study hospital	247	90.48	206	91.56
Infants still in study				
at age 6 months	155	56.78	132	58.76
at age 12 months	133	48.72	104	46.22
Reasons for loss[a]				
Could not locate	38	13.92	27	12.00
(moved or false address)				
Moved out of Nashville	30	10.99	28	12.44
Refused after birth	21	7.69	31	13.78
Did not deliver at study hospital	23	8.42	19	8.44
Fetal or nursery death	11	4.03	5	2.22
Refused after interview, before birth	8	2.93	5	2.22
Mother relinquished child	10	3.66	2	0.89
(voluntary or court order)				
Deliver before data collection started	7	2.56	0	0.00
False pregnancy	4	1.47	0	0.00
Death after nursery discharge	1	0.37	2	0.89

[a] As of June 1978.

the only difference in the mothers in the two groups was the percentage of primigravida, which was higher in the low-risk sample. This suggests that some of the responses to the interview may have reflected inexperience and/or the anxiety that sometimes accompanies first pregnancies. The only infant characteristic that differentiated the two groups was in the proportion of infants weighing more than 9 pounds at birth; we have no reasonable explanation for the higher rate of heavy babies in the high risk group. Average birthweight did not differ for the two groups.

Findings

Effectiveness of the Interview

The first question we asked of the data was, How well did our interview predict maltreatment? We examined outcomes for NFT and for abuse or neglect separately (see Altemeier et al., 1979).

We were interested in the proportion of infants at any age who were diagnosed as NFT. Overall, 14% of the high-risk group were found to have NFT while only 4.2% of the low-risk group were so diagnosed. This

TABLE 4.4. Description of High- and Low-Risk Subjects

	High risk	Low risk
Mothers	N = 273	N = 225
Mean age	21.1	20.7
% White	73	68
% Married	51	59
Weeks pregnant at interview	21.1	20.7
% Primigravida	39	55**
Years education	10.1	10.4
Infants	N = 228	N = 200
Birth weight (grams)	3220	3163
Proportion weighing > 9 lb	18/227	5/200*
Proportion weighing < 9 lb	16/227	11/200
Apgar score at 1 minute	8.2	8.3
% Male	50	43

* $p < .05$. ** $p < .01$.

was statistically significant at all ages examined below 10 months. Unfortunately, not all infants were weighed at every age due to variable attendance at pediatric examinations. Nevertheless, for the data available, it seemed that the prenatal interview was more effective than chance in predicting NFT.

Maltreatment reports to protective services were independent of our follow-up. We compared the rate of such reports in the high-risk group to that in the other 1,127 families where the mothers had been interviewed prenatally. Protective services reports were reviewed monthly. Each report made for a study subject was reviewed by one of the authors who had no knowledge of group designation. Any reports that were judged to have insufficient documentation were discarded. We found that more than 10% of the high-risk group were judged to be bona fide abuse or neglect reports, compared to about 2% of the rest of the sample ($p < .01$). If we add the NFT subjects who were not abused or neglected, almost 19% of the infants of the high-risk group experienced maltreatment. This is clear evidence that the prenatal interview, even in its form at the time of the study, was much more effective at identifying cases of maltreatment than chance.

There are important issues to be addressed regarding the 80% of the high-risk group who were not diagnosed with maltreatment using the criteria we used (false positive cases). Most recently, Altemeier has continued to refine the interview in order to reduce the high rate of false positives. Some of the issues raised by this problem of false positives are discussed later.

TABLE 4.5. Original Variables in Multiple Regression Analysis

	Period of observation			
	Prenatal	Birth	1 month	3 months
Risk status	x			
Maternal stress	x			
Birth weight		x		
NBAS clusters		x		
Birth complications		x		
Interaction variables				
Maternal visual gaze		x		
Maternal initiation		x	x	x
Maternal continuation		x	x	x
Maternal stopping		x	x	x
Maternal joining (contingent)		x	x	x
Maternal stopping (contingent)		x	x	x
Infant Temperament Questionnaire			x	x

Prediction of Maltreatment: The Transactional Analysis

In this analysis we attempted to apply the transactional approach proposed by Sameroff and Chandler to examine how well we could predict outcome, defined as either abuse, neglect, or NFT (Vietze, Falsey, Sandler, O'Connor, & Altemeier, 1980). The variables used as predictors in a regression analysis are shown in Table 4.5. We selected variables from the prenatal period and from the postnatal period by age. The sample size for this analysis was 404, of whom 72 had been maltreated according to our criteria. The results of the regression analysis indicated that the best predictor of maltreatment was risk status, which was determined primarily by responses on the prenatal questionnaire. All together, eight predictors constituted the "best set" and included five interactional variables from the neonatal and 1-month periods. In addition, the "perception of infant temperament" at 3 months also contributed to the significant regression equation. This set predicted 19% of the variance ($R = .433$, $R^2 = .187$).

Antecedents of Maltreatment

Child Abuse. In order to obtain a more complete picture of the profile of women who actually abused their children, we examined the interview responses of the original sample (Altemeier, O'Connor, Vietze, Sandler, & Sherrod, 1984). Of these 1,400 women, 23 had been reported for having abused one of their children within 24 months of the interview.

In order to determine the pattern of responding on the interview for these 23 women, we compared them with the 1377 not reported for abuse.

Recall that there were eight categories in the interview; differences between abusers and nonabusers showed up in seven of the eight categories. There were no differences between the two groups regarding knowledge of or expectations about child development norms. In their perception of nurture as a child, the abusers were more likely to have lived in foster care at some time, less likely to get along with their own mothers, more likely to feel their parents were displeased with them in general, and more likely to have received unfair severe punishment. They did not report being abused significantly more than the nonabusers did. However, they did have significantly poorer self-images than the nonabusers, but this difference was not striking (39% vs. 17%). The only difference in the social support category was in the closeness of their relationship with the father of the index child. In the area of parenting, five of the seven questions showed significant differences between the two groups. Those reported for abuse were more likely to have lost a child to foster care or avoidable death, more likely to fear hurting her child, reported having recently attacked a child or adult violently, reported feeling anger toward a screaming child, and refused to reveal a reaction to an irritating child. In relation to their pregnancy, the abusers reported not wanting to continue the pregnancy, reported that the pregnancy was unplanned or planned for selfish purposes, wished not to be pregnant, and felt depressed, lonely, or grouchy. With regard to family stress, mothers in the group reported for abuse described their child as having a medical or social problem more often than did nonabusers.

Three of the life stress events discriminated the two groups. Almost a third of the abusers had a prior birth the year before, compared to 6% of the nonabusers. The abusers were more likely to have moved frequently and less likely to have quit a job recently. A number of demographic factors differentiated the two groups. The abusers were more likely to have more than one child and more than one child under 5 years of age. They were also more likely to have been married at some time. There were no differences in age, race, education, or week of pregnancy at the interview.

The pattern of these results suggests a more complex picture than is often reported in the literature. The pattern is one of conditions likely to lead to increased stress with decreased resources for handling stress. This pattern is supported by the transactional analysis reported earlier.

Failure to Thrive. A similar analysis was performed for the outcome of NFT (Altemeier, O'Connor, Sherrod, & Vietze, 1985), in that we examined the antecedent factors, as measured by our questionnaire, that might predict NFT. Of the six subscores on the prenatal history questionnaire, only the score for the mother's report of her own childhood nurturance was significantly related to whether a child suffered from NFT. In addition, the number of life stress events reported by the mother for herself or for the father also predicted NFT. Four specific stressful events predicted NFT significantly for the mother—arguments with the baby's father, separation from the father, reconciliation with the father, and death of a friend—and two did so for the father—loss of job and an arrest. The correlations are not high, but they are all significant. There were also certain perinatal complications that seemed to differentiate the NFT group from the comparison group. These results indicated that women who failed to obtain adequate nurturance during their own formative years and who experience stress during pregnancy are more likely to have infants with NFT.

The Child's Role in Maltreatment

One aspect of the transactional approach is a consideration of the way in which the child might influence the caregiver to maltreat him or her. This was evaluated by examining antecedents of NFT and the relationship between illness and maltreatment.

Infant and Interactional Antecedents to NFT. One of the important questions concerning child maltreatment is whether the child who is a victim is different from the child who is not. Since this was a prospective study and since we observed and tested infants prior to their being maltreated, it was possible to examine data on the infant's status and behavior at birth and to observe mother-infant interactions during the newborn period (Vietze, Falsey, O'Connor, Sandler, Sherrod, & Altemeier, 1980). All infants eventually identified as having NFT were selected from the 498 infants being followed as the index group for these analyses. A comparison group of infants who had no NFT was selected at random from the remaining group. There were no differences between these two groups on the NBAS or on any demographic factors. In addition, the only birth information that distinguished the two groups was that the NFT infants had lower mean birth-weights and significantly shorter gestational periods than the comparison group, although both variables were well within the normal range. There were some behavioral differences between the groups during interaction with the mothers at feeding time.

Although there were no differences between the groups with regard to infant behavior, the mothers of the NFT infants showed significantly less visual attention during interaction; that is, they looked at their infants less than did the mothers of the comparison infants. In addition, measures of dyadic interaction differentiated the male NFT infants from the male comparison infants, but this was not so for the females. The nature of the finding was that the mothers of NFT boys tended to stop responding to their infants in comparison to the other group and to drop out of mutual responding. This suggests a lack of sensitivity to the infant's needs and social cues. Thus, it could be said that the infants who later had NFT did not show any behavioral differences at birth, though they tended to weigh less and be born earlier. The mothers of these infants, however, showed early signs of social withdrawal from interactions with their infants.

Relationship Between Illness and Maltreatment. The fact that the NFT infants were lighter and born earlier than the comparison group suggests that they may have been less capable of surviving due to subtle defects at birth. One consequence of this is that such an infant may be more prone to illness, more irritable, and therefore more at risk for maltreatment if the mother is stressed. There are suggestions in the literature that children who are maltreated may have higher rates of childhood illness than those children who are not victims of maltreatment. This analysis sought to clarify the relationship between childhood illness and maltreatment (Sherrod, O'Connor, Vietze, & Altemeier, 1984).

In order to conduct the analysis 56 children who had nonoverlapping determinations of child maltreatment and 24 randomly selected comparison children who had not been maltreated were compared with regard to prevalence of illness between 3 and 36 months. The medical records of these 80 children were evaluated to determine the reason for visits to the pediatric clinic. The visits were categorized as follows: well-child visit, infectious illness, accidents, anatomic anomalies, family dysfunction, hospitalizations. Each maltreatment group was compared with the comparison group for prevalence of the clinic visits. There were no differences in well-child visits across groups. However, the abuse and NFT groups showed significantly more illnesses than the comparison group. The abuse group showed significantly more accidents, regardless of type of accident, than the comparison group; the other two groups of maltreated children did not show more accidents than the comparison group. Finally, both abuse and NFT groups showed significantly more family dysfunction and hospitalizations than did the comparison group. The neglect group was not different from the comparison group on any measure. The results generally supported the notion that the prevalence of illness in these three groups was higher very early in their lives. We suggest that high prevalence of illness early in life could be considered as a way of identifying potential maltreatment. The differences are less striking as the children get older.

SUMMARY

The findings from the Early Screening Project suggest that conditions of the mother's childhood development and experience may be the most powerful precursor of child maltreatment. The infant's role in the dynamics of maltreatment may be limited to slight physical immaturity. There is little evidence that infants exhibit early atypical behaviors that are precursors of later maltreatment. Most of the evidence points to an accumulation of circumstances resident in the mother and her living conditions that conspire to interrupt the normal caregiving functions and lead instead to the child's endangerment.

One of the oft-cited limitations of longitudinal studies is that research methods may rapidly become obsolete (see Black, Chapter 6, this volume). Fortunately, that was not the case in our study. We selected instruments and tools that are still valid today. Of course, the ways in which measures are used may change over time. This was the case with the Neonatal Behavioral Assessment Scale (NBAS). At the start of our project the NBAS was typically administered a single time during the first month of life. The current practice is to administer it periodically during this period in order to track recovery from the birth process.

Finally, our study centered on lower income families. There is ample reason to believe that child maltreatment is not limited to people from impoverished homes. We chose some expedient solutions. It may be time to choose reality rather than expediency.

REFERENCES

Ainsworth, M. D. S. (1973). The development of infant–mother attachment. In B. M. Caldwell & H. N. Ricciuti (Eds.), *Review of child development research: Vol. 3. Child development and social policy* (pp. 1–94). Chicago: University of Chicago Press.

Altemeier, W. A., Vietze, P. M., Sherrod, K. B., Sandler, H. M., Falsey, S., & O'Connor, S. (1979). Prediction of child maltreatment during pregnancy. *Journal of the American Academy of Child Psychiatry, 18*, 205–218.

Altemeier, W. A., O'Connor, S., Vietze, P., Sandler, H., & Sherrod, K. (1984). Prediction of child abuse: A prospective study of feasibility. *Child Abuse & Neglect, 8*, 393–400.

Altemeier, W. A., O'Connor, S., Sherrod, K. B., & Vietze, P. M. (1985). A prospective study of antecedents for non-organic failure to thrive. *Journal of Pediatrics, 106*, 360–365.

Anderson, B. J., Vietze, P. M., Faulstich, G., & Ashe, M. L. (1978). Observation manual for assessment of behavioral sequences between infant and mother. Newborn to 24 months. *JSAS Catalog of Selected Documents in Psychology, 8*, 34 (Ms. No. 1672).

Bakeman, R., & Brown, J. V. (1977). Behavioral dialogues: An approach to the assessment of mother–infant interaction. *Child Development, 48*, 195–203.

Bakwin, H. (1949). Emotional deprivation in infants. *Journal of Pediatrics, 35*, 512.

Bowlby, J. (1969). *Attachment and Loss: Vol. 1. Attachment*. New York: Basic Books.

Brazelton, T. B. (1973). *Neonatal Behavioral Assessment Scale*. Philadelphia: Lippincott.

Casler, L. (1963). Perceptual deprivation in institutional settings. In G. Newton & S. Levine (Eds.), *Early experience and behavior* (pp. 573–626). Springfield, IL: Thomas.

Lewis, M., & Rosenblum, L. A. (Eds.). (1974). *The effect of the infant on its caregiver* (Vol. 1). New York: Wiley.

Sameroff, A. J. (1975) Early influences on development: Fact or fancy. *Merrill-Palmer Quarterly, 21*, 267–294.

Sameroff, A. J., & Chandler, M. J. (1975). Reproductive risk and the continuum of caretaking casualty. In F. D. Horowitz, M. Hetherington, S. Scarr-Salapatek, & G. Siegel (Eds.), *Review of child development research*_(Vol. 4, pp. 187–244). Chicago: University of Chicago Press.

Sears, R. R. (1951). A theoretical framework for personality and social behavior. *American Psychologist, 6*, 476–482.

Sherrod, K. B., O'Connor, S., Vietze, P. M., & Altemeier, W. A. (1984). Child health and treatment. *Child Development, 55*, 1174–1183.

Spitz, R. A. (1945). Hospitalism: An inquiry into the genesis of psychiatric conditions in early childhood. *Psychoanalysis Study of the Child, 1*, 53–74.

Starr, R. H., Jr., Dubowitz, H., & Bush, B. A. (1990). The epidemiology of child maltreatment. In R. T. Ammerman & M. Hersen (Eds.), *Children at risk: An evaluation of factors contributing to child abuse and neglect* (pp. 23–53). New York: Plenum.

Vaughan, V. C., McKay, R. J., & Nelson, E. (1975). *Nelson's textbook of pediatrics*. Philadelphia: Saunders.

Vietze, P. M., Falsey, S., O'Connor, S., Sandler, H., Sherrod, K., & Altemeier, W. A. (1980). Newborn behavioral and interactional characteristics of nonorganic failure to thrive infants. In T. M. Field (Ed.), *High-risk infants and children: Adult and peer interactions* (pp. 5–23). New York: Academic Press.

Vietze, P., Falsey, S., Sandler, H., O'Connor, S., & Altemeier, W. A. (l980). Transactional approach to prediction of child maltreatment. *Infant Mental Health Journal, l*, 248–26l.

Yarrow, L. J. (1963). Research in dimensions of early maternal care. *Merrill-Palmer Quarterly, 9*, 101–114.

5

Research Definitions of Child Physical Abuse and Neglect: Current Problems

SUSAN J. ZURAVIN
University of Maryland at Baltimore School of Social Work

"**M**easurement is essential to science, but before we can measure, we must know what it is we want to measure" (Eysenck, 1952, p. 34). This observation was made by Hans Eysenck during the early 1950s in the context of championing the need for a psychiatric classification system. Today, it is as applicable to the field of child maltreatment as it was to the field of psychiatry almost four decades ago. The limitations of current knowledge about child maltreatment, like the limitations of knowledge about psychiatric illnesses in the early 1950s, can be attributed, at least in part, to the absence of a "reliable, valid, accepted nosology for describing and classifying the phenomena subsumed under the rubric of child maltreatment" (Cicchetti & Rizley, 1981, p. 34).

Child maltreatment is a heterogeneous phenomenon. It refers to at least four different types of caretaking casualties: physical abuse, sexual abuse, physical neglect, and emotional mistreatment. To date, research on each type has been carried out by different groups of investigators and is characterized by (1) the use of different definitions for the same type of maltreatment, (2) the use of definitions for one category of maltreatment that evidence considerable operational overlap with definitions for other categories, and (3) a failure to assess for the presence of maltreatment types other than the one or two being studied. These practices have had a negative impact on the development of knowledge by making it difficult, if not impossible, to compare and integrate findings across studies and to determine if specific types as well as combinations of types vary with respect to sequelae, etiology, intergenerational transmission, and treatment response.

Currently, there is substantial agreement among researchers as well as funders that longitudinal studies are required to answer the most pressing questions about child maltreatment. The National Center on Child Abuse and Neglect (NCCAN) and other funders have begun to finance such efforts (Federal Register, 1989). Given the time and money involved in mounting and carrying out longitudinal research, it is particularly important that time be spent now identifying what it is that we "want to measure." If we fail to formulate agreed upon definitions, researchers will use their own definitions, and the field will continue to be faced with the problem of not being able to integrate findings across studies.

In the interest of promoting the development of a classification system and building knowledge about specific types of maltreatment, this chapter addresses the issue of defining physical abuse and physical neglect for *research* purposes. The main objective is to identify problems with existing conceptual and operational definitions and to recommend some options for resolving these problems. Focusing on physical abuse and neglect is justifiable on the basis of data from the most recent National Study of the Incidence of Child Maltreatment—the Second National Incidence Study (NIS-2)—as reported by the U.S. Department of Health and Human Services (USDHHS, 1988), data that indicate that abuse and neglect were the most prevalent of the four types of caretaking casualties seen by professionals during 1986.

Work on neglect is particularly important because it has received much less definitional attention and has been the focus of many fewer research efforts than the other three categories of caretaking casualties despite its greater prevalence (Wolock & Horowitz, 1984). As recently as 1987, the lack of a standard definition for neglect was recognized as a critical problem for developing a body of knowledge. Heading the list of recommendations made by NCCAN grantees engaged in neglect research was the development of a standard definition (National Center on Child Abuse & Neglect, 1987).

GENERAL DEFINITIONAL PRINCIPLES

The main aims of the section of this chapter are to elaborate some principles for formulating a system of definitions (classification system) and to identify the ramifications of these principles for defining abuse and neglect. To do this, four general principles of value for formulating a classification system and definitions and one principle that is specifically relevant for defining abuse and neglect are discussed.

Division of Categories into Subtypes

One important consideration when developing a classification system pertains to the issue of identifying categories that need to be divided into subtypes. Development of a classification system begins with the grouping of behaviors or events into categories (i.e., physical abuse, physical neglect, sexual abuse, and emotional maltreatment) on the basis of core similarities. For example, behaviors subsumed under physical abuse all involve physical aggression toward the child while behaviors subsumed under physical neglect involve omissions in care. Despite the core similarities, behaviors included in a category will frequently display considerable heterogeneity with respect to other characteristics. When a category includes diverse behaviors, division into subcategories or subtypes is necessary. Failure to formulate separate conceptual and operational definitions for subcategories will subvert the development of knowledge by making it impossible to determine if clinically diverse phenomena subsumed within a single category are a function of different etiologies, lead to distinctive sequelae, and require unique treatments.

While all of the behaviors subsumed under neglect are similar in that they involve an omission in care, the essential nature of the omissions differs. For example, failure to provide adequate supervision is a qualitatively different omission than failure to adequately feed or meet physical and mental health care needs. The same can be said for abuse: while all of the behaviors subsumed under abuse are acts of commission, they differ in essential nature and potential for immediate and severe physical consequences. For example, scalding differs from choking which differs from hitting with an object which differs from attacking with a knife which differs from spanking and slapping. In addition, behaviors differ along the dimension of chronicity; some types, like spanking, slapping, shaking, and hitting with objects, are more likely to be typical of family methods of discipline and therefore administered frequently. Other types, like scalding, choking, attacking with a knife or gun, are infrequent behaviors and may be the result of explosive outbursts on the part of the caretaker. Consequently, as we develop definitions for these two types of maltreatment, it is critically important that we develop a set of agreed-upon subtypes.

Conceptual Clarity

Another critically important consideration when developing a classification system pertains to the formulation of conceptually clear definitions for each category and subcategory. To achieve conceptual clarity it is necessary to clearly specify every criterion that a behavior must meet in order to be classified in a category and to make sure that at least one criterion differs for each category or subcategory. When definitions of maltreatment are under-conceptualized—that is, when there is a failure to identify distinctive criteria and/or a failure to include all relevant criteria—two serious problems with operational translations will arise (McGee & Wolfe, in press). Researchers will be unable to develop discrete operational definitions for each type and subtype of maltreatment, or they will develop operationalizations for a specific type or subtype with diverse kinds of parental behaviors—behaviors that do not have any conceptual similarity. In other words, the behaviors that operationalize a particular type of maltreatment might be equally applicable to another type. Both problems will obstruct the development of knowledge by making it impossible to determine whether the four types of maltreatment and their respective subtypes differ relative to sequelae, etiology, or treatment. Thus, it is extremely important that we begin the effort to develop a classification system for child maltreatment by formulating conceptual definitions that are as complete and as distinct from each other as possible with respect to classification criteria.

Measurability of Operational Translations

A third important definitional consideration pertains to the "measurability and observability" (McGee & Wolfe, in press) of the behavior or events used to operationalize the conceptual definitions. If the behavioral translations of a conceptual definition are vague—that is, if we fail to use behaviors that are observable and measurable with respect to degree, and fail to specify precisely how frequently the behavior must occur or how long it must endure—interrater reliability will be low. In other words, the accord between raters within and between studies with respect to classifying a particular behavior as maltreating or not will be poor. Inconsistent classification of a behavior will confound findings and increase the probability of contradictory results among studies, thus subverting the building of knowledge. Therefore, as we build a classification it is mandatory that we operationalize conceptual definitions with observable behaviors that are measurable in terms of degree, frequency and duration.

Purpose of the Definition

One essential element to consider when formulating conceptual and operational definitions is the specific objectives the definition must serve. Like theories, definitions are never assessed as true or false but, rather, as useful or not useful in attaining a goal. "Therefore, when a (definitional) system is devised, its purposes should be explicitly stated so that the system can be evaluated in terms of its success or failure in attaining these objectives" (Zigler & Phillips, 1961, p. 614).

According to Ross and Zigler (1980) the current lack of agreement about definitions of maltreatment can be explained, at least in part, by failure to recognize that no single definition is capable of "fulfilling all of the functions that social scientists and social service professionals would like" (p. 293). Aber and Zigler (1981) propose the development of "three different sets of definitions" (p. 12): legal definitions, case management definitions, and research definitions.

For research definitions, the issue of purpose specifically translates into identifying what we want to learn from longitudinal studies. Reviews of the literature (e.g., Cicchetti & Rizley, 1981; Egeland & Sroufe, 1981; Federal Register, 1989) suggest five important objectives: determination of (1) the short and long-term impact on the child's physical, cognitive, social, and emotional adjustment; (2) the processes through which maltreatment leads to its various sequelae; (3) effective intervention strategies; (4) causes; and (5) whether different types of maltreatment or different combinations of type vary with respect to any of these four factors.

Given these purposes, Aber and Zigler (1981) recommend the formulation of broad definitions—in which the main classifying principle is the nature of caretaker acts rather than child outcomes. In other words, definitions of the various types of maltreatment should involve little more than a "descriptive compartmentalization" of behaviors (Zigler & Phillips, 1961, p. 618). Definitions should not include or be tied to a particular etiology or type of sequelae. As McGee and Wolfe (in press) point out, "If we are interested in empirically determining the impact of specific parent behaviors on child adjustmen. . . . it is inherently tautological to construct definitions that focus on outcome" (p. 17). Thus, given our current research objectives, the main focus of a maltreatment definition should be parent/caretaker behaviors.

Age Grading of Operational Criteria

Specifically pertinent to the development of a child maltreatment classification system is the question of whether operational criteria should differ as a function of the child's age and developmental stage. This issue, raised by a number of researchers (e.g., Aber & Zigler, 1981; Cicchetti & Todd-Manly, in press; McGee & Wolfe, in press; Polansky, Borgman, & DeSaix, 1972) who are interested in the long-term sequelae of maltreatment, focuses on the possibility that "an act which may cause harm to a child at one vulnerable stage of development may not at another stage" (Aber & Zigler, 1981, p. 24). Aber and Zigler (1981) note that "severe emotional damage due to separation and loss may be particularly easy to inflict during the child's earliest years . . . while fostering delinquency

holds its greatest risk during the early school-age years when social standards are being internalized" (p. 24). They ask, "Are such acts [those
hypothesized not to result in harm if perpetrated at a particular stage of
development] to be included as cases of child maltreatment?" (p. 24).
McGee and Wolfe (in press) answer no to this question. Consistent with
the research objectives posed earlier, they recommend "treating the parent's behavior and the child's age as independent variables" and the
"child's adjustment as the dependent variable. Rather than labelling in
advance how the child of a given age will react to a specific parent behavior, we should determine this empirically" (p. 21).

However, the operational definition of specific types of physical
neglect, inadequate supervision, and custody-related issues pose some special problems that are not relevant to emotional maltreatment. As Polansky
and colleagues (1972) have so well noted, what is considered to be physically neglectful at one age is clearly infantilization at another age. For
example, leaving a 3-year-old alone for 5 hours is clearly inappropriate
whereas leaving a 12-year-old alone for the same period of time is not.
Consequently, certain types of neglect, namely, inadequate supervision,
probably require operationalizations that differ depending upon the child's
age. The key question that we need to address as researchers is, What criteria should we use for the age-grading?

This discussion of definitional principles has identified some important considerations that will be used in the following section of the chapter to guide the identification of definitional problems and establish
recommendations with respect to resolving these problems. They are summarized as follows:

1. The categories of physical neglect and abuse should be divided
   into subcategories.
2. Conceptual definitions of neglect and abuse categories and subcategories must be complete and distinctive. They must identify all of
   the criteria that a behavior must meet in order to be classified under
   the category or subtype, and at least some of the criteria for each
   category or subtype must differ from those for all others.
3. Operational translations of conceptual definitions for categories
   and subtypes must include concrete behaviors that are observable
   and measurable with respect to degree of behavior, frequency, and
   duration.
4. The content of definitions—the specific elements included in the
   definition—must be driven by a set of purposes. Research definitions should be broader than legal and case management definitions and focused on identifying (1) the impact of the mal-

treatment on the child's physical health as well as social, emotional, and cognitive development, (2) the etiology of maltreatment, and (3) effective treatments. Given these objectives, definitions need to be broad, and their main classifying principle should be parent/care-taker behaviors in relation to their children. Definitions should not be tied to specific sequelae, causes, prognosis, or treatment.

5. Age and developmental stage of the child should dictate the specific parent behaviors that are used to operationalize maltreatment, at least with respect to supervisory neglect.

EXISTING DEFINITIONS

The main aims of this section are to identify problems with existing definitions of abuse and neglect and to discuss some alternative strategies for resolving these problems. The section begins with a general discussion of the problems associated with defining physical abuse and physical neglect and is followed by identification and discussion of specific problems that we need to resolve.

The problem with respect to defining both physical abuse and physical neglect *for research purposes* has centered less around formulating conceptual definitions than on identifying acceptable and agreed-upon operational translations. While existing conceptual definitions are not without problems—they are not as complete or distinct with respect to criteria as they should be—there is at least general agreement that abuse represents acts of commission and neglect acts of omission (Giovannoni, 1971) by parents and/or caretakers that are "judged by a mixture of community values and professional expertise to be inappropriate and damaging" (Garbarino & Gilliam, 1980, p. 7). Further, there has been and continues to be consensus that physical neglect's acts of omission usually refer to the failure of parents/caretakers to perform parental duties adequately (Giovannoni, 1971) in relation to supervision and the physical needs of the child whereas the commission of acts of physical abuse specifically refers to the use of excessive and inappropriate physical force (Magura & Moses, 1986).

During the early phases of research on child maltreatment (1960s and 1970s) the difficult and thorny issue of operationalizing physical abuse and neglect was usually resolved by simply using "the label assigned to an act by responsible agencies, including hospitals, child protection agencies, police, and courts" (Giovannoni & Becerra, 1979, p. 14). For example, Giovannoni and Billingsley's 1970 study defined neglect in terms of situations reported to and documented by child protective services. Green,

Gaines, and Sandgrund's 1974 study defined abuse in terms of reports to the Bureau of Child Welfare and Family Court of New York City. Like types of mental illness prior to the formulation of the Research Diagnostic Criteria (Spitzer, Endicott, & Robins, 1978), DSM-III-R (American Psychiatric Association, 1987), and other operational definitions, neglect and abuse were anything labeled as such by a "professional"; there were no objective criteria for identifying when maltreatment had occurred. As Gelles so well noted in a 1982 paper, "There is no objective phenomenon that can be defined as 'child abuse'" (p. 1).

To get away from the many problems based on operational definitions professional opinion caused for interpreting as well as comparing findings from studies (see Giovannoni & Becerra, 1979), some researchers (but certainly not all) began to get more specific. They began to formulate operational definitions that *excluded* the professional opinion criterion (e.g., Egeland & Sroufe, 1981; Sack, Mason, & Higgins, 1985; Straus, Gelles & Steinmetz, 1980) and/or supplemented it with more specific criteria (e.g., U.S. Department of Health and Human Services, 1988; Wolfe & Mosk, 1983; Wolock & Horowitz, 1977; Zuravin & Taylor, 1987). In other words, researchers began to describe in greater detail what they meant by physical abuse and neglect.

While this growing trend toward specific operational definitions is a step in the right direction, it has not enhanced our ability to integrate and compare findings from different studies because few, if any, researchers have used exactly the same operational translations. In addition, definitions have violated many of the principles elaborated in the first section of this chapter. They have differed from study to study with respect to at least one, and usually more than one, of six dimensions: (1) consequence(s) of the behavior for the child, (2) maltreatment subtypes, (3) frequency of the behavior, (4) perpetrator identity, (5) perpetrator intent/culpability, and (6) age grading of operational criteria.

The following paragraphs compare a selected group of conceptual and operational definitions with respect to the aforementioned six dimensions for the purpose of identifying problems and differences. To facilitate the problem identification process, the most highly operationalized definitions—those that include the most specific information about types of behavior that are considered maltreating—were examined (see Tables 5.1, 5.2, 5.3, and 5.4). The point of this is not to criticize or find fault with the definitions but rather to facilitate the identification of existing differences that require resolution and to illustrate how definitions violate the principles identified earlier. As might be expected, given the meager amount of attention paid to defining neglect, a search of the research literature for definitions revealed many for physical abuse but few for physical neglect.

Consequence of Behavior

Identification of Issues

Consequence of behavior is a criterion that must be included in the conceptual definition of maltreatment. It refers to two issues that are pertinent to the maltreating behavior's impact on the child. The first issue pertains to whether endangerment of the child or demonstrable harm to the child is required to apply the label of abuse or neglect. The second issue pertains to instances where endangerment rather than demonstrable harm is the criterion and addresses the problem of the immediacy and degree of endangerment. Demonstrable harm definitions require that the child have suffered injuries or impairments as a result of the perpetrator's omissions or commissions whereas endangerment definitions require that the act need only increase the child's *risk* of injury or impairment. As can be noted from examining definitions of abuse in Table 5.1 and definitions of neglect in Tables 5.2, 5.3, and 5.4, a demonstrable harm requirement is exclusively characteristic of physical abuse. Neglect, regardless of subtype, is defined in terms of endangerment. Comparison of the two types of definitions for physical abuse reveals that the demonstrable harm definitions focus on the injury to the child while the endangerment definitions focus on perpetrator behavior.

While most endangerment definitions of abuse (NIS-2 is an exception) do not make a point of explicitly addressing the issue of degree and immediacy of endangerment, positions with respect to this issue are obvious from examining the definitions (see Table 5.1). For example, the Gelles and Straus (1986) definition of abuse is restricted to physical assaults—behaviors that have a high likelihood of leading to immediate and very serious injury—whereas the other endangerment definitions include not only physically assaultive behaviors but also behaviors that are less likely to result in serious physical injury (i.e., spanking, slapping, pushing, grabbing, shoving, etc). Such behaviors might be viewed as more likely to have a long-term effect on the child's mental and social health (i.e., impair ability to relate to others). Generally speaking, definitions of neglect—all of which use endangerment as the minimum criteria—vary little with respect to immediacy and degree of endangerment. Examination of the operational criteria for neglect reveals instead serious omissions in care—those that have a very high likelihood of resulting in immediate and fairly severe consequences.

Questions

This brief review of the "consequence of behavior" dimension suggests two important questions to consider as we begin to formulate agreed-upon

TABLE 5.1. Physical Abuse Definitions

Demonstrable Harm Definitions

Altemeier and colleagues (1984): An abused child is one who has incurred injuries (bruises, abrasions, cuts, burns, fractures, bites, and loss of hair) as a result of parental actions.

Starr (1982): An abused child is one who has incurred injuries as a result of parental actions.

Zuravin and Taylor (1987): A physically abused child is one who has sustained injuries that *at a minimum* include any of the following—bruises, welts, cuts, abrasions, or first degree burns—as a result of inappropriate and excessive physical force by a parent or temporary caretaker.

Endangerment Definitions

Second National Incidence Study (1987): Child abuse is physical assault with or without a weapon by a parent or temporary caretaker. It includes hitting with a stick, strap, or other hard object, as well as scalding, burning, poisoning, suffocating, and drowning. It also includes slapping, spanking with hand, hitting with fist, biting, kicking, shoving, shaking, throwing, nonaccidental dropping, stabbing, and choking (U.S. Department of Health and Human Services, 1988).

Gelles and Straus (1986): Child abuse includes the following behaviors directed at a child by a parent *at least once* during the year preceding the interview: kicking, biting, or hitting with a fist; beating up; using a knife or a gun.

Wolock and Horowitz (1977): Child abuse includes the following behaviors: bearing with hands, beating with instruments, burning, locking or tying up, stabbing or slashing, feeding child harmful substances. The perpetrator is the caretaker, someone living with the caretaker, the child's father, mother's paramour (whether living in the home or not), and anyone to whom the mother delegated responsibility for the child.

McGee, Wolfe, and Wilson (1989): Child abuse includes the following behaviors: burns or scalds, shakes intensively, hits with an object, bites, hits, punches or kicks, intensively spanks, slaps, pushes/grabs/shoves, throws against something, and throws something at child.

---

definitions: (1) Should demonstrable harm or endangerment dictate application of the label of abuse or the label of neglect? (2) If endangerment is chosen as the guiding criterion, where should we set the cutoff in terms of degree and immediacy of endangerment?

Recommendations for Resolving the Differences

On the basis of the guidelines established in the first section "General Definitional Principles," demonstrable harm definitions are not recommended for *research* definitions. Given the importance attached to deter-

TABLE 5.2. Physical Neglect Definition
The Second National Incidence Study (NIS-2)

Neglect consists of seven categories of behaviors that endanger the child's well-being. The perpetrator of the first five types must be the parent whereas the perpetrator of the last two types may be the parent or some other caretaker.

Refusal of health care: failure to provide or obtain needed assessment or treatment in accord with recommendations by a competent health care professional for an apparent physical injury, illness, condition, or impairment.

Delay in health care: failure to seek timely and appropriate medical care for a serious health problem *that* any reasonable layman would have recognized as needing professional medical attention.

Abandonment: desertion of a child without arranging for reasonable care and supervision; includes cases where children were not claimed within 2 *days* and where children were left by parents/substitutes who gave no (or false) information about their whereabouts and did not return or otherwise claim custody within 2 days.

Expulsion: blatant refusals of custody, such as permanent or indefinite expulsion of a child from the home without adequate arrangement for care by others, or refusal to accept custody of a returned runaway.

Other custody issues: custody-related forms of inattention to the child's needs other than those covered by abandonment or expulsion; includes repeated shuttling of a child from one household to another due to apparent unwillingness to maintain custody, chronically and repeatedly leaving a child with others for days/weeks at a time, leaving a child with a person clearly unable to care for the child (i.e., elderly invalid, mentally retarded person, etc.).

Inadequate supervision: child left unsupervised or inadequately supervised for extended periods of time or allowed to remain away from home overnight without the parent knowing (or attempting to determine) the child's whereabouts.

Inattention to physical needs: conspicuous inattention to physical hazards in the home or grounds (i.e., exposed wiring, broken glass, filth, unhygienic pets, etc), the child's needs for nutritious foods, adequate clothing and/or adequate personal hygiene; other forms of reckless disregard (i.e., driving with child while intoxicated, leaving young child unattended in motor vehicle, etc.).

From *Study of National Incidence and Prevalence of Child Abuse and Neglect* (pp. 4-11, 4-12) by U.S. Department of Health and Human Services, 1987, Arlington, VA: National Clearinghouse on Child Abuse and Neglect Information.

mining the longer-term impact of abuse and neglect on cognitive, social, and emotional adjustment, a demonstrable harm definition is clearly too restrictive and narrow. Physical harm need not be present for a behavior to have significant adverse effects at some later date on cognitive, social, and emotional adjustment.

The most appropriate definitions, given current research objectives, are those that use endangerment as a criteria, those that are broad in

TABLE 5.3. Child Neglect Definition

Neglect is the failure to provide basic necessities for the child that *may* or does result in damage to the physical, emotional, or intellectual development and well-being of the child. The perpetrator is the caretaker, someone living with the caretaker, the child's father, mother's paramour (whether living in the home or not), and anyone to whom the mother delegates responsibility for the child. Neglect is conceptualized into three subtypes.

Health care, hygiene, and physical needs neglect: e.g., dirty clothing and inadequate personal hygiene, child not fed properly, medical/dental/mental health problems untreated, inadequate clothing for weather

Environmental and physical care neglect: filthy home (client-induced), including dirty dishes, food laying open, smells of urine; inadequate housing or facilities (not client-induced), including no heat or hot water, broken windows, falling plaster; and failure to provide a permanent shelter

Supervision neglect: e.g., inadequate supervision, including left alone for period inappropriate to age, left with caretaker without material support, left with inadequate babysitter/caretaker, sick child left alone; inappropriate supervision, including children handled inconsistently, children put out of house when caretaker drunk or entertaining, criminal behavior by adults committed in front of children; inattention to schooling needs, including children not in school or children late to school; child exploited, including made to stay home and take care of home and parents, sent out to beg, and made to assume household responsibilities way beyond capabilities

From *Factors Relating to Level of Child Care among Families Receiving Public Assistance in New Jersey* by I. Wolock and B. Horowitz, 1977. Final report to the National Center on Child Abuse and Neglect (DHEW Grant 90-C-418).

scope with respect to hypothesized degree of endangerment posed by caretaker behaviors, and those that do not focus on immediate physical endangerment. With respect to physical abuse, this means the definition should include not only physically assaultive behaviors (those that have a high probability of leading to immediate, serious physical injury) but also physically aggressive ones like throwing something at the child, pushing, grabbing, shoving, hitting, slapping, and spanking. Such behaviors, while not likely to physically harm the child, may well affect the child's social and emotional development. If they are not included in the definitions of abuse and neglect we will never know if they have an adverse effect or the extent of this effect. With respect to physical neglect, it is probably not necessary to broaden the definitions. Research (Zuravin, Masnyk, & Smith, 1990) on each type of neglect reveals that fewer than 10% of the children suffered immediate physical harm, destroyed property, or harmed others as a result of the various subtypes of neglect. This finding suggests that the behaviors are broad enough to allow us to assess their longer-term effects on adjustment.

TABLE 5.4. Child Neglect Definition

Neglect includes eight types of omissions in care by parents or permanent caretakers that *may* or do result in physical, emotional, social, and/or cognitive harm to the child *or* harm to others or their property (as a result of the child's actions).

Physical health care: failure to obtain or delay in obtaining medical attention for acute illnesses, injuries, physical disabilities, and chronic problems, *or* failure to comply with professional recommendations (medical, school, or social work) regarding treatment.

Mental health care: failure to obtain or delay in obtaining professional attention for *obvious* mental health problems and developmental problems; *or* failure to comply with professional recommendations regarding treatment.

Supervision: inadequate supervision of child activities both inside and outside of the home—parent is in the home with the child but is not monitoring the child's activities closely enough to keep the child from behaving in ways that could have negative consequences for the child, others, and/or property *or* parent is not aware enough of the child's activities when he/she is out of the home to assure that the child is not at risk for negative personal consequences or engaging in behaviors that could harm others or other's property; includes truancy, being consistently late for school, and failure to enroll in school; *Age-Graded* (see Appendix).

Substitute child care: abandons child, leaves child alone to fend for himself, leaves child in the care of an inappropriate caretaker, leaves child with any caretaker for more than 48 hours without either telling the caretaker in advance that the child would remain for 2 days or calling during the first 2 days; *Age-Graded* (see Appendix for operational definitions).

Housing hazards: e.g., leaking gas from stove or heating unit, hot water/steam leaks from radiators, dangerous substances (household cleaning agents, insect and rodent poisons, medications, anything that if swallowed could cause death or serious illness), and dangerous objects (guns and knives) stored in unlocked lower shelves or cabinets, under sink, or in the open, etc.).

Household sanitation: garbage is not kept in a receptacle but instead is strewn around the house or kept in bags that are rarely taken away; perishable foods are not refrigerated and are frequently found spoiling; roaches, mice, and/or rats are frequently seen in the home; toilets are not functioning, with human excrement spilling on floor; animal excrement is visible around the house, etc.

Personal hygiene: constant and consistent inattention to child's personal hygiene (e.g., child's hair is matted or tangled and dirty; child's skin is dirty; child's teeth are encrusted with green or brown matter; infant/toddler's soiled diapers are not changed for hours/days; child's clothes, which are soiled and stained beyond cleaning, are worn for days).

Nutrition: failure to provide regular and ample meals that meet basic nutritional requirements (meals have not been provided at all for several days, children eat spoiled food or nonfood items like starch, dog food, or cat food, or are frequently seen begging for food) *and* failure to provide the necessary rehabilitative diet to a child with particular types of physical health problems (lead poisoning, severe diarrhea, etc.)

From *Family Planning Behavior and Child Care Adequacy* by S. Zuravin and R. Taylor, 1987. Final report submitted to the U.S. Department of Health and Human Services, Office of Population Affairs (Grant FPR 000028-01-1).

Subcategories of Neglect and Abuse

Neglect: Identification of Issues

Two issues are pertinent to the subtyping of physical neglect: (1) the clarity of conceptual definitions for the subcategories and (2) the appropriateness of specific behaviors for operationalizing each subtype.

Examination of the neglect definitions (see Tables 5.2 to 5.4) reveals substantial differences pertaining to the clarity with which subtypes are conceptualized. The Wolock and Horowitz (1977) definition, which includes only three subtypes, is the least precise conceptually. It lumps together several different kinds of neglect under each of the three subtypes. The remaining two definitions, while clearer conceptually, each has some clarity problems. NIS-2 (USDHHS, 1988) is much more precise conceptually than Zuravin and Taylor (1987) with respect to health care (there are two subtypes—refusal and delay) and custody-related issues (three subtypes—abandonment, expulsion, and other custody issues). On the other hand, Zuravin and Taylor are more precise conceptually than NIS-2 with respect to physical needs (they recognize four subtypes—housing hazards, housing sanitation, personal hygiene, and nutrition). NIS-2 groups together all physical types of neglect.

Despite these differences in conceptual clarity, comparison of the three definitions reveals more general areas of agreement than disagreement with respect to what constitutes neglect. For all three, neglect involves parental/caretaker failures with respect to physical health care, supervision, custody-related matters, conditions in the home, nutrition, and personal hygiene. They disagree with respect to two subtypes:

1. Expulsion (blatant refusal of custody and refusal to accept custody); NIS-2 includes this as a subtype, the other two do not.
2. Obtaining mental health care; both Zuravin and Taylor, and Wolock and Horowitz include this as a type of physical neglect while NIS-2 identifies it as a type of emotional neglect.

In addition to differences relative to conceptual clarity, the definitions also vary with respect to operational criteria for the subtypes. Careful examination of the specific behaviors included under each subtype reveals the following six differences:

1. Reckless disregard (driving with child while intoxicated, leaving young child in car unattended). NIS-2 includes this as supervisory neglect; the other two do not it include at all.
2. Exploitation (child made to stay home and take care of house and/or other children; child made to assume household responsi-

bilities way beyond capabilities; and child sent out to beg): Wolock and Horowitz classify exploitation as supervisory neglect; the other two references do not include it at all.

3. Exposure of child to inappropriate adult behavior (criminal behavior committed by adult in front of child). Wolock and Horowitz classify this as supervisory neglect; the other two references do not include it at all.

4. Education (truancy and failure to enroll): NIS-2 classifies this in a separate category called educational neglect; the other two references include it under supervisory neglect.

5. Failure to provide a permanent shelter: Wolock and Horowitz include this under environment/physical care neglect; the other two references do not include it at all.

6. Children handled inconsistently: Wolock and Horowitz include this under supervisory neglect; the other two do not include it at all.

Questions

This review of the type of maltreatment dimension suggests two important questions. (1) How much conceptual clarity is necessary for subtyping physical neglect—that is, should we develop a new conceptual scheme that includes more subtypes? (2) Should any of the following parent behaviors be construed as physically neglectful: blatant custody refusals, failure to obtain mental health care, educational neglect (failure to enroll child in school, failure to get child off to school in morning, allowing child to remain out of school, etc.), abandonment/desertion, failure to provide a permanent residence, reckless disregard, exploitation, exposure of child to inappropriate adult behavior, and inconsistent handling of the child? If so, should they be included as separate subtypes or operationalizations of existing subtypes?

Resolving the Differences

As noted in the section "General Definitional Principles," conceptual clarity is exceptionally important for research definitions, particularly those formulated for the purpose of identifying short- and long-term sequelae. Given that few children are subjected to all of the various types of neglect (Zuravin, Masnyk, & Smith, 1990), it will not be possible to determine if consequences vary as a function of subtype if the distinction between subtypes is blurred. Refusal of health care and delay in obtaining health care should be conceptualized as two different subtypes. Even though they may result in equally serious physical consequences for the child, they represent very different issues and may have different effects on emotional/social adjustment.

Educational neglect, custody refusals, refusal to provide mental health care, delay in providing mental health care, and failure to provide a permanent residence should all be conceptualized as specific subtypes of neglect. Because their hypothesized consequences are more likely to be emotional, social, or cognitive in nature is not sufficient justification for classifying them as other types of maltreatment (education for NIS-2) or psychological maltreatment (custody refusals, mental health care). They do represent omissions in care. Failure to provide a permanent residence, conceptualized by Wolock and Horowitz (1977) as supervisory neglect, is not an appropriate operationalization of this concept; it is an example of using many very different kinds of parental behaviors to operationalize a single concept. Clearly, this behavior does not appropriately operationalize any other concept; however, it is common enough and possibly serious enough in terms of consequences that it should stand alone as a subtype.

Abandonment/desertion, exploitation, exposure of the child to inappropriate adult behavior, and inconsistent handling of the child are all behaviors that have been used to operationalize psychological maltreatment. On the basis of McGee and Wolfe's (in press) operational definition of psychological maltreatment— "negative parent–child *communications* that may potentially damage the child psychologically, given his or her special vulnerabilities" (p. 31)—the latter two behaviors are not physically neglectful behaviors. Exploitation, a behavior not considered by McGee and Wolfe, is also ruled out; it is a commission and is more clearly a type of psychological maltreatment than an instance of physical neglect. Abandonment/desertion, a type of behavior that has been considered as psychological maltreatment (Garbarino, Guttman, & Seeley, 1986; Hart, Germain, & Brassard, 1987 McGee & Wolfe, in press) should be established as its own subtype. It is clearly different from supervisory neglect, custody refusals, and other custody-related problems.

Reckless disregard, an operationalization of supervisory neglect used by NIS-2, presents somewhat of a problem. It includes two types of behavior: leaving a young child unattended in the car and driving with a child while intoxicated. The former behavior clearly fits with the other operational criteria for supervisory neglect while the latter does not. Despite this, the concept fits well enough with supervisory neglect that it probably should be used as an operational definition.

Given the importance of being able to determine if different subtypes of maltreatment vary with respect to their effects, a conceptual scheme for physical neglect that includes 14 subtypes may be established. These are listed in Table 5.5. Particularly relevant to defining physical neglect is avoidance of overlap with emotional maltreatment. Review of definitions for emotional maltreatment (e.g., Garbarino, Guttman, & Seeley, 1986; Hart, Germain, & Brassard, 1987; McGee & Wolfe, in press) revealed only

TABLE 5.5. Neglect Subtypes

Refusal to provide physical health care	Abandonment/desertion
Delay in providing physical health care	Failure to provide a permanent home
Refusal to provide mental health care	Personal hygiene neglect
Delay in providing mental health care	Housing hazards
Supervisory neglect	Housing sanitation
Custody refusal	Nutritional neglect
Custody-related neglect	Educational neglect

one—that of McGee and Wolfe (in press), whose conceptual and operational definitions are quite distinct from those of neglect. Conceptually, McGee and Wolfe (in press) restrict emotional maltreatment to "negative parent–child *communications* that may potentially damage the child psychologically, given his or her special vulnerabilities (particularly his or her developmental level)" (p. 31). Operationally, McGee, Wolfe, and Wilson (1989) define psychological maltreatment in terms of 23 parent behaviors.

Abuse Subtyping: Identifying and Resolving Issues

Unlike neglect, there are no existing models for subtyping abuse. Consequently, the main issue centers around how to subcategorize this type of maltreatment. As noted earlier, abusive behaviors differ in three ways: (1) potential of the behavior for leading to serious immediate injuries, (2) the type and nature of the behavior, and (3) whether the behavior is fairly frequent and typical of the discipline used by the caretaker or is infrequent and episodic. It might be best to divide abuse into two subtypes: discipline behaviors and behaviors that are episodic and due to explosive outbursts.

Identity of the Perpetrator

Identification of Issues

"Identity of the perpetrator" is an element that needs to be part of the conceptual definition of maltreatment. The issue regarding this element pertains to whether the label of abuse or neglect should be applied to acts committed by a wide or narrow range of perpetrators. Narrow definitions identify the perpetrator as the primary caretaker (parent or guardian), wider definitions include a variety of others (e.g., temporary caretakers like baby-sitters, mother's boyfriend). Examination of the sample definitions does not reveal any predominant patterns. Of the six abuse definitions, three use a narrow definition, two a very wide definition, and the sixth does not specify a definition. Of the three neglect definitions, one construed perpetrator very narrowly (Zuravin and Taylor, 1987), one (NIS-2; see USDHHS, 1987) semi-narrowly (five types were restricted to the parent and two types to parent or temporary caretaker), and one (Wolock & Horowitz, 1977) very widely.

Questions

The perpetrator issue suggests three important questions. (1) Should we construe perpetrator broadly or narrowly? (2) Should this dimension differ by type of maltreatment or subtype of neglect? (3) If it should be construed broadly, who should be included as perpetrators?

Resolving the Issues

Physical abuse should take a broad definition of perpetrator. Regardless of who does the abusing the child may be endangered physically, socially, and emotionally. Furthermore, consequences with respect to a child's adjustment could vary as a function of the abuser's identity. As Widom (1988) notes, "There has been little systematic research into the causes or consequences of abuse by a variety of perpetrators" (p. 262). All of the following may be included as perpetrators: the child's permanent caretaker/parent(s), adults other than the caretaker living in the same household as the child, the child's father/mother (not living in the household), mother/father's paramour or boyfriend/girlfriend (regardless of whether they live in the household), someone else to whom the caretaker delegates responsibility for the child or someone with whom the caretaker leaves the child, teachers, licensed day-care providers, and staff of residential centers. While the last three perpetrators differ conceptually (professional vs. lay) from the others, abuse by a professional (a person who occupies roles of responsibility and is trusted by the child) may be as likely to have harmful consequences as abuse by persons in the child's informal network. At the very least, it is important to test the hypothesis empirically.

An interesting problem and potential area of overlap between physical neglect and physical abuse is the situation in which the child's caretaker/parent has delegated responsibility for the child or dropped the child off without any formal delegation of responsibility to an inappropriate substitute caretaker (a person who is mentally retarded, mentally ill, or known by the mother to be abusive or who has abused the child in the past). If the inappropriate caretaker physically or sexually abuses the child, is this situation to be classified as both neglect and abuse? The answer is yes, because use of an inappropriate caretaker is one of the core operational criteria for custody-related physical neglect. If the child was not harmed, the label of neglect would be applied. Thus, why would it *not* be applied if the child *was* harmed? Moreover, in this type of situation, neglect could be construed as an important etiological factor for the abuse.

With respect to physical neglect, the issue of perpetrator needs to be treated differently than it was for abuse. *In most instances*, the perpetrator should be restricted to the child's parent(s)/permanent caretaker. After all, parents are legally responsible for providing daily care for their children. If the parent delegates responsibility to an inappropriate caretaker, drops the child off somewhere, and so forth and the child is at risk for harm or is actually harmed (because of physical or sanitation hazards in the caretaker's home or, for example, because the caretaker does not take the child for health care or does not feed the child) the parent, *not* the caretaker, is the perpetrator. The parent had an obligation to make sure that the child was being left with a responsible person. On the other hand, if the parent makes every effort to ensure that the child is being left with a responsible temporary caretaker but the child turns out to be at risk for harm or is actually harmed as a result of any of the various types of neglect, then the temporary caretaker is the perpetrator.

Behavioral Frequency/Chronicity/Time Period

Identification of Issues

"Behavioral frequency" is an operational problem that centers around the issue of how often the act of maltreatment must occur or how long it must continue before the label of "physical abuse" or "neglect" is applied. Some definitions do not address the issue of frequency/chronicity/time period for either physical abuse or neglect. Examination of those that do reveals a range of patterns with differences being dependent on one or more of five factors: (1) the type of behavior, (2) the potential of the behavior for harm, (3) whether the child has suffered demonstrable harm, (4) the severity of the harm, and (5) the child's age. As noted earlier, those definitions that require "a recurrent or chronic pattern" do not operationally define what this means. How many times does the maltreatment have to occur before it is classified as chronic or recurrent? Moreover, none of the definitions distinguish between "chronic behavioral patterns and infrequent explosive episodes" (Widom, 1988, p. 263).

With respect to physical abuse two patterns are evident. Zuravin's definition of physical abuse, which is dependent on evidence of physical harm, requires only one incident of inappropriate and excessive force regardless of how severe the harm. The same is true for definitions by Altemeier and associates (1984) and by Starr (1982). Gelles and Straus' (1986) endangerment definition, which includes behaviors with a very

high potential for resulting in injury, also requires on¹
Wolock and Horowitz's (1977) definition of abuse is de,
severity of injury and chronicity. If the injury is severe, one i..
sufficient. If the injury is not severe (bruises) or there are no injuries, the..
a recurrent pattern is required.

With respect to neglect, each of the three definitions uses a somewhat different method of handling the issue of frequency and chronicity (see Tables 5.2–5.4). Wolock and Horowitz (1977) use the same method that they use for abuse (see previous paragraph): if a severe injury or illness results, only one episode is required; otherwise, chronicity is required. NIS-2 uses a variety of methods. To be labeled as deserting a parent must be away for at least 2 days without notifying the temporary caretaker of her/his whereabouts. Custody-related neglect is operationalized as *repeated* shuttling of a child from one household to another due to apparent unwillingness to maintain custody and/or chronically and repeatedly leaving a child with others for days or weeks at a time. Supervisory neglect involves leaving a child unsupervised or inadequately supervised for extended periods of time or allowing the child to remain away from home overnight without the parent knowing (or attempting to determine) the child's whereabouts.

Zuravin and Taylor (1987) also use a variety of methods to deal with the issue of frequency and chronicity, methods similar to Wolock and colleagues: if the neglect leads to injury or illness, establishment of a chronic pattern is not necessary; otherwise it is. Like NIS-2, they require 2 days to establish desertion. With respect to supervisory and caretaker-related neglect, time periods vary as a function of the child's age (see Appendix). With respect to educational neglect a child must be absent from school for a minimum of 20 days without legitimate reason (illness) or the parent *never* enrolled the child in school.

Questions

The frequency/chronicity/time period issue suggests a number of interesting and important questions. (1) If the behavior results in an injury/illness/impairment, is the need to establish chronicity eliminated? Should the severity of the injury/illness make a difference? (2) With respect to physical abuse, should the highly assaultive types of behavior (i.e., use of a knife or gun, scalding, burning, poisoning, suffocating, drowning, choking, etc.), those likely to result in very serious injury, require chronicity? (3) Which subtypes of neglect should require a chronicity/frequency criterion? (4) How should we operationalize chronicity? How many times or for how long a time does a type of behavior have to occur before it is considered chronic?

Resolving the Issues

Any abusive or neglectful behavior that results in an injury/ illness/ impairment, regardless of severity, should be considered maltreatment and eliminate the need to establish chronicity. Because the short-term effect of an act is confined to a minor injury/illness/impairment (Wolock & Horowitz, 1977) does not automatically rule out a longer term effect on social and emotional adjustment. Clearly, we need to test empirically whether acts resulting in minor versus severe immediate consequences differ with respect to both etiology and longer-term impact. With respect to degree of assaultiveness, those behaviors with a very high likelihood of causing serious injury should be considered abuse even if they occur only one time.

Of the 14 subtypes of neglect (see Table 5.3) at least 5 should probably require establishment of a chronic pattern *if* they do not result in immediate harm. They are custody-related neglect, supervision, child's personal hygiene, education, and failure to provide a permanent home—all have been defined by one or more of the existing definitions as requiring chronicity. The problem with chronicity lies in specific operationalization of the concept. As noted earlier, none of the definitions specifically define how long or how many times the behavior must occur. As we formulate agreed-upon definitions, this is an issue that is probably best decided by consensus. Generally speaking, the subtypes are operationalized in terms of specific, concrete behaviors. However, there are some problems with respect to issues of frequency and time periods. For example, what does "constant inattention" (Zuravin and Taylor, 1987) mean with respect to housing hazards, housing sanitation, and the child's personal hygiene? What does "extended periods of time" (NIS-2) mean with respect to supervision?

Perpetrator Intent to Harm/Culpability for Behavior

Identification of Issues

"Intent to harm" and culpability for behavior are conceptual problems. The former refers to the issue of whether the perpetrator purposely meant to harm the child while the latter concept refers to the issue of whether the perpetrator can legitimately be blamed for the behavior. An intention to harm, a criterion that has been used mainly for physical abuse, is not a part of any of the more recent research definitions of abuse or neglect. On the other hand, the concept of culpability, is currently being used as a qualifier with respect to defining the physical types of neglect. NIS-2 (USDHHS, 1987) specifies that, in cases where parents cannot financially provide generally safe hygiene conditions, hazardous housing conditions cannot be called neglectful. Wolock and Horowitz (1977) employ the same type of qualifier with respect to housing. For housing sanitation problems (spoiled foods, dirty dishes, etc.) to qualify as neglect, they must be parent induced. For inadequate housing (no heat or hot water, broken windows, falling plaster) to qualify as neglect, they also must be parent-induced.

Questions

The issue of intent to harm or culpability for behavior raises one important question: Should either be required to classify a particular type of behavior as either abusive or neglectful? With respect to neglect, this issue translates into the question: Are some parents so poor that neglect—particularly in terms of health care and housing conditions—is unavoidable and thus cannot be considered an omission in care on the part of the parents? With respect to abuse, the issue can be translated into two specific questions. Must the motive for the behavior be an intent to harm, or can discipline that gets out of hand qualify as abuse? The second question, one identified by researchers (e.g., Fisher & Berdie, 1978) who are working with adolescent abuse, pertains to the issue of provocation. They ask, If the teen provokes the abuse, is the parent culpable? In other words, considering of the teenager's larger size, greater strength, and greater independence, should the parent be blamed for the abuse when the teenager is provocative?

Resolving the issues

Neither the concept of intent nor the concept of culpability should be used as a definitional criterion. First and foremost, it is exceptionally difficult, if not impossible, to operationalize either of these terms. Second, even if we could operationalize them, it would be unwarranted to eliminate from the definition behaviors that are unintended, behaviors for which the parents are not culpable, or behaviors that are provoked. We are interested in determining the effects of parent/caretaker behaviors on child/teen adjustment, in identifying etiologies, and in determining treatments. In addition, it does not seem likely that any of the qualifiers would attenuate the effects of unsanitary and inadequate housing, delay/refusal in providing health care, blatant custody refusals, or assaultive behaviors. Thirdly, with respect to neglect, survey studies (Giovannoni & Billingsley, 1970; Wolock & Horowitz, 1977; Zuravin & Taylor, 1987) that have compared very low income (mainly or exclusively AFDC—Aid to Families of Dependent Children—recipients) neglectful and nonneglectful families have found that the neglectful families are significantly poorer with respect to material things (housing, possessions, etc.) than their comparably poor counterparts. I interpret these findings to mean that the neglectful mother's housing and sanitary problems are not a reflection of her poverty—as NIS-2 and Wolock and Horowitz suggest—but, rather, a reflection of her poor management of financial and other material resources. If, in fact, these problems are due to poor management, then they are involved in the etiology of certain types of neglect. The last thing we would want to do would be to rule out a potential etiological factor. A similar point can be made with respect to provocation by a child or teen— the type of parent–child interaction where children are provocative is very likely to represent a significant etiological issue as well as an important treatment concern.

Age of Child

Identification of Issues

The age of the child is an operational consideration when age-graded criteria need to be elaborated for certain types of parent/caretaker behavior. In other words, should the labeling of certain types of caretaker behaviors as maltreating be dependent on the child's age? As noted earlier, this issue is more relevant to neglect than abuse. Of the three definitions, Zuravin and Taylor's (1987) is the only one that establishes explicit age-related standards. The two maltreatment subtypes that they age-grade have to do with supervision and child care arrangements (see Appendix). The other two definitions of neglect do not treat the issue of age-grading in an explicit fashion. Wolock and Horowitz's (1977) definition of supervisory neglect mentions "age appropriateness" but does not include explicit criteria. NIS-2 does not address the issue at all except with respect to leaving young children alone in a car.

Questions

Three questions are raised by this issue. Should we age-grade operational definitions of various types of neglect? If so, which subtypes should be age-graded? And what factors should drive the age-grading?

Resolving the Issues

There is no doubt that certain subtypes of neglect require age-grading. I concur with Polansky and colleagues (1972) that what is considered neglect at one age can be seen as infantilization at another. Review of the 14 neglect subtypes listed in Table 5.5 identifies only two that would be appropriate for age-grading: supervision and custody-related neglect (see NIS-2 for definitions of both). Zuravin and Taylor (1987), who age-graded both, did so on a rational-intuitive basis. As we formulate agreed-upon definitions for neglect subtypes, decisions about specific age-graded operationalizations should be made by consensus.

SUMMARY

One of the major problems impeding the development of knowledge about child maltreatment is the lack of a reliable, agreed-upon taxonomy. In the absence of such a taxonomy, researchers have used different definitions for the same type of maltreatment, have failed to collect information about the presence of other types of maltreatment when studying one particular type, and have used definitions of one type of maltreatment that overlap with definitions of other types. In the interest of developing standard *research* definitions for abuse and neglect, this chapter focuses on (1) identifying conceptual and operational problems with existing definitions and (2) making recommendations on how to resolve these problems. Specific recommendations are made for conceptually and operationally defining the two types of maltreatment with respect to six parameters: consequences of the behavior, types of behavior, perpetrator, chronicity, perpetrator intent/culpability, and age of child. These recommendations, some of which differ for the two types of maltreatment, are summarized below.

1. *Consequence of behavior.* Endangerment of the child's health and welfare rather than demonstrable harm to the child should be the criterion for applying the labels of physical abuse and physical neglect. It should be an element of the conceptual definition for each type of maltreatment and should be operationally translated by specific parent/caretaker behaviors.

2. *Type of behavior.* Neglect should be divided into 14 subtypes of behavior (see Table 5.5) that pertain to health care, supervision and custody issues, education, and physical care issues. Each subtype needs to be conceptually defined and its operational translations need to be distinct, that is nonoverlapping with those of other subtypes and with definitions of emotional mistreatment. Abuse should be divided into two subtypes: discipline behaviors and behaviors that are infrequent and the result of explosive outbursts.

3. *Perpetrator.* The perpetrators of abuse should be defined very broadly and include permanent caretakers, persons living in the same household, temporary caretakers, and professionals who have roles of responsibility and are trusted by the child. The perpetrators of neglect should be defined very narrowly and include the permanent caretaker as well as any supposedly responsible person to whom the caretaker delegates responsibility for the child. The range of perpetrators is a conceptual issue and needs to be an element of the conceptual definition.

4. *Chronicity*. Of the 14 subtypes of neglect (see Table 5.5) at least five should require establishment of a chronic pattern *if* they do not result in immediate harm (regardless of severity). They are custody-related neglect, supervision, personal hygiene, education, and failure to provide a permanent home. With respect to abuse, any highly assaultive behavior should be considered abusive even if it occurs only one time. Less assaultive behaviors (grabbing, shaking, spanking, etc.) require chronicity *unless* they result in an injury (regardless of severity). Chronicity—an operational issue that has not yet been defined—needs to be considered as we formulate agreed-upon definitions.

5. *Perpetrator intent to harm/culpability for harm*. Neither perpetrator intent to harm, culpability for harm, or provocation by the child should be a criterion for defining a behavior as abusive or neglectful.

6. *Age of child*. The age of the child should *not* be a consideration with respect to defining abuse. It is, however, important with respect to defining at least two subtypes of neglect: supervision and custody-related neglect. The operational definitions for both should be age-graded so that criteria for labeling a type of behavior as neglectful vary with the age of the child.

In summary, if we truly want to develop a sound knowledge base about physical abuse and neglect, it is mandatory that we undertake the difficult task of developing standard definitions for these two types of maltreatment. While one researcher can make recommendations regarding the resolution of existing problems, it is unlikely that we will ever standardize our definitions unless we come together as a group and hammer out our differences. With respect to using groups to arrive at definitions, we can take a lesson from the American Psychiatric Association. This organization convened groups of experts on a variety of mental disorders to undertake the awesome task of developing standardized definitions for 180 mental disorders. By comparison, the four types of maltreatment we have to define seem approachable. Researchers and practitioners, therefore, must advocate for the National Center on Child Abuse and Neglect to do the same thing for maltreatment that the American Psychiatric Association did for mental illness.

APPENDIX

Supervisory Neglect Age Graded Criteria

Neglect in this area refers to inadequate supervision of child activities both inside and outside of the home by the mother or other primary caretaker. More specifically, it refers to two types of situations:

1. The primary caretaker is in the home with the child but is not monitoring the child's activities closely enough to keep the child from behaving in ways that could have negative consequences for himself, others, and/or others' property.

2. The primary caretaker is not aware enough of the child's activities when child is out of the home to ensure that she/he is not at risk for negative personal consequences or engaging in behaviors that could harm others or others' property.

It is important to note that the specific types of supervisory omissions that define neglect in this area differ by age of the child. Obviously, what is inadequate supervision for a 3-year-old may not be inadequate supervision for a 12-year-old. The age-graded operational definitions are as follows:

1. *Inadequate supervision inside the home* includes but is not limited to the following activities for children of various age ranges (all examples are cumulative, meaning that what is true for a child under 12 is automatically true for a child under 3):

  a. Children under 12: (1) playing with matches, the stove, the space heater, electrical outlets, heated irons, medications, and household cleaning agents; (2) playing on fire escapes, steep stairways, windowsills; (3) locking playmates in closets or other closed in spaces; and (4) hanging out windows.

  b. Children under 3: (1) sitting unattended in a high chair or tub full of bathwater or (2) lying on a bed without sides.

2. *Inadequate supervision outside the home* includes but is not limited to the following activities for children of various age ranges (examples are cumulative):

  a. Children under 16: (1) caretaker is completely unaware of child's whereabouts when child is out of the house, i.e., doesn't know where child is or who child is with; (2) child remains out all night without informing caretaker of whereabouts or companions; (3) child is gone for days at a time without caretaker knowing his whereabouts or companions; (4) truancy (child is absent from school for a minimum of 20 days without legitimate reason , e.g., illness); (5) Not enrolling a child in school (primary caretaker never bothers to register a child for school, regardless of the reason).

  b. Children under 12: (1) child remains outside after dark with no supervision.

  c. Children under 7: (1) child wanders outside the home alone and plays unsupervised; (2) child wanders off, gets lost, and is unable to find caretaker without help.

Substitute Child Care: Age-Graded Criteria

Neglect in this area refers to failure on the part of the primary caretaker to arrange safe and appropriate substitute child care when caretaker needs to be away from the child for a period of time. This kind of neglect refers to three general types of situations. The primary caretaker:

1. leaves child alone to fend for self
2. leaves child in the care of an inappropriate caretaker
3. deserts child

Operational definitions of the three types of inadequate substitute child care vary with the age of the child. The age-graded operational definitions are as follows:

1. *Inappropriate caretakers* include strangers, children under 13 for purposes of baby sitting for a few hours with other children under 13, children under 16 for purposes of overnight caretaking of other children under 16, individuals with alcohol and drug problems, individuals who are known to have sexually victimized and/or physically abused children, individuals with serious mental health problems (severe depression, mania, and/or schizophrenia), individuals who are mentally retarded, and individuals with physical handicaps (blind, deaf, wheelchair-bound).

2. *Desertion* pertains to two situations: leaving children under 16 to (1) fend for self for more than 48 hours or (2) with any caretaker for more than 48 hours without either telling the caretaker in advance that the child would remain for 2 days or calling during the first 2 days to explain the delay and to specify how much longer return would be delayed.

3. *Age level definitions of inappropriate child care arrangements*:

   a. *Children under 8*: leaving children under 8 alone or with an inappropriate caretaker for any amount of time is neglectful.

   b. *Children 8 to 12*: Leaving children 8 to 12 years old alone for short periods of time (3 or 4 hours), provided they have been instructed about how to obtain help in an emergency, provided they know where mother is and when she is returning, and provided mother is responsible about returning on time is NOT considered neglect.

      1. Leaving children in this age range alone for 3 or 4 hours and NOT instructing them about where and how to obtain help, NOT notifying them when return is going to be delayed, and NOT telling them where mother is going is considered neglect.

      2. Leaving children in this age range with an inappropriate caretaker for any period of time is considered neglect.

   c. *Children 13 to 15*: Leaving children alone or with an inappropriate caretaker overnight or longer is considered neglect.

REFERENCES

Aber, L., & Zigler, E. (1981). Developmental considerations in the definition of child maltreatment. *New Directions in Child Development, 11,* 1–29.

Altemeier, W., O'Connor, S., Vietze, P., Sandler, H., & Sherrod, K. (1984). Prediction of child abuse: A prospective study of feasibility. *Child Abuse & Neglect, 8,* 393–400.

American Psychiatric Association. (1987). *Diagnostic and Statistic Manual of Mental Disorders* (3rd ed., rev.). Washington, DC: Author.

Cicchetti, D., & Todd-Manly, J. (in press). Problems and solutions to conducting research in maltreating families: An autobiographical perspective. In I. Siegel & G. Brody (Eds.), *Research on families.* New York: Pergamon Press.

Cicchetti, D., & Rizley, R. (1981). Developmental perspectives on the etiology, intergenerational transmission, and sequelae of child maltreatment. *New Directions for Child Development, 11,* 31–55.

Egeland, B., & Sroufe, A. (1981). Developmental sequelae of maltreatment in infancy. *New Directions for Child Development, 11,* 77–91.

Eysenck, H. (1952). *The scientific study of personality.* London: Routledge & Kegan Paul.

Federal Register. (1989, June). Program announcement # 13670–891, 54(104): 23566–23587.

Fisher, B., & Berdie, J. (1978). Adolescent abuse and neglect: Issues of incidence, intervention, and service delivery. *Child Abuse & Neglect, 2,* 173–192.

Garbarino, J., & Gilliam, G. (1980). *Understanding abusive families.* Lexington, MA: Lexington Books.

Garbarino, J., Guttman, E., & Seeley, J. (1986). *The psychologically battered child.* San Francisco: Jossey-Bass.

Gelles, R. (1982). Problems in defining and labeling child abuse. In R. H. Starr, Jr. (Ed.), *Child abuse prediction: Policy implications* (pp. 1–29). Cambridge, MA: Ballinger.

Gelles, R., & Straus, M. (1986). Societal change and change in family violence from 1975 to 1985 as revealed by two national surveys. *Journal of Marriage and the Family, 48,* 465–479.

Giovannoni, J. (1971). Parental mistreatment: Perpetrators and victims. *Journal of Marriage and the Family, 33,* 649–657.

Giovannoni, J., & Becerra, R. (1979). *Defining child abuse.* New York: The Free Press.

Giovannoni, J., & Billingsley, A. (1970). Child neglect among the poor: A study of parental adequacy in families of three ethnic groups. *Child Welfare, 49,* 196–204.

Green, A. H., Gaines, R., & Sandgrund, A. (1974). Child abuse: Pathological syndrome of family interaction. *American Journal of Psychiatry, 131*(8), 882–886.

Hart, S., Germain, R., & Brassard, M. (1987). The challenge: To better understand and combat psychological maltreatment of children and youth. In M. Brassard, R. Germain, & S. Hart (Eds.), *Psychological maltreatment of children and youth* (pp. 3–24). New York: Pergamon Press.

Magura, S., & Moses, B. (1986). *Outcomes measures for child welfare services.* New York: Child Welfare League of America.

McGee, R., & Wolfe, D. (in press). Psychological maltreatment: Towards an operational definition. *Development and Psychopathology.*

McGee, R., Wolfe, D., & Wilson, S. (1989). *Development of a record of maltreatment experiences (ROME) device.* Unpublished manuscript, Department of Psychology, University of Western Ontario, London, Ontario and the Institute for the Prevention of Child Abuse, Toronto, Ontario.

National Center of Child Abuse and Neglect. (1987). Proceedings of the neglect grantees meeting. Washington, DC, August 17–19, 1987.

Polansky, N., Borgman, R., & DeSaix, C. (1972). *Roots of futility.* San Francisco: Jossey-Bass.

Ross, C., & Zigler, E. (1980). An agenda for action. In G. Gerbner, C. Ross, & E. Zigler (Eds.), *Child abuse: An agenda for action* (pp. 293–304). New York: Oxford University Press.

Sack, W. H., Mason, R., & Higgins, J. (1985). The single-parent family and abusive child punishment. *American Journal of Orthopsychiatry, 55,* 252–259.

Spitzer, R., Endicott, J., & Robins, E. (1978). Research diagnostic criteria: Rationale and reliability. *Archives of General Psychiatry, 35,* 773–782.

Starr, R. H., Jr. (1982). A research-based approach to the prediction of child abuse. In R. H. Starr, Jr. (Ed.), *Child abuse prediction: Policy implications* (pp. 105–134). Cambridge, MA: Ballinger.

Straus, M., Gelles, R., & Steinmetz, S. (1980). *Behind closed doors: Violence in the American family.* Garden City, NY: Anchor/Doubleday.

U.S. Department of Health and Human Services. (1988). *Study Findings: Study of national incidence and prevalence of child abuse and neglect.* Arlington, VA: National Clearinghouse on Child Abuse and Neglect Information.

Widom, C. (1988). Sampling biases and implications for child abuse research. *American Journal of Orthopsychiatry, 58,* 260–270.

Wolfe, D., & Mosk, M. (1983). Behavioral comparisons of children from abusive and distressed families. *Journal of Consulting and Clinical Psychology, 51,* 702–708.

Wolock, I., & Horowitz, B. (1977). *Factors relating to levels of child care among families receiving public assistance in New Jersey.* Final report to the National Center on Child Abuse and Neglect (DHEW Grant 90-C-418). Washington, DC: National Clearinghouse on Child Abuse and Neglect Information.

Wolock, I., & Horowitz, B. (1984). Child maltreatment as a social problem: the neglect of neglect. *American Journal of Orthopsychiatry, 54,* 530–543.

Zigler, E., & Phillips, L. (1961). Psychiatric diagnosis. *Journal of Abnormal and Social Psychology, 63,* 607–618.

Zuravin, S., Masnyk, K., & Smith, C. (1990). *Maternal age: Its relationship to types and severity of child neglect.* Unpublished manuscript, University of Maryland School of Social Work, Baltimore, MD.

Zuravin, S., & Taylor, R. (1987). *Family planning behaviors and child care adequacy.* Final report submitted to the U.S. Department of Health and Human Services, Office of Population Affairs (Grant FPR 000028-01-1).

6

Longitudinal Studies in Child Maltreatment: Methodological Considerations

MAUREEN BLACK
University of Maryland School of Medicine

Child maltreatment is a complex behavior that defies basic societal principles of protection and nurturance toward children. Although evidence of child abuse has existed throughout history (Aries, 1962; Ross, 1980), sanctions against harmful family practices, coupled with institutional procedures for protecting children, have only been in effect during the past two or three decades. With an estimated incidence of more than 10% of parents admitting that they committed violent acts against their children in the previous year (Straus & Gelles, 1986), the magnitude of the problem is substantial.

As the responsibility for protecting children has become a societal concern, rather than merely a private matter within families, our understanding of the determinants of child maltreatment has expanded. Systems models, particularly family systems, have enabled us to recognize that child maltreatment is more likely to occur as a pattern of family dysfunction than as an isolated event (Gelles, 1973). Similarly, risk factors for child maltreatment extend beyond single-factor theories to include family functioning and societal influences, as well as temperamental attributes associated with the child (Friedrich & Boriskin, 1976).

Integrated, multifactorial theoretical models have been proposed to reflect the factors and processes associated with both the etiology and the perpetuation of harmful behavior within maltreating families (Belsky,

1980; Cicchetti & Rizley, 1981). Since these models require that attention be given to processes within the family and their potential impact on maltreatment over time, they require more complex research approaches than the cross sectional designs that characterized much of the initial empirical research in child maltreatment (Aber & Cicchetti, 1984).

In this chapter the application of longitudinal study designs to issues of child maltreatment is addressed by reviewing the components of longitudinal study design, types of longitudinal designs, the advantages of longitudinal designs, and the biases and disadvantages that can compromise implementation and interpretation.

LONGITUDINAL STUDY DESIGN

Longitudinal research permits the study of patterns of behavior over time (Goldstein, 1979). Unlike cross sectional research, in which subjects are sampled at a single point, subjects in a longitudinal project are recruited and followed over a predetermined period with either time-dependent or event-dependent data collection points (Baltes & Nesselroade, 1979). By collecting information from subjects with a set of measures repeated at multiple time periods, researchers minimize error variance, and small behavioral changes may be readily detected (Feinstein, 1977). Cross sectional designs can be extremely useful in describing group characteristics and in generating hypotheses about age-related or event-related changes in behavior. However, without the temporal sequencing of measurements inherent in longitudinal designs, cross sectional designs lack the explanatory power to test hypotheses adequately or to identify causal agents.

In the 1920s and 1930s several longitudinal studies were initiated to measure changes in the physical, physiological, and mental growth of children. Many of the original projects have continued and have been extended into multigenerational explorations of personality variables, interpersonal relationships, and caregiving practices (Garmezy, 1988). The shift in emphasis from physical changes to psychological changes required that increased attention be paid to the multiple environmental factors that contribute to psychological development. The major strides in the development of longitudinal methodology and analysis made by the fields of life span development and gerontology (Campbell, Mutran, & Parker, 1987; Patrick & Borgatta, 1981) have enhanced the feasibility of using longitudinal designs in the study of the impact of psychosocial risk factors, such as child maltreatment, on children's adaptation and development (Rutter, 1988).

Behavioral outcome is influenced by the competing influences of normative age-graded, normative history-graded, and nonnormative determinants (Baltes, 1979). Normative age-graded determinants are developmental factors that are associated with age, such as the onset of puberty or the initiation of school attendance. Normative history-graded determinants are variables that influence the members of a group, with less regard for age (Baltes, Reese, & Lipsitt, 1980). For example, economic changes can have a profound impact on child and family development through both direct and indirect influences (Elder, 1979). Nonnormative determinants of behavior change occur selectively in the population and may include both negative events, such as incidence of child maltreatment, and positive events, such as effective intervention programs. The addition of normative history-graded and nonnormative determinants of behavior change has broadened the traditional age-graded longitudinal models into models that can be used to investigate the developmental implications of psychosocial risk factors associated with child maltreatment.

TYPES OF LONGITUDINAL DESIGNS

In order to gather information across time, investigators must focus on previous events, future events, or a combination of past, current, and future events. Garmezy (1988) has outlined four types of longitudinal designs useful in studies of children at risk:

1. *Retrospective data collection* is frequently used by clinicians in their investigation of the relationship between previous events and present behavior. Similarly, researchers may ask subjects to recall events in their past. For example, much of our knowledge about child sexual abuse has come from retrospective surveys of adults (Finkelhor, 1979, 1984). While retrospective study designs can be extremely enlightening and economical in terms of collecting data over a long period of time, they are subject to the possibility of recall bias as more recent events and perceptions interfere with the accurate recollection of past events.

2. *Follow-back designs* are similar to retrospective designs in that they focus exclusively on events in the past and assume a continuity of development. The difference is that in follow-back designs the investigator attempts to reduce recall bias by relying on formal records, such as school reports. However, follow-back investigations are limited to available formal data and provide no information on processes or linkages between earlier information and current findings. Moreover, unless the historical data were collected systematically, group comparisons may be difficult. When the goal of the investigation is to explore antecedents to behavior that is currently maladaptive, both retrospective and follow-back designs are enhanced by the inclusion of a control group (Cook & Campbell, 1977).

3. *Follow-up designs* also take advantage of previous records, but they differ from follow-back studies in their direction. In follow-up studies the investigator begins with previous records and attempts to locate the individuals to collect information on present behaviors. Theoretical linkages are then made from previous records to current behavior; however, again there is no information available on the processes connecting behavior during the two time periods. While follow-up studies are useful in defining the range of outcome options that may result from specific risk factors, unless they include follow-up of a control group of individuals who did not experience the risk factor, they are limited in their generalizability. Despite a lack of studies on the impact of maltreatment on children's social and psychological adjustment (Lamphear, 1985), much of the available information comes from controlled, follow-up designs (Zimrin, 1986)

4. *Follow-through or longitudinal-developmental designs* are an improvement over the previous three types of designs. They begin with at least two groups of children: one experiencing the risk factors under question and the other a control group who did not experience the risk factors. Both groups are followed at regular intervals with data collection designed to measure outcome variables, as well as mediating and moderating variables that may influence the link between risk status and outcome. This type of design is necessary to evaluate intervention programs (Hornick & Clarke, 1986) and has contributed to an understanding of the causes and consequences of child maltreatment (Cicchetti & Rizley, 1981; Egeland, Sroufe, & Erikson, 1983).

ADVANTAGES OF LONGITUDINAL STUDIES

Rutter (1988) has defined the major advantages to longitudinal projects as precision in the timing and measurement of experiences, heterogeneity of outcome, subdivision of disorders by age of onset, intraindividual change, and causal chain analyses. While these categories can be applied to the field of child maltreatment, each advantage must be weighed against the associated costs.

Precision in Timing and Measurement

Researchers interested in the stability or change of behaviors over time can use carefully designed prospective study strategies. For example, Egeland and Sroufe (1981) followed a sample of 267 high-risk primiparous women for 24 months and identified four patterns of maltreating behavior. In a subsequent study (Egeland et al., 1983) they continued the fol-low-through design through the children's preschool years. By identifying a control group of children from families with no identified patterns of maltreating behaviors, the researchers were able to demonstrate deficits in social competence and problem-solving skills among the maltreated children. Moreover, they identified processes that differentiated coping strategies among maltreatment groups. The importance of maternal emotional support was noted at each age (Farber & Egeland, 1987). Through precision in timing in their carefully controlled study, the investigators were able to provide specific information about the impact of types of maltreating families on development among preschoolers.

Timing becomes a critical consideration in the study of the antecedents of child maltreatment. Families must be recruited before the negative behaviors occur, giving rise to both logistical and ethical dilemmas. Since the incidence of child maltreatment ranges from 2% to 14%, depending on the definition of child maltreatment (Wolfe, 1988), one may have to recruit and follow a large number of families in order to obtain a sample of maltreated children. For example, in a prospective study among 1,400 pregnant women in Nashville, 275 high-risk women were identified. By age 3, 25 of the high risk children had been reported for child abuse or neglect and 31 had experienced nonorganic failure to thrive (Altemeier et al., 1979). These rates are consistent with expectations based on national reporting figures.

Heterogeneity of Outcome

The analysis of risk factors has enabled researchers to identify individuals who may be more likely than the general public to experience negative outcomes. However, risk factor analysis sometimes assumes a linear relationship between risk factors and outcome variables with little consideration of intervening variables that may alter the course of events. The transactional nature of child and caregiver interactions and their ability to influence one another's behavior has led researchers away from linear models and toward more interactive models in which multiple routes may be available between risk and outcome (Sameroff & Chandler, 1975; Seifer & Sameroff, 1987). In order to understand how the paths leading to heterogenous outcomes are activated, risk factors have to be operationalized into risk mechanisms (Rutter, 1988).

Children who experience the challenge of risk factors, yet escape the negative sequelae are thought to be invulnerable and perhaps buffered by protective mechanisms. Although Farber and Egeland (1987) present a rather pessimistic view, with few children avoiding the diminished competence associated with early exposure to abuse and neglect, some children may be less vulnerable to these adverse family patterns. By studying the escape routes used by these less vulnerable children, we gain insight into the family processes that influence adaptation in children raised in maltreating environments (Rutter, 1988).

The linkage between risk factors and outcome can be clarified by examining the roles of moderator and mediator variables (Baron & Kenny, 1986). *Moderator variables* influence or clarify the relationship between the predictor and outcome variables. They usually occur at the same time or level as predictor variables and may in fact function as predictor variables. For example, socioeconomic status may be a moderating variable between family behavior and child maltreatment (Pelton, 1978) such that children raised in dysfunctional families who are also poor are more likely to experience maltreatment. Interaction effects between moderator variables and predictor variables also occur, as can be demonstrated using age as an example. Despite at least an equal incidence in maltreatment between adolescents and children, younger children are more likely to be reported for maltreatment than are adolescents (Garbarino, 1989). Thus, knowing the socioeconomic status of a dysfunctional family increases the ability to predict if maltreatment will occur, but knowing the age of the child increases the ability to predict if child maltreatment will be reported.

Mediator variables modify the relationship between the predictor and outcome variables by a transformation process that replaces the direct relationship (Baron & Kenny, 1986). Through mediator variables external factors are transformed into psychological processes that impact behavior. For example, protective factors such as social support decrease the likelihood of maltreatment by altering the relationship between family behavior and child outcome (Garbarino, 1976). Mediational issues are important in understanding how other external variables influence the parent-child relationship. By translating risk factors into actual behaviors, researchers move toward a closer understanding of why certain families become maltreating and others escape that negative route. Since some risk factors may be extremely difficult to change (e.g., poverty), an understanding of mediator variables facilitates the transition from descriptive or inferential research into programmatic recommendations and intervention or prevention research.

Subdivision of Disorder by Age of Onset

Just as longitudinal studies of divorcing families have illustrated the differential impact of divorce based on the age and gender of the child (Hetherington, 1989), studies indicate that both the risk for child maltreatment and the consequences of maltreatment can vary as a function of character-istics of the child (see review by Wolfe, 1988). For example, among young children maltreatment is associated with poverty and limited parental edu-cation (Pelton, 1978). However, among adolescents those associations do not hold, and maltreatment is more broad-based in the population (Gar-barino, 1989). As investigators, service providers, and public policy mak-ers become more informed about the dimensions of child maltreatment, they will be better able to develop programs specifically designed for at-risk populations, rather than generic programs that may not meet the needs of any one group.

Intraindividual Change

Longitudinal studies provide a critical advantage over cross-sectional stud-ies, since the data can be analyzed either to assess changes between groups of individuals or changes within individuals over time. The assembly of a cohort is a central concept in longitudinal research. A cohort is a group of people sharing an age-graded, history-graded, or nonnormative event, who are followed over time and subjected to similar measurement proce-dures. In the examples from life span development or growth studies, cohorts are often selected based on age. In this way each member of a cohort has an equal time opportunity to experience the events under investigation. Data on the outcome and mediator variables of interest are collected during at least two measurement periods. Although *cohort* designs enable the investigator to describe the intraindividual and interindividual changes that occur within the cohort, generalizability may be limited by the presence of cohort bias or cohort differences (Elder, 1975; Gergen, 1980). For example, a longitudinal study of classroom pun-ishment from the 1960s would have significant cohort differences with a study from the 1980s, since the attitudes and policies toward corporal punishment in the classroom have changed.

Schaie (1965) recognized the potential problem with cohort effects and proposed a General Developmental Model incorporating age, cohort, and time of measurement. He recommended recruiting at least two cohorts separated in time, so one could assess the impact of cohort differ-ences on developmental change. These recommendations have sparked debate, and Schaie and Baltes (1975) have agreed that when describing developmental change the ideal matrix for data collection is a bifactorial age-by-cohort model in which at least two cohorts are recruited. Thus, investigators can compare changes in behavior both within and between cohorts with the objective of describing intraindividual change, within cohort interindividual change, and between cohort interindividual changes (Baltes, 1979).

Causal Chain Analyses

Complex social behavior is determined not by single factor main effects models, but by transactions, interactions, and interrelationships among variables (Sameroff & Chandler, 1975; Seifer & Sameroff, 1987). With longitudinal studies designed to assess theoretical models, investigators can move beyond the descriptive stage of design and analysis to the experimental stage.

Although descriptive designs are useful for theory building and hypothesis generation, experimental designs are necessary for hypothesis testing. In an experimental design an antecedent is introduced that precedes the outcome behaviors. The impact of the antecedent condition on intraindividual change and interindividual differences in intraindividual change can then be evaluated. The pattern of intraindividual change can include either changes in the frequency of behaviors across time or in the type of behavior that occurs. For example, if a prevention program for families of newborns were introduced (antecedent condition), investigators could evaluate the impact of the program on the development of parenting practices within individual families, as well as group comparisons between participating and nonparticipating families.

BIASES IN LONGITUDINAL STUDIES RELEVANT TO CHILD MALTREATMENT

While the advantages of longitudinal methodology are significant, one must consider the potential biases that threaten interpretations from longitudinal projects (Feinstein, 1977). In addition to recall bias in retrospective designs, there are several serious biases that are particularly relevant to projects investigating child maltreatment.

When cohort designs are used to investigate the impact of events (e.g., child maltreatment), the cohort may be selected using an event criterion (exposure to child maltreatment) rather than an age criterion. This selection procedure introduces the threat of chronology bias (Feinstein, 1977). Since the children may have experienced child maltreatment for differing lengths of time, estimations of the severity or chronicity of other factors (e.g., behavior changes, stressful events) within the cohort are confounded by the variability in time exposure. The threat of chronology bias is a serious consideration because it is difficult to define exactly when a child began to be maltreated, particularly since the actual maltreatment may precede the identification of maltreatment based on reporting practices. Thus, most investigations of the consequences of child maltreatment include mixed-age cohorts of children with varying degrees of exposure to child maltreatment. Although the potential for chronology bias can not be eliminated, Feinstein (1977) recommends that investigators select and follow multiserial cross-section groups in which the differential time exposure effect is considered. Time-dependent comparisons based on the duration of time since the occurrence of child maltreatment would not be accurate unless clear evidence were available on maltreatment patterns. However, there are other relevant questions investigators could ask regarding exposure to life in a dysfunctional family, behavioral changes since the report was made, and behavioral adjustment since intervention.

Transition bias is a second common research problem and can occur when the cohort is recruited, during the follow-up period, or during the measurement phase (Feinstein, 1977). Transition bias occurs when subjects no longer represent their reference population, thus jeopardizing the generalizability of the findings. If a high risk sample is chosen, then the ability to generalize to other lower risk groups may be compromised. The processes leading to maladaptive outcome in a high risk sample are not necessarily the same as in a lower risk sample. If subjects are not equally eligible for recruitment, then bias may be introduced by those who are approached or by those who agree to participate. For example, without replication studies, findings from studies that involve children who have experienced sexual abuse can not be generalized to other groups of victimized children or to the general population of children. Moreover, the selection process itself introduces transition bias as participants recognize themselves as study participants and thereby different from nonparticipants.

During the follow-up or intervention phase, transition bias takes the form of differential participation. If the participants do not have equal exposure to the intervention or to the event under investigation, then the findings can not even be generalized back to the study cohort. Subject retention and equivalent participation are major considerations in longitudinal projects, particularly among high risk families who may have other environmental pressures more compelling than the demands of completing tasks designed by a researcher (Osofsky, Culp, & Ware, 1988).

During the measurement phase of a project, transition bias may be introduced if the participants do not have an equal opportunity to demonstrate the target behavior. For example, if one group of high risk families has close contact with a service program and a comparison group has no contact, those receiving the services may actually have a higher incidence of reports for maltreatment because the service providers are more familiar with the daily behavior of the families.

Although some forms of transition bias are impossible to eliminate, Feinstein (1977) provides several recommendations for reducing transition bias. The selection of a cohort is a critical first step. The more representative the cohort is of the corresponding group in the general population, the greater the generalizability of the findings. However, if the event under investigation occurs with relatively low frequency, the size of the cohort may have to be prohibitively large in order to detect adequate numbers of people who have experienced the event. The balance between the goal of generalizability and the goal of studying the event is a critical issue to be considered during the design phase of a project.

A third research consideration is selection of an adequate control or comparison group. In order to determine the impact of an intervention or an event, a comparison process is necessary in which one group experiences the event and the other group does not. The lack of an adequate control group has been a concern in much of the child maltreatment literature (Aber & Cicchetti, 1984). Moreover, when testing the efficacy of an intervention, the assignment of group membership should be based on a randomization procedure in order to eliminate systematic bias (Feinstein, 1977). Each participant should have equal opportunity to be assigned to the study group or to the control group. Within the study group each participant should have an equal opportunity to experience the experimental procedure or intervention. For example, in a study of the effectiveness of two intervention programs for maltreated children, the children could be assigned to groups using a randomization procedure. The intervention would then vary by group. As a safeguard, researchers should verify that the intervention has actually occurred and determine the intensity of the intervention for each child. As a final precaution, each participant in the project must have an equal opportunity to exhibit the outcome.

While many of these potential biases to longitudinal methodology can be reduced with careful planning, there are basic disadvantages that remain and should be considered prior to initiating a longitudinal project:

1. In longitudinal projects, data collection can extend over a long period of time with few intermediate rewards. The extended time period required increases the cost of maintaining both the cohort and the research team. For example, the Kauai study enabled researchers to describe how the delicate balance among risk factors, environmental stress, and protective mechanisms evolved and led to varying levels of developmental adaptation among children raised in high risk environments (Werner & Smith, 1982). While the study made many valuable contributions to our understanding of developmental adaptation under environmental stress, it took over 20 years to complete. Adaptations of the multiserial cross-section longitudinal strategy proposed by Schaie and Baltes (1975) and subsequently recommended by Feinstein (1977) might allow researchers to reach a compromise. Cohorts could be stratified into age clusters and followed, so that the 20-year developmental period could be described in fewer years. For example, rather than recruiting only a birth cohort, researchers could recruit four cohorts (newborns, and chil-

dren of ages 5, 10, and 15 years) and follow them for five years. While this plan reduces the problems of subject and researcher attrition, error variance may be increased by the lack of subject continuity, since subjects no longer serve as their own controls throughout the project period.

The duration of the project and the timing of the observations are dependent upon the theory under study. For example, if the relationships among variables are thought to be linear, fewer observations are required than would be necessary to test a nonlinear or multidirectional theory (Nesselroade & Baltes, 1979). However, since ecological theories of child maltreatment are multifactorial and often transactional, and since behavioral adaptation among maltreated children does not appear to follow clear linear trends (Farber & Egeland, 1987), developmental continuity over extended periods can not be assumed.

2. Projects that extend over many years face the risk of using outdated procedures as more sophisticated measurement tools become available. A move toward theory-driven research and a reliance on multiple measurements of the variables under investigation should offer some protection against advances in measurement tools.

Similarly, as the state of art in the theory changes, new variables may be introduced. Pilot projects, careful reviews of recent literature, and a combination of longitudinal and cross-sectional methodology (Aaronson & Kingry, 1988) guard against the threat of becoming outdated but do not eliminate the possibility.

3. Continuity of measurements may also present a problem because many measurements are age-dependent. For example, assessments of cognition, temperament, and academic achievement vary by age. If a same-age cohort is recruited, then intraindividual comparisons may include measurement changes. On the other hand, if a cohort is selected by event rather than age, different measurement tools may be required to measure the same construct because the ages of the children will differ. Thus, during the analysis of both intraindividual and interindividual comparisons, investigators must be aware of the possibility of measurement changes.

Problems associated with measurement change can be eliminated if the investigator chooses a constricted age cohort (e.g., abuse among children under 3 years of age) or measurements that are not age-dependent. In cases where age-dependence can not be eliminated, the investigator should ensure that the measurements are assessing the same components of a construct. Using multiple measurement tools and multiple sources of information offers some protection against measurement changes. Furthermore, when normative data are available, standard scores can be used to facilitate comparisons across ages.

4. There are natural changes or history-graded events that may influence either the entire cohort or groups of families within the cohort.

Changes at the societal level, such as changes in the reporting laws for child protective services, can influence families' willingness to participate in projects and to share information about their daily lives. Similarly, changes in family structure can influence family behavior independent of the design of the project. The recommendation for a combined longitudinal and cross-sequential cohort design in which same-age or same-event cohorts are assembled at two points in time (Schaie & Baltes, 1975) reduces the risk of cohort effects and enables researchers to analyze the impact of natural changes.

5. Attrition of either the study participants or the staff can cause major problems. Subject attrition may not be random, thus introducing potential bias into the follow-up components of the design and complicating the analysis and interpretation (Feinstein, 1977). For example, if the highest risk families are lost to follow-up, the findings may be truncated and no longer represent the spectrum of child maltreatment under investigation. Even if families do not drop out of the project, compliance may be variable, particularly among at risk families in intervention projects (Osofsky et al., 1988). The content of the intervention may also contribute to differential rates of subject retention. In their intervention programs with pregnant and newborn mothers who had low social support, Barnard and colleagues (1988) reported an 80% retention rate among women participating in the mental health program and a 53% retention among women in the information/resource group. Strategies to avoid subject attrition and increase compliance include sensitivity regarding the respondent burden associated with the measurements, flexibility in scheduling, reminders, taxi service, babysitting, and payment of families.

Staff attrition is also a major concern in longitudinal projects, since it threatens continuity and introduces another source of error variance. Strategies to reduce staff attrition and associated problems include careful documentation, systematic supervision and feedback, and intermediate rewards.

6. Studies may be longitudinal in design but not in analysis. Analytic strategies are emerging that account for missing data, particularly when they are not random. However, these strategies incorporate multivariate models and are not simple (Campbell et al., 1987). The recent study by Herrenkohl, Herrenkohl, Egolf, and Wu (Chapter 3, this volume) provides an example of using a multivariate analysis strategy to investigate the developmental consequences of child abuse. Investigators who rely on univariate or bivariate analyses lose the power of a longitudinal design. Analytic strategies should be incorporated into the design of the study before data collection begins to ensure that an adequate sample size is recruited and that the assumptions of the analysis are met.

The disadvantages and potential biases in longitudinal research are so substantial that Garmezy (1988) warns that although longitudinal studies are vital to the understanding of developmental processes and adaptation, particularly in risk research, they should be not be implemented before the final phases of a research program. Nevertheless, longitudinal research is a necessary process in our quest to understand the relationships between risk factors and developmental outcome.

Carefully controlled longitudinal studies can be an effective means to test the importance of factors and processes proposed in the transactional models of child maltreatment (Belsky, 1980; Cicchetti & Rizley, 1981). Moreover, if these models lead to an identification of accurate predictors of risk (Vietze, Falsey, Sandler, O'Connor, & Altemeier, 1980), longitudinal strategies will be necessary to evaluate prevention and intervention programs. Primary prevention programs to reduce the incidence of child maltreatment and secondary prevention programs to reduce the negative sequelae for children raised in maltreating families are needed urgently, and as responsible investigators and service providers we need the methodological strategies to propose effective programs and to evaluate their impact on children and families.

REFERENCES

Aaronson, L. S., & Kingry, M. J. (1988). A mixed method approach for using cross-sectional data for longitudinal inferences. *Nursing Research, 37,* 187–189.

Aber, J. L., & Cicchetti, D. (1984). The socio-emotional development of maltreated children: An empirical and theoretical analysis. In H. Fitzgerald, B. Lester, and M. Yogman (Eds.), *Theory and research in behavioral pediatrics* (Vol. 2, pp. 147–205). New York: Plenum.

Altemeier, W. A., Vietze, P. M., Sherrod, K. B., Sandler, H. M., Falsey, S., & O'Connor, S. (1979). Prediction of child maltreatment during pregnancy. *Journal of the American Academy of Child Psychiatry, 18,* 205–218.

Aries, P. (1962). *Centuries of childhood.* New York: Vintage Books.

Baltes, P. B. (1979). Life-span developmental psychology: Some converging observations on history and theory. In P. B. Baltes & O. G. Brim (Eds.), *Life-span development and behavior* (Vol. 2) (pp. 256–279). New York: Academic Press.

Baltes, P. B., & Nesselroade, J. R. (1979). History and rationale of longitudinal research. In J. R. Nesselroade & P. B. Baltes, (Eds.), *Longitudinal research in the study of behavior and development* (pp. 1–39). New York: Academic Press.

Baltes, P. B., Reese, H. W., & Lipsitt, L. P. (1980). Life-span developmental psychology. *Annual Review of Psychology, 31,* 65–110.

Barnard, K. E., Magyary, D., Sumner, G., Booth, C. L., Mitchell, S. K., & Spieker, S. (1988). Prevention of parenting alterations for women with low social support. *Psychiatry, 51,* 248–253.

Baron, R. M. & Kenny, D. A. (1986). The moderator-mediator variable distinction in social psychological research: Conceptual, strategic, and statistical considerations. *Journal of Personality and Social Psychology, 51,* 1173–1182.

Belsky, J. (1980). Child maltreatment: An ecological integration. *American Psychologist, 35*, 320–335.

Campbell, R. T., Mutran, E., & Parker, R. N. (1987). Longitudinal design and analysis: A comparison of three approaches. *Research on Aging, 8*, 480–504.

Cicchetti, D., & Rizley, R. (1981). Developmental perspectives on the etiology, intergenerational transmission, and sequelae of child maltreatment. *New Directions for Child Development, 11*, 31–55.

Cook, T. & Campbell, D. T. (1977). *Quasi-experimentation design and analysis issues for field settings.* Boston: Houghton Mifflin.

Egeland, B., Sroufe, L. A., & Erikson, M. (1983). The developmental consequence of different patterns of maltreatment. *Child Abuse & Neglect, 7*, 459–469.

Egeland, B., & Sroufe, L. A. (1981). Developmental sequelae of maltreatment in infancy. In R. Rizley & D. Cicchetti (Eds.), *New directions for child development: Developmental perspectives in child maltreatment* (pp. 77–92). San Francisco: Jossey Bass.

Elder, G. H., Jr. (1979). Historical changes in life patterns and personality. In P. B. Baltes & O. G. Brim (Eds.), *Life-span development and behavior* (Vol. 2), pp. 118–159). New York: Academic Press.

Farber, E. A., & Egeland, B. (1987). Invulnerability among abused and neglected children. In E. J. Anthony & B. J. Cohler (Eds.), *The invulnerable child* (pp. 253–288). New York: The Guilford Press.

Feinstein, A. R. (1977). *Clinical biostatistics.* St. Louis: Mosby.

Finkelhor, D. (1979). *Sexually victimized children.* New York: Free Press.

Finkelhor, D. (Ed.). (1984). *Child sexual abuse: New theories and research.* New York: Free Press.

Friedrich, W. N., & Boriskin, B. A. (1976). The role of the child in abuse. *American Journal of Orthopsychiatry, 46*, 580–590.

Garbarino, J. (1976). A preliminary study of some ecological correlates of child abuse: The impact of socioeconomic stress on mothers. *Child Development, 47*, 178–185.

Garbarino, J. (1989). Troubled youth, troubled families: The dynamics of adolescent maltreatment. In D. Cicchetti & V. Carlson (Eds.), *Child maltreatment: Theory and research on the causes and consequences of child abuse and neglect* (pp. 685–706). Cambridge: Cambridge University Press.

Garmezy, N. (1988). Longitudinal strategies, causal reasoning and risk research: A commentary. In M. Rutter, (Ed.), *Studies of psychosocial risk: the power of longitudinal data* (pp. 29–44). Cambridge, UK: Cambridge University Press.

Gelles, R. (1973). Child abuse and psychopathology: A sociocultural critique and reformulation. *American Journal of Orthopsychiatry, 43*, 611–621.

Gergen, K. J. (1980). The emerging crisis in life-span developmental theory. In P. B. Baltes & O. G. Brim, Jr. (Eds.), *Life-span development and behavior* (Vol. 3). New York: Academic Press.

Goldstein, H. (1979). *The design and analysis of longitudinal studies.* New York: Academic Press.

Hetherington, E. M. (1989). Coping with family transitions: Winners, losers, and survivors. *Child Development, 60*, 1–14.

Hornick, J. P. & Clarke, M. E. (1986). A cost/effectiveness evaluation of lay therapy treatment for child abusing and high risk parents. *Child Abuse & Neglect, 10*, 309–318.

Lamphear, V. S. (1985). The impact of maltreatment on children's psychosocial adjustment: A review of the research. *Child Abuse & Neglect, 9*, 251–263.

Nesselroade, J. R., & Baltes, P. B. (1979). *Longitudinal research in the study of behavior and development.* New York: Academic Press.

Osofsky, J. D., Culp, A. M., & Ware, L. M. (1988). Intervention challenges with adolescent mothers and their infants. *Psychiatry, 51*, 236–241.

Patrick, C. H., & Borgatta, E. F. (1981). Available data bases for aging research. *Research on Aging, 3*, 371–503.

Pelton, L. H. (1978). Child abuse and neglect: The myth of classlessness. *American Journal of Orthopsychiatry, 48*, 608–617.

Ross, C. J. (1980). The lessons of the past: Defining and controlling child abuse in the United States. In G. Gerber, C. J. Ross, & E. Zigler (Eds.), *Child abuse: An agenda for action* (pp. 63–81). New York: Oxford University Press.

Rutter, M. (1988). Longitudinal data in the study of causal processes: Some uses and some pitfalls. In M. Rutter, (Ed.), *Studies of psychosocial risk: The power of longitudinal data* (pp. 1–28). Cambridge: Cambridge University Press.

Sameroff, A., & Chandler, M. (1975). Reproductive risk and the continuum of caretaking casualty. In F. Horowitz (Ed.), *Review of child development research* (Vol. 4, pp. 187–244). Chicago: University of Chicago Press.

Schaie, K. W. (1965). A general model for the study of developmental problems. *Psychological Bulletin, 64*, 92–107.

Schaie, K. W. & Baltes, P. B. (1975). On sequential strategies in developmental research: Description or explanation? *Human Development, 18*, 384–390.

Seifer, R. & Sameroff, A. J. (1987). Multiple determinants of risk and vulnerability. In E. J. Anthony & B. J. Cohler (Eds.), *The Invulnerable Child* (pp. 51–69). New York: The Guilford Press.

Straus, M. A., and Gelles, R. J. (1986). Change in family violence from 1975–1985. *Journal of Marriage and the Family, 48*, 465–479.

Vietze, P., Falsey, S., Sandler, H., O'Connor, S., & Altemeier, W. A. (1980). Transactional approach to prediction of child maltreatment. *Infant Mental Health Journal, 1*, 248–261.

Werner, E. E., & Smith, R. S. (1982). *Vulnerable but invincible.* New York: McGraw Hill.

Wolfe, D. (1988). Child abuse and neglect. In E. J. Mash & L. G. Terdal (Eds.), *Behavioral assessment of childhood disorders* (pp. 627–669). New York: The Guilford Press.

Zimrin, H. (1986). A profile of survival. *Child Abuse & Neglect, 10*, 339–349.

7

Discovery-Oriented, Qualitative Methods Relevant to Longitudinal Research on Child Abuse and Neglect

JANE F. GILGUN
University of Minnesota

"Does not inquiring into murder prove very like the scientific in vestigating of Nature, in which one observes close, questions hard, gathers facts, discovers correlations, condenses them to a truth?"

A fictionalized Ben Franklin in HALL (1988, p. 71)

"You ought to be a journalist or a politician," he said. "The way you make a plausible story and lose the facts that don't suit you. I wonder that sort of thing doesn't hamper you in your research."

The fictionalized Inspector Mitchell
in BELL (1939/1988, p. 215)

"When you get a pattern . . . facts fall into place like a chorus line on cue, and they all start kicking their legs in unison."

Kate Fansler in CROSS (1989, p. 140)

The analysis of qualitative data is like solving a murder mystery. In fact, those who know Miss Marple, Lord Peter Wimsey, and Kate Fansler may already be qualitative methodologists or are in their hearts. The murder mystery begins with a corpse. The detective's job is to piece together seemingly divergent or irrelevant bits of information to discover patterns that lead to the discovery of who did it. The fictionalized Ben Franklin, quoted above, describes the process of inquiry, while Inspector Mitchell warns of the pitfalls of letting preconceived notions determine what counts as facts. When the investigator discounts facts or is unable to discover them, someone gets away with murder, and an innocent person may be prosecuted. Yet when the researcher discovers the pattern, facts fall into place, just as Kate Fansler describes them.

Research using qualitative methods, like any research, often begins with a problem. The investigator's job is to define the problem and discover relationships among factors that contribute to the problem. Discounting or overlooking facts leads to incomplete understanding. Consequences vary for incomplete understanding of scientific problems, but when the issue is a problematic human condition such as child abuse and neglect, the consequences are a perpetuation of human suffering.

The purpose of this chapter is to define a place for qualitative research methods in the design of longitudinal research on child abuse and neglect. There are many excellent books and articles on qualitative research and data analysis (Bogdan & Biklen, 1982; Denzin, 1978; Gilgun, in press; Glaser & Strauss, 1967; Miles & Huberman, 1984; Strauss, 1987; Van Maanen, 1983). Van Maanen is editing a Sage series on qualitative research methods. Little help, however, is available on the ways qualitative approaches might fit into a comprehensive research design.

A secondary purpose of this paper is to show that qualitative methods have a place in the canon of scientific methods. Well-trained researchers understand the shortcomings and the strengths of quantitative approaches. They also are well versed in the limitations of some types of qualitative approaches. Rarely do they have an appreciation of the strengths of qualitative approaches. The fictionalized Ben Franklin quoted earlier was referring to scientific investigations as cognitive and not necessarily as mathematical processes. He also was seeing scientific investigations as based on empirical data. Qualitative methods encompass both; that is, they involve cognitive processes brought to bear on the empirical world. As Cook and Campbell (1979) pointed out, qualitative judgments underlie all science. Gephart (1988) developed this idea in his conceptualization of ethnostatistics, which explores the qualitative foundations of quantitative methods.

The approach of this chapter is practical; it is written for quantitatively trained researchers who are interested in learning ways of incorporating qualitative methods into a research design. Specialized terminology is avoided, and philosophical issues are discussed insofar as these issues support the goal of demonstrating the application of qualitative methods. (Cook & Campbell, 1979; Diesing, 1971; Feyerabend, 1975; Gephart, 1988; Knorr-Cetina & Mulkay, 1983; Mishler, 1986; Mullen, 1985; and Silverman, 1985, contain helpful discussions of some of these important philosophical issues.)

DEFINITION OF QUALITATIVE RESEARCH

In this chapter, qualitative methods are defined as a set of cognitive processes used to discover and to make sense of the data of the empirical world. The data themselves are represented by words and not by numbers, although some qualitative approaches quantify data. Cognitive processes include ways of conceptualizing, analyzing, and interpreting data and decisions about how to write up results. Basing their approach on an anthropological and sociological tradition of interacting directly with subjects in their own language and on their own turf, qualitative researchers primarily use the data collection methods of participant observation, in-depth interviewing, and document analysis, including film and video.

There are many types of qualitative research. Each has its own perspectives and approaches to the empirical world. The types of qualitative approaches a researcher incorporates into a research design depends upon the research question, as do all design issues. The framing of the question in turn, however, is based on personal ideology and theory.

QUESTIONS ANSWERABLE BY QUALITATIVE APPROACHES

Qualitative approaches can be helpful in answering many types of questions, such as the following:

1. focused questions that lead to hypothesis testing and may or may not be concerned with causality;
2. broadly framed questions that lead to hypothesis development;
3. questions that seek to understand the social context of a phenomenon;
4. questions that seek to understand the perspective of insiders; and
5. questions that seek to understand processes.

A comprehensive research project that is investigating a poorly understood area might include all five types of research questions. Investigations into poorly understood areas also would be enhanced by a flexible research design, that is, one that allows for the development of new questions, hypotheses, and investigative methods during the course of the research. In this chapter, childhood maltreatment is viewed as a poorly understood phenomenon. The development of comprehensive knowledge of childhood maltreatment would require a flexible research design and several types of research questions, and the present chapter is written from this perspective. (See Marshall and Rossman, 1989, for an extended discussion of qualitative design issues.)

In the design of longitudinal research on childhood maltreatment, investigators need to be able to do two things: to cast a wide net in order to gather as many facts as possible and and then to have a method of deciding which facts are relevant.

TRIANGULATION

Qualitative methods are not likely to be used as the sole method in longitudinal research. Although a completely qualitative approach could result in an important advance in knowledge, funding would be difficult. Few funding sources accept qualitative methods to the extent that they accept quantitative approaches. While qualitative methods are as dependent on the scientific method as quantitative methods, they frequently are not viewed this way. When researchers use qualitative methods, then, these methods would be used in conjunction with quantitative approaches. Such triangulation of method could represent a "wide net" and could "capture" a great deal of relevant data (Connidis, 1983; Denzin, 1978; Cook & Reichardt, 1979; Fielding & Fielding, 1986; Jick, 1983; Webb et al, 1981). A qualitative component can add important elements to a design, including the following:

1. providing validity and reliability checks on quantitative findings;
2. providing a means of estimating the validity of the design itself;
3. providing a flexible research design capable of responding to the discovery of new information; and
4. providing a multivariable, microview of phenomena that quantitative approaches can represent only by a limited number of variables.

Focused Questions and Triangulation

When using a mix of qualitative and quantitative methods, the researcher has many alternatives from which to chose; there are various ways to mix methods. Sometimes two or more methods can focus on the same issues, and the substantive domains of each method intersect. This approach would fit a focused research question and would have implications for reliability and validity of measurement. For example, if a survey looks at the subjects' ability to express feelings, then the qualitative component also could look at this issue. The qualitative component could involve participant observation of the subject or open-ended interviewing, and use already existing data sources, such as school, social service, and correctional records.

This type of triangulation is well known and important in research because it provides a means of increasing both reliability and validity of findings. If the use of two or more different methods yields similar results, then confidence in these results increases. If two different methods yield dissimilar results, then the facts need to be reassembled and tested in new ways. Two different methods may reveal complementary but somewhat divergent aspects of the same phenomenon, adding to the construct validity of findings.

Triangulation and Complementary Questions

A second type of triangulation of method has each method doing different jobs, one testing hypotheses and the other developing them. This approach is suitable to broadly framed questions examining process, context, and questions that lead to the development of new knowledge. Analysis of archival data and other documents, open-ended life history interviews (Watson & Watson-Franke, 1985), and participant observation could provide information on the social context of the variables investigated by the quantitative component.

For example, a study could be concerned with the effect of high-risk neighborhoods on the development of children maltreated in childhood. The quantitative component could be composed of standardized instruments related to development and to social context (such as social support). Open-ended interviewing of subjects, interviewing of informants in the neighborhood, and participant observation of the neighborhood would add to the understanding of maltreated children's development. The participant observation and use of informants are ethnographic (Fetterman, 1989), generally defined as "empirical accounts of the culture and social organization of a particular human population" (Ellen, 1984, p. 7). A participant observer is likely to note the presence or absence of facilities such as playgrounds, pools, youth centers, schools, and libraries. It is possible that the simple availability of such facilities could be associated with a maltreated child's resilience and with the interruption of a potentially negative developmental pathway. The observer might also note drug dealing, domestic abuse, sexual violence, muggings, and gang activity. These activities are likely to be correlated with more negative developmental pathways than occur in neighborhoods where these activities are not observed.

The other qualitative components would add to the richness of the data. An informant could provide information about the physical and social organization of the neighborhood that the observation might not uncover. Obtaining a life history from one or more subjects from the neighborhood would be another way of understanding the impact of social context on human development. Each of these three methods—participant observation, informant interviewing, and the life history—would add important contextual information to the variables used in the quantitative analysis.

Triangulation and Flexible Research Designs

These three methods could also lead to discovery of new information and a change in the research design. For example, the aforementioned hypothetical study originally might have been conceptualized quite generally. As the research proceeded, the relationship between maltreatment, neighborhood, and developmental pathway might have become increasingly delineated. The instrumentation originally planned to investigate social context may no longer fit the newly emerging understandings rendered by qualitative analysis. The investigators could add questions based upon the qualitative findings to the interview schedule to investigate these findings more closely. They could also develop new instruments to test the relationships discovered in the qualitative component, and items for the instruments can be taken from the qualitative data. Thus, the instruments would be tailored to the specific domain under investigation. Another choice is to develop instrumentation from some of the qualitative findings and to let other findings remain qualitative.

To summarize, then, the mixed strategy approach can lead to incorporating new elements into the design as the research progresses. As analysis and interpretation proceed on data gathered through open-ended interviewing, participant observation, or written records, new questions may develop and be added to the interview schedule and new instrumentation may be introduced. An example from my current research provides another illustration of how qualitative components can lead to a change in the design. One year into a retrospective study, using qualitative methods, of persons maltreated in childhood, I discovered that the presence of someone to talk to and feel accepted by were associated with good peer relationships, respectable academic records, and lack of acting out and delinquency. The lack of a confidant was associated with isolation, perpetration of various forms of abuse including sexual abuse, and some delinquency (Gilgun, 1991). Because of this new information, the interview schedule with which the research began was changed by incorporating questions that explore the presence or absence of confidants and their correlates (Gilgun, in press).

Hypothesis-Generating Questions and Triangulation

A third type of triangulation of qualitative and quantitative method focuses exclusively on hypothesis generation. The quantitative component involves administering several types of instruments measuring variables thought to be related to childhood maltreatment during the time period when open-ended interviewing and/or participant observation on the same variables are being conducted. Both methods can be considered exploratory, and each has the goal of "condensing" empirical data to a hypothesis or empirical generalization—or a truth, to paraphrase the fictionalized Ben Franklin cited earlier.

Cook and Campbell (1979) strongly endorse qualitative methods as complementary to quantitative approaches and as important in determining a study's validity. If, for example, the research question is causal, the qualitative component can help discover and/or rule out threats to internal validity and can clarify the nature of the causal and outcome variables in relation to construct validity. Specific time-, place-, and subject-bound threats to validity can be estimated through qualitative methods. Confusing or unusual outcomes suggested by statistical analysis can be clarified through qualitative approaches.

Triangulation of Perspective

Using a mixed method is not the only choice researchers have when seeking to triangulate. Triangulation of perspectives also casts a wide net and can lead to the discovery of significant data and to changes in research design. Triangulation of perspective in a longitudinal study would involve investigating both the individual's perspective and the perspectives of others on the individual. For example, a study could focus on all the siblings of a family where maltreatment has occurred; subjects in the study would be the siblings. Standardized instruments could be administered and open-ended questions asked asked of each of the siblings, their parents, foster parents, and teachers. The instrumentation and interviews could focus on the subjects' point of view on their own lives and also on how they see their siblings. Interviews and instruments administered to parents and teachers could focus on each of the siblings. Participant observation of classroom, family life, or other social scenes are ways to increase the number of perspectives. Multiple viewpoints on the same subjects using different methods would result in a major array of facts on subjects: the validity and reliability of findings would be exemplary.

The incorporation of qualitative methods into a research design, then, adds several important components: theory development, checks on the reliability and validity of findings, clarification of the validity of major elements of the design, contextual information that aids in the interpretation of quantitative results, a flexible research design responsive to evolving understanding of the phenomena under investigation, multiple perspectives, and the development of instrumentation that fits the particular situation under investigation.

Types of Triangulated Designs

Using participant observation, in-depth interviewing, archival data, and instrumentation in a longitudinal study on child maltreatment would be very expensive and would require much in terms of human ingenuity and resources. With unlimited financial and human resources this type of design would be the design of choice. More modest designs can be developed out of the principles discussed earlier. The following are examples of other types of triangulated designs that require fewer resources:

1. instrumentation administered at regular intervals with participant observation, in-depth interviewing, and the use of archival data done on a subsample of the entire sample at the same intervals;
2. instrumentation administered at regular intervals with participant observation, in-depth interviewing, and the use of archival data done on the entire sample at relatively infrequent intervals;
3. instrumentation administered at regular intervals using only participant observation, or in-depth interviewing, or archival data;
4. participant observation, in-depth interviewing, and analysis of archival data done at regular intervals for the first two years of the study, with instrumentation developed from the qualitative findings gradually being introduced; in the following years, the balance could shift to an equal emphasis on qualitative and quantitative data collection and analysis;
5. participant observation, in-depth interviewing, and analysis of archival data done at regular intervals and instrumentation administered on the entire sample in less frequent intervals;
6. participant observation, in-depth interviewing, analysis of archival data done at regular intervals and instrumentation administered on a subsample at less frequent intervals; and
7. the use of qualitative methods alone.

Given what qualitative approaches have to offer, the use of one of these models would enhance a longitudinal study of childhood maltreatment.

DECIDING WHICH FACTS ARE RELEVANT

Casting a wide net through the incorporation of qualitative components generates a great deal of data. Theory is the key to the management of qualitative data. Two types of theory guide data management: theory developed in situ and previously developed theory. Some ethnographies are written with no reference to previous research and theory. They stay at the first-order descriptive level in an attempt to allow the accounts to speak for themselves and to allow readers to draw their own conclusions. Theory is central to analytic induction and the constant comparative method, two major approaches to qualitative data analysis and interpretation. Each uses theory in different ways.

Previous Research and Theory and Analytic Induction

Analytic induction is a type of qualitative research that seeks to verify and test theory and to identify universal propositions. Analytic induction usually begins with a set of hypotheses developed from previous research and theory. Often causal in nature, these hypotheses are tested and verified on a case-by-case basis. The inquiry remains focused on the testing and revision of one hypothesis or a set of interrelated hypotheses. The researcher uses purposeful sampling and seeks negative cases that would disconfirm the theory. When the data of the case do not fit the hypotheses, the hypotheses are modified. The end product is a theory tested and verified on a wide range of cases, theory that fits the data of each of the cases. Analytic induction reaches toward universality of propositions by demonstrating the wide range of cases to which the theory has been applied. The framework provided by theory guides data analysis and interpretation. The theory being tested is like a grid. The researcher puts together a second grid of the empirical findings. When the two grids do not match, then the conceptual grid is changed to fit the empirical pattern. Cressey (1953), for example, began his study of embezzlers with a hypothesis developed from previous research. This hypothesis suggested that embezzlers saw their acts as technical violations but not as illegal or wrong. After interviewing a few convicted embezzlers, all of whom said they knew embezzling was wrong and illegal, Cressey revised his hypothesis. In fact, he revised his hypothesis four more times. He tested the final revision on 200 cases collected by another researcher and on additional cases of his own. Finding no data that contradicted the final formulation of his theory, he believed his theory approached universality. (See Taylor and Bogdan, 1984, for a useful discussion of analytic induction.)

Researchers who use analytic induction are free to incorporate previous research and theory at any time during the research process. After the initial formulation of their hypotheses, however, many find they have little need to do so, given the focused nature of their work. With its wide-ranging method of inquiry, the constant comparative method of Glaser and Strauss (1967) assigns pivotal roles to previous research and theory during data analysis and interpretation. The role of research and theory prior to data collection continues to emerge and appears to depend upon the purpose and type of research.

Previous Research and Theory and Constant Comparison

The constant comparative method is used to develop concepts and theory grounded in the empirical world. Grounded theorists are not specifically seeking to develop universal propositions but to discover and define concepts and develop hypotheses. Concepts are defined "from the ground up"; that is, the dimensions of a concept are developed from empirical data. The relationships among concepts are also determined "from the ground up," meaning the piecing together of concepts to form a pattern is done empirically. As Kate Fansler, quoted earlier, stated so eloquently, when the researcher sees the pattern, the facts fall into place and start "kicking their legs in unison" like "a chorus line on cue" (Cross, 1989, p. 140). The relationships among concepts or patterns are abstractions or empirically based hypotheses, and they represent "condensations" of carefully gathered facts and their correlations. The constant comparative method begins in an open-ended way. After being in the field and observing patterns in the data, the researcher chooses one or more patterns on which to focus. This constant comparison approach is much different from analytic induction because initial theory is developed in situ from empirical data while in analytic induction the initial theory is based on previous knowledge. Theoretical sampling guides the researcher to select cases on the basis of the potential to expand the scope of concepts and hypotheses and to refine them. Theoretical saturation occurs when the addition of new cases no longer adds to the definition of concepts or disconfirms emerging hypotheses, and marks the point when the research may stop. In practice, theoretical sampling and purposeful sampling work in similar ways. Once the major themes of the investigation are chosen, the sweep of the inquiry usually narrows. The approach to data using the constant comparative method is often compared to a funnel: the inquiry begins in an open-ended way and gradually focuses on a limited number of themes.

The matching of the patterns discovered in each successive case is similar to analytic induction. As mentioned earlier, in the constant comparison method, the initial conceptual framework is constructed from empirical data and then tested against patterns found in successive cases. When data contradict the emerging hypotheses, the hypotheses are modified. Each produces pattern theory (Kaplan, 1964). Like analytic induction, the constant comparative method can make some claims of breadth of applicability, depending on the range of cases involved in concept and hypothesis formulation. Generalizability is not a major issue for constant comparison method because its hypotheses are much more useful in a pattern-matching, idiographic application to individual cases (Gilgun, 1989).

Although the constant comparison method develops its initial framework in situ from data and not from previous knowledge, previously developed theory and research have a major role in data analysis. Because of the emphasis on in situ theory development, controversy exists over whether the investigator should do a literature review prior to entry into the field. Those who argue against this are concerned with the irrelevancy of prior constructions, with problems related to the imposition of the researcher's framework on the data, and with missing important facts because of ideological or theoretical blindness. These concerns are related to the investigator's goal of understanding the subjective viewpoint of persons and of settings under study.

Many qualitative researchers interested in discovery have found that prior constructions often are not relevant. An open-ended approach is designed to discover and develop perspectives the literature review could not have anticipated. A prior review, then, risks wasting effort. Furthermore, these researchers have found that they are not sure of what questions to ask until they have become familiar with the persons and settings they are studying. Preconceived ideas of what is relevant may be "naive, misleading, or downright false" (Taylor & Bogdan, 1984, p. 16).

Understanding the viewpoints of persons and settings under study is difficult because of the human tendency to see what we expect to see and to overlook what is unexpected. Many qualitative researchers believe that a prior literature review feeds into these tendencies. These researchers attempt to be as open as possible to the empirical data, including data that contradict previously formulated theory. Researchers interested in descriptive studies and who are ethnographically oriented rather than motivated to generate theory probably are the strongest proponents of not doing a prior review.

The desire to avoid pitfalls induced by prior constructions and unexamined personal ideology also is strong in those who argue for reviews of the literature prior to entry into the field. Besides doing a literature review, these investigators advocate the writing down of personal beliefs and conceptualizations related to the phenomena to be investigated; this is meant to help the investigator become aware of personal ideology and biases. Upon entering the field, the researcher puts in brackets previous knowledge and ideology in order to take a fresh look at the situation and to formulate questions that are relevant to the situation.

Once the inquiry is under way, previous research and theory become important in theory-generation. The empirically derived statements can be linked to other research and theory, just as the murder investigator links clues to prior knowledge. Because findings can lead the researcher into unfamiliar areas of inquiry, it is important that the grounded theorist have knowledge of many different fields—or can consult with individuals who do.

The balance between openness to new data and the use of prior knowledge is difficult to achieve and requires a tolerance of ambiguity or a prolonged "I don't know" stage. For example, early in my current research, the presence of confidants appeared to differentiate subjects who were not perpetrators of child sexual abuse from persons with similar backgrounds who were perpetrators of child sexual abuse. This was an unexpected finding. The presence of this relationship was replicated in about 30 cases consisting of men who were perpetrators and women and men who were not perpetrators. The "I don't know" stage lasted at least a year. The next step was a review of the literature on resilience and protective mechanisms (Cicchetti, 1987; Garmezy, 1987; Masten, 1989; Rutter, 1987; Werner & Smith, 1982). This literature was not part of the original literature review. The study of resilience suggests that the presence of at least one supportive person is associated with resilience while the lack of supportive persons is associated with major maladjustment such as mental illness and the perpetration of child physical abuse. My research, then, linked two different bodies of research, and enhanced the credibility of both. So far, my research is linked to five different bodies of theory and research. The credibility of empirical findings is enhanced by links to other bodies of knowledge (Gilgun, in press).

Caveats: Ethics and Emotional Reactions

Qualitative researchers working in the area of maltreatment may observe or hear about instances of maltreatment. This dilemma is often encountered in qualitative fieldwork. There are several ways to deal with it. One choice is for researchers to report all instances of abuse their investigations uncover, regardless of the consequences to the research. A second choice involves advising subjects about their Fifth Amendment right not to incriminate themselves. In this instance, researchers may advise subjects not to go into detail about the maltreatment they have perpetrated because if they do, the researcher will have to report them. Yet another choice is not to report instances of maltreatment. This can be done in two ways. In the United States, the federal government issues certificates of confidentiality exempting researchers from reporting instances of child maltreatment discovered in the research process. Yet another choice involves not having a certificate of confidentiality and also not reporting instances of maltreatment. In this case, the researchers are liable to charges of failure to report. The procedures the researcher will follow when instances of maltreatment arise must be part of informed consent. Taylor (1987) and Taylor and Bogdan (1984) contain an extended discussion of ethical dilemmas in fieldwork and ways these dilemmas can be handled.

Another area in which the researcher may discover dilemmas is emotional reactions to maltreatment. In my research there was a point when I was ready to give it up because I could not bear the pain of the stories I was hearing. Instead of giving up, I marshaled a host of supportive persons to help me through a very difficult period. Having emotional reactions and even crises of identity and meaning are common in anthropological fieldwork. The investigator enters into a world that is totally different from what she or he has known before. The challenge to the sense of self can be devastating and overwhelming. Wengle (1988) describes a fascinating and significant study of the emotional cost and the shedding of the self that may occur when a fieldworker ventures into an unfamiliar culture.

CONDENSING THE DATA

Condensing is not a term commonly used in the management of qualitative data, but it is the term the fictionalized Ben Franklin (Hall, 1988) used. It has a ring to it that fits qualitative analysis better than does the more commonly used term *reduction*, which connotes dieting and also is associated with quantitative research. In this chapter, the expression *condensing data* is used instead of *data reduction*.

Coding

Coding is the second method of managing qualitative data. (Using previous research and theory to organize findings was the first method of managing qualitative data, as discussed earlier.) Most often in the analysis of qualitative data, the text to be coded is composed of words, although various photographs and nontranscribed audiotapes can also be coded. The texts may be archival texts, field notes, or transcriptions of tape-recorded interviews. Coding is a means of organizing the content of texts; hence the term *content analysis*, which is what researchers are doing when they are coding a text. (Weber, 1985, and Bogdan and Biklen, 1982, contain an extended discussion of *content analysis*.)

Coding categories are developed from empirical data and from previous research and theory. Coding is another method of managing and "condensing" qualitative data. In fact, data collection, piecing data together to form patterns, pattern matching, developing definitions and linking hypotheses to other knowledge (when this is done at all), and coding are all done contemporaneously. Each of these individual processes influences all of the other processes. Overall data analysis, then, becomes interactive and consists of mutually supportive and corrective feedback loops. Ethnographies involve many of the same processes, as does analytic induction, although here the focus is less on concept development and more on ascertaining whether patterns found in individual cases fit the emergent theory.

Coding is done simultaneously with the other tasks of qualitative analysis because it provides structure to the analysis. Data collection using constant comparison and analytic induction leads to further questions as the research proceeds, and each question asked is tailored to the individual and the situation of interest. Being without an external structure, qualitative data gathering requires an internal structure. This structure is provided by theory, as discussed earlier, but the development of coding categories during data collection is another way of structuring data analysis and interpretation.

Coding also can be done after data collection is complete. This is probably only practical when the questions being coded are open-ended but structured (that is, they are asked in the same way of every subject).

Deciding on Names

Codes are names. The names of codes usually arise quite naturally. Developing codes requires familiarity with the text. To stay involved in and to facilitate the recursive, interactive process of data analysis, the investigator who does the data collection is involved in the development of codes. If other persons are doing the mechanical coding of the text, the investigator continually discusses the coding, the definitions of codes, and the emerging categories with them. This continual discussion increases understanding of the data, leads to the formulation of new questions, helps the investigator see where gaps in the interview schedule might be, and continues the process of concept development. As the inquiry proceeds, the names of the codes, the connections among codes, and the definitions of the codes may change.

In my current research, I am the only interviewer. So far, three different research assistants have helped me code the transcripts. With each new assistant, I spend several weeks coding the text. In that way the assistant learns how to code and learns the names and the content of codes. Once I am satisfied that the assistant and I are calling the same bits of data by the same names, then I code only occasionally with the assistant, although I spend at least two hours per week talking to the assistant about what I am learning in the interviews and what the assistant is learning in the text.

Memos and Observer Comments

Memos and observer comments are useful in data analysis and interpretation when the researcher is writing fieldnotes (see, Bogdan & Biklen, 1982). They represent a third way of managing qualitative data. Observer comments are any thoughts, feelings, and hunches that the researcher writes down while recording the fieldnotes. Rather than waiting until the end of the account of that day's observations and risking the loss of important insights, the observer sets personal comments in brackets and labels them as observer comments with the text. Memos are statements the researcher makes at the end of the day's notes. In the memos the researcher summarizes the day's findings, ties together ideas from the observer comments, and is begins to formulate the emerging theory. Memos provide a time for reflection. Thus, memos and observer comments can be incorporated into fieldnotes, which are tape-recorded and then transcribed.

Memos and observer comments are also important in open-ended interviews that are tape-recorded. During the interview, when the interviewer has an important insight, the interviewer can tell the subject that she or he would like to say something into the tape recorder. The interviewer then makes the comment in the subject's presence. I have done this many times, and interviewees have never had a problem with this. In this way, I do not lose those insights that seem important at the time, and subjects obtain insights into my interpretations.

I also use memos in open-ended interviews. They have the same function as in fieldnotes, but this is also a place where I can express my feelings. During the interview, when I feel like saying, "You did what?" —such as when a subject describes sodomizing a 6-year-old—I can't shout out my feelings as I would like and continue to foster a dialogue. So any feelings I may have controlled in the interview I state in the memo, along with any additional thoughts I have about emerging theories. Memos and observer comments are part of code development.

Transcription

Transcribing tapes is time-consuming and expensive. The transcriptions should be done literally, with pauses marked by ellipsis points and with all the "ums" and "ahs" present. If there is a long pause, then the transcriptionist should note how long the pause was. Literal transcription is important in capturing the interview. If fieldnotes are to be coded using a computer program, it would be most efficient for the fieldworker to type the notes directly into a computer file, following the format required by the program.

Computers and Coding

Before computer programs, it was customary to have four copies of the text. One copy was locked away somewhere safe, such as a bank vault or a refrigerator, a second copy was cut up by code and made into stacks, and the other two copies were used to relocate the context of coded segments and for ongoing reading and recoding. The analyst's nightmare was a gust of wind scattering the paper scraps. With the availability of computer programs, the mechanics of coding have been simplified.

The computer program acts like a clerk or a series of file cards. The first step in the process is to transcribe tapes or text onto a computer disk. The transcriptions should be in the form that the program can read, so format is important. Once the transcriptions are on disk, they are printed. Codes are written directly onto the transcriptions, whose format leaves a large margin on the right side of the page. After hand-coding, the codes are entered into a computer file. Once the transcripts are coded on the computer, the investigator can then simply tell the computer which coded segments are to be printed and out they come. The computer program Ethnograph (Seidel & Clark, 1984; Seidel, Kjolseth, & Clark, 1985) performs these data management tasks in an exemplary way. Having the help of the computer in coding, in storing the coded segments, and in assembling the coded segments has greatly facilitated qualitative data analysis.

Quantifying Data

The quantification of qualitative data can result from focused questions which are asked in a similar if not the same way for each subject. Subject responses are then coded, counted, and subjected to appropriate statistical analysis (Weber, 1985). This approach would not be useful in construct development and in developing grounded theory but would be helpful in verification and testing. Besides descriptive statistics, multiple regression, and analysis of variance, which are possible with quantified data, mathematical analysis of qualitative data includes clustering and multidimensional scaling with ethnographic data (Roberts, Williams, & Poole, 1982), logit and probit with qualitative dependent variables (Aldrich & Nelson, 1986), and key words in context and word retrieval (Pfaffenberger, 1988; McTavish & Pirro, 1984; Weber, 1985).

For many qualitative researchers, quantitative analysis of qualitative data is not qualitative research, which they would define as seeking to understand persons and settings in natural as opposed to mathematical language. If, however, quantification can advance knowledge, then it has a claim on legitimacy.

Validity of Constructs

The validity of qualitative findings can be high when the multiple dimensions of a construct have been delineated. Construct validity in qualitative work can be enhanced through multiple interviews where similar questions are asked of the same individual over time and through multiple interviews with a series of different subjects. A similar result can be obtained through multiple observations, or through reading multiple texts. Each time a question is asked in the same or in a slightly different way, a bit more information usually emerges.

A construct that is being developed can be thought of initially as a large, empty space. The empty space slowly is filled in as information relevant to the construct is developed. An example from my own research is the definition of the term *confidant*. This definition has been emerging for about three years. In another year or more, I could probably write an entire paper on confidants as protective factors for persons who have experienced childhood maltreatment; a research assistant and I did write an entire paper on isolation and the adult male perpetrator of child sexual abuse (Gilgun & Connor, 1990). (Lincoln and Guba, 1985, and Marshall and Rossman, 1988, contain extended discussions of the logic, validity, and reliability of qualitative approaches.)

Reliability of Qualitative Findings

For the same reasons that the constructs of qualitative research can approach validity, the stability of the constructs and the relationships among constructs can be quite high. Each time a question is asked—the same questions are asked of the same and different subjects many times in most qualitative studies—not only does new information emerge but some of the same information is given again. Over multiple interviews with multiple persons at different times and settings, the replication of findings mounts up, leading to confidence in findings. As stated earlier, qualitative findings are best suited to be used in an idiographic or pattern-matching way, where the patterns in an individual case are fitted to the patterns of the theory.

WRITING UP THE RESULTS

Writing up the results of a qualitative study takes training and practice. Developing a focus—using a theme, a coding category, or a pattern discovered in the data—is the key part of this process, as it is in any other type of writing. General statements followed by specific supporting quotes are the rule in reporting results. Bogdan and Biklen (1982) contain an excellent discussion of writing research reports based on qualitative inquiry.

SUMMARY AND DISCUSSION

The purposes of this chapter are to define a place for qualitative methods in longitudinal studies of childhood maltreatment and to show that qualitative methods have a place in the canon of scientific research methods. I used the analogy of the methods of solving murder mysteries to help explain the logic of qualitative data analysis and interpretation. I also intended for this analogy to make qualitative inquiry more familiar and less exotic, "down home" yet intriguing and challenging.

Analytic induction and constant comparison are two major forms of qualitative inquiry, each with its own purposes and procedures yet also having some procedures in common. Doing ethnographies, participant observation, life histories, intensive and open-ended interviewing, and document analysis using constant comparison or analytic induction will greatly enhance the depth and breadth of longitudinal studies. Constant comparison leads to discovery of new knowledge, to flexible research designs, and to the development of instrumentation that fits the situations under study. Analytic induction can greatly aid the theory-testing component of a study. Contextual information, so important in aiding understanding as well as providing reliability and validity checks, can be developed through interviewing, participant observation, and document analysis. Triangulation, with its tie to replication, is a central feature of scientific inquiry. Triangulation using qualitative and quantitative approaches upgrades the quality of a research project. Qualitative research, then, is a reliable and valid way of generating theory, testing hypotheses, and enhancing the quality of research findings.

Acknowledgments. Support for this paper was through the Minnesota Agricultural Experiment Station, Edwards Memorial Trust, F. R. Bigelow Foundation, First Bank Saint Paul, Mardag Foundation, Minneapolis Star and Tribune/ Cowles Media Company, the St. Paul Companies, and the Saint Paul Foundation.

REFERENCES

Aldrich, J. H., & Nelson, F. D. (1986). Logit and probit models for multivariate analysis with qualitative dependent variables. In W. D. Berry & M. S. Lewis-Beck (Eds.), *New tools for social scientists* (pp. 115–156). Beverly Hills, CA: Sage.

Bell, J. (1988). *Curtain call for a corpse.* New York: Harper & Row. (Original work published 1939).

Bogdan, R. C., & Biklen, S. K. (1982). *Qualitative research for education.* Boston: Allyn & Bacon.

Cicchetti, D. (1987). Developmental psychopathology in infancy: Illustrations from the study of maltreated youngsters. *Journal of Consulting and Clinical Psychology, 55,* 837–845.

Connidis, I. (1983). Integrating qualitative and quantitative methods in survey research on aging: An assessment. *Qualitative Sociology, 6,* 334–352.

Cook, T. D., & Campbell, D. T. (1979). *Quasi-experimentation design and analysis for field settings*. Boston: Houghton Mifflin.

Cook, T. D., & Reichardt, C. S. (1979). *Qualitative and quantitative methods in evaluation research*. Sage Research Progress Series in Evaluation, Vol. 1. Beverly Hills, CA: Sage.

Cressey, D. (1953). *Other people's money: A study in the social psychology of embezzlement*. Glencoe, IL: Free Press.

Cross, A. (1989). *A trap for fools*. New York: Dutton.

Denzin, N. K. (1978). *The research act*. New York: McGraw-Hill.

Diesing, P. (1971). *Patterns of discovery in the social sciences*. Chicago: Aldine.

Ellen, R. F. (Ed.). (1984). *Ethnographic research: A guide to general conduct*. New York: Academic Press.

Fetterman, D. M. (1989). *Ethnography step by step*. Newbury Park, CA: Sage.

Feyerabend, P. (1975). *Against method*. New York: Schocken.

Fielding, N. G., & Fielding, J. L. (1986). *Linking data*. Sage University Paper Series on Qualitative Research Methods, Vol. 4. Newbury Park, CA: Sage.

Garmezy, N. (1987). Stress, competence, and development: Continuities in the study of schizophrenic adults, children vulnerable to psychopathology, and the search for stress-resistant children. *American Journal of Orthopsychiatry, 57*, 159–174.

Gephart, R. P., Jr. (1988). *Ethnostatistics: Qualitative foundations for quantitative research*. Sage University Paper Series on Qualitative Research Methods, Vol. 12. Newbury Park, CA: Sage.

Gilgun, J. F. (1989, March). Starting where the practitioner is: Toward a conceptual framework for social work research. Paper presented at the Annual Program Meeting of the Council on Social Work Education Symposium on Philosophical Issues in Social Work, Chicago.

Gilgun, J. F. (in press). Hypothesis generation in social work research. *Journal of Social Service Research*.

Gilgun, J. F. (1991). Resilience and the intergenerational transmission of child maltreatment. In M. Q. Patton (Ed.), *Family sexual abuse: Frontline research and evaluation* (pp. 93–105). Newbury Park, CA: Sage.

Gilgun, J. F., & Connor, T. M. (1990). Isolation and the adult male perpetrator of child sexual abuse. In A. L. Horton, B. L. Johnson, L. M. Roundy, & D. Williams (Eds.), *The incest perpetrator* (pp. 74–87). Newbury Park, CA: Sage.

Glaser, B. G., & Strauss, A. L. (1965). Discovery of substantive theory: A basic strategy underlying qualitative research. *American Behavioral Scientist, 9*, 5–11.

Glaser, B. G., & Strauss, A. L. (1967). *The discovery of grounded theory: Strategies for qualitative research*. New York: Aldine.

Hall, R. L. (1988). *Benjamin Franklin takes the case*. New York: St. Martin's Press.

Jick, T. (1983). Mixing qualitative and quantitative methods. In J. Van Maanen (Ed.), *Qualitative methodology* (pp. 135–148). Beverly Hills, CA: Sage.

Kaplan, A. (1964). *The conduct of inquiry*. San Francisco: Chandler.

Knorr-Cetina, K. D., & Mulkay, M. (Eds.). (1983). *Science observed: Perspectives on the social study of science*. Beverly Hills, CA: Sage.

Lincoln, Y., & Guba, E. (1985). *Naturalistic inquiry*. Beverly Hills, CA: Sage.

Marshall, C., & Rossman, G. B. (1989). *Designing qualitative research*. Newbury Park, CA: Sage.

Masten, A. (1989). Resilience in development: Implications of the study of successful adaptation for developmental psychopathology. In D. Cicchetti (Ed.), *Rochester symposium on developmental psychopathology* (Vol. 1, pp. 260–294). Hillsdale, NJ: Erlbaum.

McTavish, D. G., & Pirro, E. B. (1984, April). *Contextual content analysis*. A revised version of a paper presented at the Pacific Sociological Association Meeting, Seattle. (Available from Donald G. McTavish, Department of Sociology, University of Minnesota, Minneapolis, MN 55455.)

Miles, M. B., & Huberman, A. M. (1984). *Qualitative data analysis: A sourcebook of new methods*. Beverly Hills, CA: Sage.

Mishler, E. G. (1986). *Research interviewing: Context and narrative*. Cambridge, MA: Harvard University Press.

Mullen, E. J. (1985). Methodological dilemmas in social work research. *Social Work Research and Abstracts, 21*(3), 12–20.

Pfaffenberger, B. (1988). *Microcomputer applications in qualitative research*. Sage University Paper Series on Qualitative Research Methods, Vol. 14. Newbury Park, CA: Sage.

Roberts, J. M., Williams, M. D., & Poole, G. C. (1982). Used car domain: An ethnographic application of clustering and multidimensional scaling. In H. C. Hudson & Associates (Eds.), *Classifying social data* (pp. 13–38). San Francisco: Jossey-Bass.

Rutter, M. (1987). Psychosocial resilience and protective mechanisms. *American Journal of Orthopyschiatry, 57*, 316–331.

Seidel, J. V., & Clark, J. A. (1984). The ETHNOGRAPH: A computer program for the analysis of qualitative data. *Qualitative Sociology, 7*, 110–125.

Seidel, J. V., Kjolseth, R., & Clark, J. A. (1985). *The ETHNOGRAPH*. Littleton, CO: Qualis Research Associates.

Silverman, D. (1985). *Qualitative methodology and sociology*. Brookfield, VT: Gower. Strauss, A. L. (1987). *Qualitative analysis for social scientists*. Cambridge: Cambridge University Press.

Taylor, S. J. (1987). Observing abuse: Professional ethics and personal morality in field research. *Qualitative Sociology, 10*, 288–302.

Taylor, S. J., & Bogdan, R. (1984). *Introduction to qualitative research methods* (2nd ed.). New York: Wiley. Van Maanen, J. (Ed.). (1983). *Qualitative methodology*. Beverly Hills, CA: Sage.

Watson, L. C., & Watson-Franke, M. B. (1985). *Interpreting life histories : An anthropological inquiry*. New Brunswick, NJ: Rutgers University Press.

Webb, E. J., Campbell, D. T., Schwartz, R. D., Sechrest, L., & Grove, J. B. (1981). *Nonreactive measures in the social sciences* (2nd ed.) Boston: Houghton-Mifflin.

Weber, R. P. (1985). *Basic content analysis*. Sage University Paper Series on Quantitative Applications in the Social Sciences, Vol. 49. Beverly Hills, CA: Sage.

Wengle, J. L. (1988). *Ethnographers in the field: The psychology of research*. Tuscaloosa: University of Alabama Press.

Werner, E., & Smith, R. S. (1982). *Vulnerable but invincible*. New York: McGraw-Hill.

8

Measuring Parental Personality Characteristics and Psychopathology in Child Maltreatment Research

JOEL S. MILNER
Northern Illinois University

Assessments of perpetrator, familial, and societal factors are all needed in child maltreatment research; the focus of this chapter is on the measurement of perpetrator characteristics. A literature review indicates a recent proliferation of personality measures. Unfortunately, the increased rate of measure development has not uniformly advanced our understanding of child maltreatment because many measures are of questionable or unknown psychometric quality. If inadequate measures are used, results may be meaningless or misleading. Given the effort and expense required to conduct child maltreatment research, the development and selection of appropriate measures are critical. This review begins with a discussion of some basic measurement issues that should be considered when developing or choosing personality measures. Next, different types of personality measures are described, and then reviews of personality measures are cited.

GENERAL MEASUREMENT ISSUES

Nomothetic and Idiographic Approaches to Measurement

Most researchers in the child maltreatment field maintain a nomothetic view of personality which assumes that measurable personality dimensions exist across individuals. Nomothetic tests are used to measure basic personality characteristics upon which different groups, such as abusive and comparison parents, are thought to vary. Properly developed nomothetic measures have been subjected to psychometric evaluations and tend to meet scaling assumptions that allow for traditional statistical analysis. Well-known questionnaire measures like the Minnesota Multiphasic Personality Inventory-2 (MMPI-2, Hathaway & McKinley, 1989) and the Millon Clinical Multiaxial Inventory-II (MCMI-II, Millon, 1987) have been developed to obtain nomothetic data. In contrast, the idiographic view assumes that each individual has unique personality characteristics and that universal personality factors do not exist or if they do exist they fail to adequately describe the individual personality (Nunnally, 1970). Thus, idiographic measures focus on unique characteristics of the individual. These measures often are not subjected to traditional psychometric evaluations and frequently do not yield data that are appropriate for group analyses. Projective tests, such as the Rorschach (Rorschach, 1942) and the Thematic Apperception Test (Morgan & Murray, 1935; Murray, 1943), are used to obtain idiographic data.

Although idiographic data are usually difficult to analyze on a group basis, Kline (1979) suggests that a content analysis of idiographic data can be used to convert the individualized personality data to a nomothetic form. This involves evaluating the idiographic data for the presence or absence of a selected personality characteristic, resulting in a dichotomous score (e.g., 0 if not present and 1 if present) for the characteristic for each subject. Of course, the criteria for determining the presence or absence of the personality characteristic should be available prior to the analysis of the idiographic data. In addition, several raters should be used to determine interrater reliability.

Conceptualization of the Constructs to be Measured

A wide variety of child maltreatment perpetrator characteristics have been studied. A representative, albeit not exhaustive, list of perpetrator characteristics from both the physical and sexual child abuse literature is presented in Table 8.1. Reviews of physical and sexual child abuse perpetrator characteristics are available elsewhere (e.g., Bolton & Bolton, 1987; Hamilton, 1989; Milner & Chilamkurti, in press; Milner & Robertson, 1987; Starr, 1988; Walker, Bonner, & Kaufman, 1988; Wolfe, 1985, 1987). When investigators begin the process of studying a personality variable, they should define the construct and select a measure that provides an adequate evaluation of the construct, assuming that such a measure exists. As part of the definitional process, investigators should decide whether the personality constructs are continuous or latent class variables.

A *continuous variable* changes in a partial or graded fashion on a dimension. Most personality characteristics, from anxiety to coping skills,

TABLE 8.1. Examples of Perpetrator Personality Characteristics Measured and Reported in Child Maltreatment Research

---

Historical variables
　　Childhood history of abuse (receipt and/or observation); poor parent, sibling, and peer relationships; isolation; history of emotional problems; history of adjustment problems; academic problems

Physiological variables
　　Somatic complaints; physiological reactivity to child and non-child related stimuli

Self-concept
　　Self-esteem; ego-strength; self-image; self-concept; adequacy; personal worth; self-alienation

Stress
　　Life stress (events); perceived stress; life hassles and uplifts; personal distress; perceived ability to handle stressful situations

Gregariousness
　　Perceived isolation; perceived lack of social support; withdrawal; shyness; loneliness; fear of rejection; jealousy

Beliefs
　　Belief that personal pain and misery are beneficial; belief in the value of punishment; inappropriate (distorted) beliefs related to parent–child and/or adult-child relationships; unrealistic expectations of children

Sexual problems
　　Rigid moral standards; sexual expectations; sexual identity; sexual functioning fears; sexual dysfunction; sexual estrangement

Parenting styles
　　Perceived problems in their children; perceived child compliance; quality of child attachments; availability to child; responsiveness to child's behavior; need for control; use of physical punishment; use of rewards; use of induction techniques

Social skills
　　Competency; personal resourcefulness; general communication skills; adaptability; self-control; empathy; cognitive, mastery, and coping skills; cognitive rigidity; impulsiveness; proneness to temper outbursts; assertiveness; aggressiveness; assaultiveness

Depressed affect
　　Moodiness; frustration; worry; pessimism; expressiveness; life satisfaction; dependency; unhappiness; depression

Other characteristics
　　Anxiety; guilt; apprehensiveness; tenseness; restlessness; touchiness; reactiveness; irritableness; frustration tolerance; sensitivity to anxiety-evoking stimuli; emotional lability; impulse control; disorganized thought patterns; unique perceptions; attributional style; self-centeredness; locus of control; denial and defensiveness

---

Note. Many of these categories and examples of characteristics overlap.

are viewed as continuous variables. In contrast to the quantitative characteristics of a continuous variable, a *latent class variable* varies qualitatively
in a relatively all-or-none fashion. For example, some evidence exists that
Type A-B behavior represents a latent class variable (Strube, 1989). That
is, either a person is a Type A or a Type B personality. In the conceptualization of the latent class variable, the concept of threshold is often used:
when the threshold is reached, a different type of behavior or condition is
expected. The threshold concept suggests that the measurement tool
should provide a dichotomous classification of the construct under study.

Strube (1989) notes that the continuous versus latent class variable
distinction is important because continuous variable models usually suggest diffuse etiology with numerous antecedent factors contributing in
varying amounts to the condition. In contrast, latent class variable models
often assume that the class variable results from a limited number of
antecedent factors. Further, when observing change in longitudinal studies, a continuous variable model assumes that different degrees of change
occur across time and that even small changes can be measured and are
meaningful. In contrast, a latent class variable model usually assumes that
a class variable is more difficult to change because several factors must be
substantially impacted for change to occur; relatively small changes are
not viewed as meaningful. When change occurs, it is expected to be relatively dramatic. It should be obvious that when a measure is selected, the
measure should represent the continuous or latent class variable under
investigation. Gangestad and Snyder (1985) point out that failure to
appropriately match the variable to the measure can result in statistical
and interpretive problems. In situations where the match between the construct definition and the construct measured is not exact, the use of a measure may require redefinition of the construct under study. In such cases,
the investigator should modify the study definition to indicate what is
actually measured. If the modification is unacceptable in terms of what is
specified in the study model, the measure should not be used.

Measurement of Trait and State Personality Characteristics

A *personality trait* is some measurable personality attribute that is a relatively stable and enduring personality dimension. In contrast, a *personality
state* is some personality attribute that is observed for only brief periods,
usually in a specific context. In this conceptualization, the same personality
dimension may exist both as a personality state and as a trait (e.g., state
and trait anxiety).

Investigators should carefully evaluate the psychometric characteristics of trait and state measures. A trait measure should be stable across
time, whereas a state measure usually shows variability across time. Thus,

trait measures should have high temporal stability (i.e., test-retest reliabilities). Since personality states are defined as unstable, state measures are not expected to have high levels of temporal stability. In longitudinal research, trait measures should have adequate temporal stability across time periods similar to the periods used in the study. In addition, the mean trait scores and standard deviations should be about the same at each testing interval because in longitudinal research it is desirable to use trait measures with modest gain scores (i.e., the tendency of test scores to increase at retesting).

Descriptive Name of Measure

Some measures are named with general titles, such as the Mental Health Index (MHI, Veit & Ware, 1983), while other measures are named with titles that describe the methodology (e.g., client rating scale) and/or the content domain (e.g., parental expectations questionnaire). Any scale with a general title must be carefully assessed to determine what constructs are actually measured. Likewise, when scales include terms that indicate multidimensional measures, for example, MMPI-2 (Hathaway & McKinley, 1989) or California Psychological Inventory (CPI, Gough, 1975), it should be determined which specific scales are included and if each scale adequately measures what it purports to measure.

Even when scales indicate that specific constructs are assessed (e.g., self-esteem), validity data must be evaluated to determine what is actually measured. For example, although self-esteem may appear to be a unitary construct, factor analytic studies suggest that self-esteem is a hierarchical, multifaceted construct. According to one hierarchical model (Shavelson, Hubner, & Stanton, 1976), global self-esteem is at the apex. Global self-esteem is divided into two components: academic and nonacademic self-esteem. Both of these components are further subdivided. The non-academic self-esteem is divided into physical, social, and emotional components. So it must be determined if the study constructs are unitary and, if not, the investigator must determine if the construct component defined in the study model is the same as the construct component measured.

In summary, regardless of the title of the measure, the challenge for the investigator is to determine if sufficient psychometric data exist to indicate that the measure is appropriate for the intended use. In addition, because of measurement error, the investigator should consider obtaining two measures of each construct. It is also desirable to select a second measure that uses a different assessment methodology (e.g., self-reports combined with direct observations). Although the use of a second measure of each construct is time consuming and can complicate the data reduction process, this approach can increase the reliability and validity of the study results.

Validation Populations

In the selection of a measure, it should be remembered that the validity and reliability of a scale will vary as a function of the population under study. Thus, the investigator should note not only the general validity data but should determine if specific validity data exist for the study population. A measure may be an appropriate construct measure for one group with one set of characteristics (e.g., demographics, pathology) but inappropriate for another group with different characteristics. This can be a special problem in the measurement of personality characteristics because a number of scales have been developed for use with deviant populations. Except in instances where the measure has subsequently been validated for use with general population subjects, these measures should not be used with general population individuals. If testing of general population individuals is required, the use of a parallel scale that is designed for use with nonpathological groups is required. A major problem is that there often is no alternative measure for nondeviant populations. In child maltreatment research the abuse group may or may not be conceptualized as pathological on a specific dimension. If they are viewed as pathological, then a measure must be found that can be used appropriately with both deviant and nondeviant groups.

A problem in longitudinal child abuse research is that psychopathology may exist at one point in time but not at another point in time. Again, to avoid problems, it is preferable to find a measure that is valid for both deviant and nondeviant groups. Even when such a scale is found, the scale should be checked for *homoscedasticity*, which means that scores show the same variation for target subjects as for comparison subjects. If heteroscedasticity exists for a measure selected to study child abusers, abusers will show more or less score variation at one or both ends of the scale relative to comparison subjects. This means that the standard error of measurement will not be the same for both groups.

Population Base Rates

In determining the utility of a measure, the base rate of the construct in the population under study must be estimated. The *base rate* refers to the frequency of occurrence of a condition or behavior in the population under study. Measures provide maximal incremental validity when base rates are approximately 50%. If the base rate is assumed to be 50% because equal numbers of abusers and matched comparison parents are used, then base rates are not a concern for the researcher. However, when the personality characteristic does not exist in about 50% of the cases, base rates can be a major problem because the number of false positive classifications will increase as the base rates decrease.

Low base rates are of special concern when latent class variables are under investigation. If base rates are low for a condition and an all-or-none classification measure is used, then the low base rates will produce many false-positive classifications. Even when continuous variables are used with adjustable cutting scores, increases in classification error due to low base rates will add dramatically to the experimental error, producing excessive numbers of false-positive classifications.

Response Distortions

Another major measurement concern in child maltreatment research is the issue of response distortions (i.e., faking good, faking bad, and random responding). It is widely known that individuals often distort their responses on self-report measures. In addition, response distortions are a potential problem when observational techniques are used because the individual can still censor his behavior.

Unfortunately, most parent measures do not assess response distortions. If response distortion (validity) scales are available, these scales should be used to detect individuals who distort responses. If response distortion scales are not available, some measure of response distortion should be added to the personality measurement package to detect response distortions. For example, the Marlowe-Crowne Social Desirability Scale (M-C SDS, Crowne & Marlowe, 1964) can be added to the measurement package to detect subjects' efforts to respond in a socially desirable manner. However, when observational measures are used, the investigator is presented with a special challenge to find methods to detect subjects who distort their responses. Other types of personality measures (e.g., projective tests) are designed to make response distortion difficult because there are no obvious appropriate responses to the test stimuli. Still, respondents can engage in response distortions by giving what they believe are common responses, and they can give a reduced number of responses.

In longitudinal research an added problem is that the degree of response distortion can vary at each measurement period. That is, across time, intervening variables may increase or decrease the likelihood of response distortions. For example, subjects may be less defensive as they become familiar with the research project and staff. Alternately, changes in the individual's personal situation may increase the need for the subject to distort responses. Valid measures are needed at each time period so that changes in scale scores reflect changes in parental personality, not variation in response distortions.

Additional Concerns

There are several remaining measurement issues that should be considered in child maltreatment research. One problem is that some acute pathological conditions may affect a subject's responses to scales that measure personality traits (Overholser, Kabakoff, & Norman, 1989). For example, it has been suggested that traits assessed during a depressive episode (Akiskal, Hirschfeld, & Yerevanian, 1983) or during the experience of anxiety (Reich, Noyes, Coryell, & O'Gorman, 1986) may not represent conditions that exist before or after the episode. Thus, the presence of one pathological condition may limit the ability of a measure to accurately assess other personality characteristics.

Another problem in personality assessment is that the relationship between ethnic characteristics and the measurement of personality has not been adequately investigated (Turner & Hersen, 1985). Investigators, therefore, should be alert to possible confounds in assessment due to ethnic differences. The demographic matching of abusive and comparison subjects may help control for this factor in a particular study, but there still may be unique child maltreatment by ethnic background by test interactions that affect personality measures and that are not avoided by the matching of groups.

TYPES OF MEASURES

This section describes and compares different procedures used to evaluate parental personality characteristics and psychopathology. Available measures include a variety of assessment approaches, including structured interviews, questionnaires, adjective checklists, projective techniques, and observational methods, to assess personality characteristics and psychopathology.

Structured Interviews

The structured interview assesses personality characteristics through the use of a planned question and answer interview format. For example, Kelly (1983) developed interview guides that obtain information on how parents view their child, and Hamilton (1986) has developed a structured interview for assessing individual depression (The Hamilton Rating Scale for Depression). The structured interview method has been used in a number of child abuse perpetrator studies (e.g., Altemeier, O'Connor, Vietze, Sandler, & Sherrod, 1982; Altemeier et al., 1979; Murphy, Orkow, & Nicola, 1985). Structured interviews attempt to provide consistent assessment methodology by using a standard list of questions and rules for guiding the interview activities. When a structured interview is used to assess personality characteristics or psychopathology, the interview is usually restricted to the assessment of particular personality characteristics or selected types of psychopathology.

The success of a structured interview depends on a number of factors. The interviewer needs substantial training in interviewing techniques including specific training and talent in the assessment of the dimensions under investigation. The interviewer must have adequate time to establish rapport with the subject and to conduct the interview. To maintain the validity and reliability of the assessment, the interviewer must adhere to the recommended structure of the interview, which at times may be difficult because the interview process is interactive.

Although attempts have been made to standardize the interview process to increase the accuracy of the information obtained, personality evaluations based on interviews tend to have low levels of reliability and validity. Although exceptions may exist (e.g., The Hamilton Rating Scale for Depression, Hamilton, 1986), the investigator should be aware of the psychometric limitations of most structured interviews. Further, when used with objective tests of personality, structured interviews may add little to the predictive validity of the objective tests (Nunnally, 1970), which indicates that the interview method may not account for any unique variance in the assessment of personality. Finally, there can be data reduction problems associated with the interview assessment method because, even though all subjects are asked the same interview questions, the subjects' responses can vary in content.

Given the time consuming nature of the structured interview method, the difficulties in establishing reliability and validity for the interviewing procedures, and the overlap with the data obtained from objective measures, assessments of personality characteristics and psychopathology using the interviewing approach may be less desirable for research than other assessment methods.

The structured interview, however, may be appropriate for obtaining personality data in designs where idiographic measurement is desired. In idiographic assessment, the opportunity to deviate from the structured interview format to obtain personality data thought to be unique to the subject would be seen as a positive aspect of the interview technique.

Questionnaires and Inventories

Self-report questionnaires and inventories typically provide the subject with a series of statements or questions in a printed format to which the subject is asked to respond. The use of self-report questionnaires and inventories is the most common approach to the assessment of parental personality characteristics and psychopathology. These measures have been used to assess a wide array of individual beliefs, values, perceptions, expectations, motives, traits, and pathology.

One questionnaire designed specifically for screening and describing parents reported for physical child abuse is the Child Abuse Potential (CAP) Inventory (Milner, 1986, 1990). In addition to a physical abuse scale, the CAP Inventory contains six descriptive factor scales and three validity indices (i.e., faking good, faking bad, and random response). The CAP Inventory also contains two special scales, the ego-strength scale (Milner, 1988) and the loneliness scale (Mazzuacco, Gordon, & Milner, 1989). Information on the applications and limitations of the CAP inventory is available elsewhere (e.g., Milner, 1989). Other questionnaires that have been frequently used with child abusers include the Michigan Screening Profile of Parenting (MSPP, Helfer, Hoffmeister, & Schneider, 1978; Schneider, 1982), the Conflict Tactics Scale (CTS, Straus, 1979; Straus & Gelles, 1990), the Adult-Adolescent Parenting Inventory (AAPI, Bavolek, 1984, 1989), and the Parenting Stress Index (PSI, Abidin, 1983).

Numerous questionnaires are available that measure abuse related characteristics, such as depression (e.g., Beck Depression Inventory, Beck, Ward, Mendelson, Mock, & Erbaugh, 1961), anxiety (e.g., State-Trait Anxiety Scale, Spielberger, Gorsuch, & Lushere, 1970), locus of control (e.g , Levenson's Locus of Control Scales, Levenson, 1981; Parental Locus of Control Scales, Campis, Lyman, & Prentice-Dunn, 1986), parenting attitudes (e.g., Parent Attitude Research Inventory, Emmerich, 1969), loneliness (e.g., the Revised UCLA Loneliness Scale, Russell, Peplau, & Cutrona, 1980), self-concept (e.g , Tennessee Self Concept Scale, Fitts & Hamner, 1969), general life stress (e.g., Holmes & Rahe, 1967), and microstressors (e.g., Hassles and Uplifts Scale, Kanner, Coyne, Schaefer, & Lazarus, 1981).

Questionnaires and inventories can be constructed using different procedures. Questionnaire items can be chosen rationally, which usually means that items are written and selected on the basis of expert opinion. Items can be selected on the basis of item analysis, that is, items are chosen because of their ability to discriminate between criterion groups that have the characteristic in question and comparison groups that do not have the characteristic. Other questionnaires are developed based on a factor-analytic item selection procedure in which the correlation of an item with an underlying factor is used as the criterion for item selection.

In child maltreatment research, questionnaire statements presented to the parents require them to indicate whether the item represents their perceptions, traits, motives, and so forth. The respondent is usually given a forced-choice response format (e.g., "yes" or "no," "true" or "false," "agree" or "disagree") or a multiple step response format (e.g., Likert scale, ranking of statements).

Although multiple step response formats allow for the possibility of more precise measurement, these formats often provide subjects with the possibility of choosing a neutral response, such as occurs on many Likert response scales. In contrast, in a forced-choice response format the subject must choose one of two alternatives. A forced-choice response may lack precision but the format eliminates the possibility of neutral responses that may be given by a respondent who is engaging in response distortion. Of course the respondent may decide to skip items to avoid the forced-choice response options.

Questionnaires and inventories that assess personality characteristics and psychopathology are typically designed as nomothetic measures of continuous variables and subjected to standard validity and reliability evaluations. Although the assumption of interval scaling in questionnaires and inventories is common and provides the basis for a wide array of statistical analyses, it is not always clear to what extent the personality scales meet the requirements of interval scaling. In some instances it appears that personality measures are ordinal measures defined by score ranges, and in other cases they may be little more than dichotomous measures. The type of information provided by a measurement device depends both on the type of construct measured and on the type of scaling achieved by the instrument.

Adjective Checklists

The adjective checklist requires subjects to select or to rate a list of adjectives that they believe are descriptive of themselves. The Semantic Differential (Osgood, Suci, & Tannenbaum, 1957), the Multiple Affect Adjective Check List (MAACL, Zuckerman & Lubin, 1965), and the Adjective Checklist (ACL, Gough & Heilburn, 1980) are examples of this type of measurement technique.

Traditional reliability and validity data are expected for adjective checklists, and some checklists appear to have adequate psychometric characteristics. Checklists have the advantage of generating personality data quickly. Obvious limitations are that the checklists are restricted to an adjectival format and the subject's responses are limited to the evaluation of the adjectives presented.

Projective Techniques

In contrast to self-report questionnaires and adjective checklists that ask subjects to describe themselves, projective techniques ask the subjects to describe and/or comment on unstructured or semistructured stimuli. An unstructured stimulus is a stimulus, such as an inkblot, that is thought to have little or no conventional meaning; a semistructured stimulus is a stimulus that has some agreed-upon meaning. With a projective technique using a semistructured stimulus, the respondent is required to provide information beyond the content of the stimulus.

Projective tests are based on the belief that the subject's responses to unstructured and semistructured external stimuli are determined by the subject's beliefs, values, attitudes, motives, expectations, and current concerns, thus revealing the respondent's personality characteristics. A variety of projective formats have been developed, including association techniques, construction methods, completion methods, and expressive techniques.

Association Techniques

These projective techniques use unstructured stimuli, such as inkblots, to obtain responses from the subject. The best known examples of this approach are the Rorschach (Rorschach, 1942) and the Holtzman (Holtzman, Thorpe, Swartz, & Herron, 1961) inkblot techniques. The inkblot techniques are believed to provide perceptual-associative data on what the respondent believes the inkblot represents. The inkblot measures give a variety of scores that are used to provide information on a number of different personality characteristics of the respondent.

Construction Methods

Projective measures using the construction technique usually provide a semistructured stimulus, such as a picture, and the respondent provides a story related to the stimulus. The Thematic Apperception Test (Morgan & Murray, 1935) is the most frequently used example of the construction technique, although a number of storytelling techniques are also used. The assumption is that the story elicited by the stimulus indicates characteristics of the respondent's personality.

Completion Techniques

In projective measures that use the completion technique, subjects are presented with a semistructured stimulus, such as a sentence stem, that they complete; or the examiner presents a picture whose outcome is provided by the respondent. The subject's response to the semistructured situation is evaluated to determine his or her personality characteristics. The Incomplete Sentence Test, of which there are various forms, is an example of this approach.

Artistic Expression Techniques

Typically, projective measures using the artistic expression technique with adults require the subject to provide some artistic production, such as a drawing of the human figure (e.g., the Draw-A-Person Test, Machover, 1949). Personality characteristics are determined through an analysis of the artistic production. A major problem is that no expressive technique has been developed that controls for the subject's level of artistic ability. Further, the validity and reliability of human drawings and other artistic productions as a method of assessing personality characteristics remain to be demonstrated (e.g., Kahill, 1984).

General Projective Test Issues

Even when psychometric data are available on the various types of projective tests, the data are often difficult to evaluate. Examiners structure the projective tasks differently. The number and order of presentation of the stimulus materials (e.g., inkblots, pictures) vary, and different scoring procedures are used. Each variation makes comparisons of the validity studies difficult. Perhaps because of the many limitations of projective techniques, there are only a few reports that have used projective techniques to study child abuse perpetrators (e.g., Derr, 1978; Lerner, 1975).

Observational Methods

Numerous observational methods have been developed for use in natural and laboratory settings. In each setting the observational technique can assess either quantitative or qualitative aspects of the personality. The advantage of these techniques is that they provide direct observations of the subject's behavior rather than assessments of attitudes and beliefs that are assumed to be related to the subject's behavior. The literature on different observational techniques is very large and is not reviewed here. Only general comments about observational methods in natural settings and in structured situations is provided.

Observations in Natural Settings

This method involves the rating of personality characteristics based on observations made in the daily life of the person under investigation. A measure that examines qualitative aspects of the parent's behavior as part of the analysis of the parent–child interaction is the Interpersonal Behavior Construct Scale (Kogan, 1972; Kogan & Gordon, 1975). A coding system that examines primarily quantitative aspects of the parent's behavior as part of the analysis of the parent–child interaction is the Dyadic Parent-child Interactional Coding System (Robinson & Eyberg, 1981).

Another example of an observational measure used in child abuse research is the Home Observation for Measurement of the Environment Inventory (HOME, Caldwell & Bradley, 1978). Despite the inclusion of observation in the title, approximately one-third of the HOME items are actually answered through parental interview and the rest of the items are answered on the basis of observation of the caretaker and child in the home. Modifying an existing technique, Wolfe, Sandler, and Kaufman (1981) describe a structured home observation of parenting practices measure that they used with abusive parents. In a study of child abuse predictive factors, Rosenberg, Meyers, and Shackleton (1982) used a rating procedure that was completed in a hospital while the parent was observed undressing his or her child.

When observational methods are used, a professional, family member, friend, or colleague rates the personality characteristics of a parent on the basis of past and/or present observations. A rating scale structures the evaluation. Typically, personality descriptors are provided on a rating form, and the rater indicates on a Likert scale a rating of the degree to which a characteristic describes the person (albeit the HOME Inventory mentioned earlier uses a yes/no format). The personality descriptors are usually of clearly positive and negative characteristics, such as friendly versus hostile and calm versus agitated.

Nunnally (1970) indicates that when daily life observational methods are used to generate ratings of personality characteristics, there is a tendency for most of the variance in the individual ratings to be due to a single general factor that reflects rater bias. This factor is the tendency of evaluators to give positive ratings. The degree of positive rating bias varies from evaluator to evaluator and may also vary as a function of the type of person evaluated. The validity of the observational rating is also related to the amount of knowledge the rater has about the person rated. Finally, any preexisting rater–subject relationship can affect the degree of rater bias. Rating bias adds to the variation found in the daily life observational measure and reduces the reliability of the observational approach. On the positive side, these observational ratings are based on evaluations of behaviors observed in the daily activities of the individual and, therefore, should have more ecological validity than other observational methods that are based on ratings obtained in restricted and/or artificially structured situations.

Observations in Structured Situations

In these measures of personality the individual is presented with a contrived situation and the subject is asked to respond to the situation. A variety of contrived situations have been used, such as providing a parenting problem and asking the subject to act out or otherwise provide a solution to the problem. The challenge is to develop situations that are as natural as possible for the person who is observed and that contain opportunities for the rater to observe the personality characteristics of interest.

As occurs with naturalistic observation, structured observational methods often have modest reliability and validity because the observer has access to only a limited sample of behavior. In addition, the structured situation should not be so structured that appropriate responses are obvious. Observational ratings depend on the subjective judgment of the rater, which, as previously noted, may be affected by a positive response set. Even though a positive response set may affect the content of the rating, this does not mean that raters are uniform in their ratings. Thus, even with careful rater training, observational methods may have only modest interobserver reliability.

Physiological Measurement Techniques

A number of physiological techniques have been used to assess parental personality. More specifically, autonomic nervous system measures, such as heart rate, blood pressure, respiration rate, and skin conductance, have been used to measure personality characteristics. For example, studies have investigated the autonomic reactivity of at-risk and physically abusive parents in response to child-related and non-child-related stressful stimuli (e.g., Casanova, Domanic, McCanne, & Milner, in press; Friedrich, Tyler, & Clark, 1985; Frodi & Lamb, 1980; Pruitt & Erickson, 1986; Stasiewicz & Lisman, 1989; Wolfe, Fairbanks, Kelly, & Bradlyn, 1983). Although not without criticism (e.g., Hall, Proctor, & Nelson, 1988), other studies have used physiological measures (e.g., penile tumescence) to study sexual child abusers' responses to visual and auditory, child and adult stimuli (e.g., Abel, Becker, Murphy, & Flanagan, 1981; Geer, 1980).

Such approaches are usually based on the assumption that physiological mechanisms are responsible for mediating emotional states. Major problems in establishing the reliability and validity of psychophysiological measures continue to plague this measurement approach. Further, the physiological measures are taken almost exclusively in laboratory settings, and even when reliable findings occur, questions of ecological validity remain.

SOURCES OF PERSONALITY MEASURES

To date, no comprehensive review of the personality scales used in child maltreatment research has been published, albeit such a focused review, funded by a grant from the National Center on Child Abuse and Neglect (#90-CA-1403), is currently under way (M. Straus & D. Finkelhor, personal communication, October 16, 1990). There are, however, numerous published reviews of general personality measures, such as *Tests in Print III* (Mitchell, 1983) and *Tests: A Comprehensive Reference for Assessment in Psychology, Education, and Business* (Sweetland & Keyser, 1986), that are widely available and regularly updated. Although these reviews tend to be broad and describe a variety of scales and instruments, including such things as aptitude and vocational tests, they can be used to locate personality measures.

There also have been notable efforts to survey and review family measures. Some of these reviews can be used to locate parental personality measures. Significant older works include *Family Measurement Techniques: Abstract of Published Instruments, 1935-1965* (Straus, 1969) and the revision, *Family Measurement Techniques: Abstracts of Published Instruments, 1935-1974* (Straus & Brown, 1978). This latter work provides brief descriptions of more than 800 measures. Another older work that examines measures of individual psychopathology, parental attitudes, and parent–child interactions is *Tests and Measurement in Child Development* (Johnson, 1976). More recent efforts to review family measures include *Family Assessment: A Guide to Methods and Measures* (Grotevant & Carlson, 1989) and the *Handbook of Family Measurement Techniques* (Touliatos, Perlmutter, & Straus, 1990).

A review of the literature indicates that a large number of more focused reviews exist. For example, there are works that review the measurement of personality characteristics by scales and inventories (e.g., Edwards, 1970), books that review scales for the measurement of attitudes (e.g., Shaw & Wright, 1967), books on methods for surveying subjective phenomena (Turner & Martin, 1984), and reviews of instruments for assessing parental attitudes toward childrearing (Holden & Edwards, 1989). In addition to the focus on content areas, other papers focus on the specific techniques reviewed in this chapter (e.g., Q sort for assessing parent beliefs [Lawton et al., 1983], Rorschach measures of family interaction [Lerner, 1975], and MMPI for sexual child abuse assessment [Hall, 1989; Hall, Maiuro, Vitaliano, & Proctor, 1986; Quinsey, Arnold, & Pruesse, 1980]). There are also a number of works describing methods used for conducting structured and semistructured evaluations using stories, vignettes, or other test stimuli.

Finally, there are comprehensive reviews of program evaluation measures (e.g., National Institute of Mental Health, 1986) that are useful in longitudinal research. However, there are few reviews of program evaluation measures in child maltreatment research. One significant attempt to review measures in this area is a work entitled *Outcome Measures for*

Child Welfare: Theory and Applications (Magura & Moses, 1986). A limitation of this book is that the review is highly selective. Only thirteen measures were chosen for review, with the remaining part of the book focusing on the Child Well-Being Scales developed by the authors.

Since at present no single review focuses solely on the measures and instruments used in the assessment of personality characteristics and psychopathology in child maltreatment research, it is incumbent upon the investigator to conduct a comprehensive literature survey to locate personality measures that assess the construct of interest. Unfortunately, many of the more commonly used lists of personality measures include only measures that are commercially available. Since many potentially useful personality measures exist only in the research literature, the investigator should locate reviews that include both commercially available and other (e.g,, research) measures of personality. Finally, a new resource that lists 4,000 instruments available from test publishers as well as those described only in journal articles is the Health Instruments File (HIF). The HIF, developed by Evelyn Perloff at the University of Pittsburgh, is updated quarterly and is available as an on-line data base at most university libraries.

Acknowledgment. The development of this chapter was supported, in part, by National Institute of Mental Health Grant NH34252.

REFERENCES

Abel, G. G., Becker, J. V., Murphy, W. D., & Flanagan, B. (1981). Identifying dangerous child molesters. In R. Stuart (Ed.), *Violent behavior: Social learning approaches to prediction, management, and treatment* (pp. 116–137). New York: Brunner/Mazel.

Abidin, R. R. (1983). *Parenting Stress Index: Manual.* Charlottesville, VA: Pediatric Psychology Press.

Akiskal, H., Hirschfeld, R., & Yerevanian, B. (1983). The relationship of personality to affective disorders: A critical review. *Archives of General Psychiatry, 40,* 801–810.

Altemeier, W. A., O'Connor, S., Vietze, P. M., Sandler, H. M., & Sherrod, K. B. (1982). Antecedents of child abuse. *Journal of Pediatrics, 100,* 823–829.

Altemeier, W. A., Vietze, P. M., Sherrod, K. B., Sandler, H. M., Falsey, S., & O'Connor, S. M. (1979). Prediction of child maltreatment during pregnancy. *Journal of the American Academy of Child Psychiatry, 13,* 205–218.

Bavolek, S. J. (1984). *Adult-Adolescent Parenting Inventory (AAPI).* Eau Clair, WI: Family Development Resources.

Bavolek, S. J. (1989). Assessing and treating high-risk parenting attitudes. In J. T. Pardeck (Ed.), *Child abuse and neglect: Theory, research, and practice* (pp. 97–110). New York: Gordon & Breach.

Beck, A. T., Ward, C. H., Mendelson, M., Mock, J., & Erbaugh, J. (1961). An inventory for measuring depression. *Archives of General Psychiatry, 4,* 561–571.

Bolton, F. G., & Bolton, S. R. (1987). *Working with violent families: A guide for clinical and legal practitioners.* Newbury Park, CA: Sage Publications.

Caldwell, B. M., & Bradley, R. H. (1978). *Home Observation for Measurement of Environment.* Little Rock: University of Arkansas.

Campis, L. K., Lyman, R. D. , & Prentice-Dunn, S. (1986). The Parental Locus of Control Scale: Development and validation. *Journal of Clinical Child Psychology, 19,* 260–267.

Casanova, G. M., Domanic, J., McCanne, T. R., & Milner, J. S. (in press). Physiological responses to non-child-related stressors in mothers at risk for child abuse. *Child Abuse & Neglect.*

Crowne, D. P., & Marlowe, D. (1964). *The approval motive.* New York: Wiley.

Derr, J. (1978). Using the Rorschach Inkblot Test in the assessment of parents charged with abuse and neglect. *British Journal of Projective Psychology and Personality Study, 23,* 29–31.

Edwards, A. L. (1970). *The measurement of personality traits by scales and inventories.* New York: Holt, Rinehart & Winston.

Emmerich, W. (1969). The parental role: A functional-cognitive approach. *Monographs of the Society for Research in Child Development, 34* (8, Serial No. 132).

Fitts, W. H., & Hamner, W. T. (1969). *The self concept and delinquency.* Nashville, TN: Marshall & Bruce.

Friedrich, W. N., Tyler, T. D., & Clark, J. A. (1985). Personality and psychophysiological variables in abusive, neglectful, and low-income control mothers. *The Journal of Nervous and Mental Disease, 170,* 577–587.

Frodi, A. M., & Lamb, M. E. (1980). Child abusers' responses to infant smiles and cries. *Child Development, 51,* 238–241.

Gangestad, S., & Snyder, M. (1985). "To carve nature at its joints": On the existence of discrete classes in personality. *Psychological Review, 92,* 317–349.

Geer, J. H. (1980). Measurement of genital arousal in human males and females. In I. Martin & P. H. Venables (Eds.), *Techniques in psychophysiology* (pp. 431–458). New York: Wiley.

Gough, H. G. (1975). *Manual for the California Psychological Inventory.* Palo Alto, CA: Consulting Psychologists Press.

Gough, H. G., & Heilbrun, A. B. (1980). *The Adjective Check List manual.* Palo Alto, CA: Consulting Psychologists Press.

Grotevant, H. D., & Carlson, C. T. (1989). *Family assessment: A guide to methods and measures.* New York: The Guilford Press.

Hall, G. C. N. (1989). WAIS-Rs and MMPIs of men who have sexually assaulted children: Evidence of limited utility. *Journal of Personality Assessment, 50,* 404–412.

Hall, G. C. N., Maiuro, R. D., Vitaliano, P. P., & Proctor, W. C. (1986). The utility of MMPI with men who have sexually assaulted children. *Journal of Consulting and Clinical Psychology, 54,* 493–496.

Hall, G. C. N., Proctor, W. C., & Nelson, G. M. (1988). Validity of psychological measures of pedophilic sexual arousal in a sex offender population. *Journal of Consulting and Clinical Psychology, 56,* 118–122.

Hamilton, L. (1989). Variables associated with child maltreatment and implications for prevention and treatment. In J. T. Pardeck (Ed.), *Child abuse and neglect: Theory, research and practice* (pp. 29–54). New York: Gordon & Breach.

Hamilton, M. (1986). The Hamilton Rating Scale for Depression. In N. Sartorius & T. A. Ban (Eds.), *Assessment of depression* (pp. 143–152). Berlin: Springer-Verlag.

Hathaway, S. R., & McKinley, J. C. (1989). *Minnesota Multiphasic Personality Inventory-2*. Minneapolis: National Computer Systems.

Helfer, R. E., Hoffmeister, J. K., & Schneider, C. J. (1978). *MSPP: A manual for the use of the Michigan Screening Profile of Parenting*. Boulder, CO: Express Press.

Holden, G. W., & Edwards, L. A. (1989). Parental attitudes toward child rearing: Instruments, issues, and implications. *Psychological Bulletin, 106*, 29–58.

Holmes, T., & Rahe, R. (1967). The social readjustment rating scale. *Journal of Psychosomatic Research, 11*, 213–218.

Holtzman, W. H., Thorpe, J. S., Swartz, J. D., & Herron, E. W. (1961). *Inkblot perception and personality*. Austin: University of Texas Press.

Johnson, O. G. (1976). *Tests and measurements in child development: Handbook I*. San Francisco: Jossey-Bass.

Kahill, S. (1984). Human figure drawing in adults: An update of the empirical evidence, 1967–1982. *Canadian Psychology, 25*, 269–292.

Kanner, A., Coyne, J., Schaefer, C., & Lazarus, R. (1981). Comparison of two modes of stress management: Daily hassles and uplifts versus major life events. *Journal of Behavioral Medicine, 4*, 1–39.

Kelly, J. (1983). *Treating child-abusive families*. New York: Plenum Press.

Kline, P. (1979). *Psychometrics and psychology*. London: Academic Press.

Kogan, K. L. (1972). Specificity and stability of mother–child interactional styles. *Child Psychiatry and Human Development, 2*, 160-168.

Kogan, K. L., & Gordon, B. M. (1975). Interpersonal behavior constructs: A revised approach to defining dyadic interactional styles. *Psychological Reports, 36*, 835–846.

Lawton, J., Coleman, M., Boger, R., Pease, D., Galejs, I., Poresky, R., & Looney, E. (1983). A Q-sort assessment of parents' beliefs about parenting in six midwestern states. *Infant Mental Health Journal, 4*, 344–351.

Lerner, P. M. (1975). Rorschach measures of family interaction: A review. In P. M. Lerner (Ed.), *Handbook of Rorschach Scales* (pp. 406–419). New York: International Universities Press.

Levenson, H. (1981). Differentiating among externality, powerful others and chance. In H. M. Lefcourt (Ed.), *Research with the locus of control construct* (pp. 15–63). New York: Academic Press.

Machover, K. (1949). *Personality projection in the drawing of the human figure*. Springfield, IL: Thomas.

Magura, S., & Moses, B. S. (1986). *Outcome measures for child welfare: Theory and applications*. Washington: Child Welfare League of America.

Mazzuacco, M., Gordon, R. A., & Milner, J. S. (1989, March). *Development of a loneliness scale for the Child Abuse Potential Inventory*. Paper presented at the meeting of the Southeastern Psychological Association, Washington, DC.

Millon, T. (1987). *Manual for the MCMI-II.* Minneapolis, MN: National Computer Systems.

Milner, J. S. (1986). *The Child Abuse Potential Inventory Manual* (2nd ed.). Webster, NC: Psytec.

Milner, J. S. (1988). An ego-strength scale for the Child Abuse Potential Inventory. *Journal of Family Violence, 3,* 151-162.

Milner, J. S. (1989). Applications and limitations of the Child Abuse Potential Inventory. In J. T. Pardeck (Ed.), *Child abuse and neglect: Theory, research, and practice* (pp. 83-95). New York: Gordon & Breach.

Milner, S. (1990). *An interpretive manual for the Child Abuse Potential Inventory.* Webster, NC: Psytec.

Milner, J. S., & Chilamkurti, C. (in press). Physical child abuse perpetrator characteristics: A review of the literature. *Journal of Interpersonal Violence.*

Milner, J. S., & Robertson, K. R. (1987). Psychological characteristics of sexual child abuse: A selected review of the literature. *Social and Behavioral Sciences Documents, 16,* 63 (Ms. No. 2780).

Mitchell, J. V. (1983). *Tests in print III.* Buros Institute of Mental Measurement. Lincoln: University of Nebraska Press.

Morgan, C., & Murray, H. (1935). A method for investigating phantasies: The Thematic Apperception Test. *Archives of Neurological Psychiatry, 34,* 289-306.

Murphy, S., Orkow, B., & Nicola, R. M. (1985). Prenatal prediction of child abuse and neglect: A prospective study. *Child Abuse & Neglect, 9,* 225-235.

Murray, H. A. (1943). *Thematic Apperception Test Manual.* Cambridge, MA: Harvard University Press.

National Institute of Mental Health. (1986). *Assessing mental health treatment and outcome measurement techniques* (DHHS Publication No. ADM 86-1301). Washington, DC: U.S. Government Printing Office.

Nunnally, J. C. (1970). *Introduction to psychological measurement.* New York: McGraw-Hill.

Osgood, C. E., Suci, G. J., & Tannenbaum, P. H. (1957). *Measurement of meaning.* Urbana: University of Illinois Press.

Overholser, J. C., Kabakoff, R., & Norman, W. H. (1989). The assessment of personality characteristics in depressed and dependent psychiatric inpatients. *Journal of Personality Assessment, 53,* 40-50.

Pruitt, D. L., & Erickson, M. T. (1986). The Child Abuse Potential Inventory: A study of concurrent validity. *Journal of Clinical Psychology, 41,* 104-111.

Quinsey, V. L., Arnold, L. S., & Pruesse, M. G. (1980). MMPI profiles of men referred for pretrial psychiatric assessment as a function of offense type. *Journal of Clinical Psychology, 36,* 410-417.

Reich, J., Noyes, R., Coryell, W., & O'Gorman, T. (1986). The effect of state anxiety on personality measurement. *American Journal of Psychiatry, 143,* 760-763.

Robinson, E. A., & Eyberg, S. M. (1981). The dyadic parent–child interaction coding system: Standardization and validation. *Journal of Consulting and Clinical Psychology, 49,* 245-250.

Rorschach, H. (1942). *Psychodiagnostics.* New York: Grune & Stratton.

Rosenberg, N. M., Meyers, S., & Shackleton, N. (1982). Prediction of child abuse in an ambulatory setting. *Pediatrics, 70,* 879–882.

Russell, D., Peplau, L. A., & Cutrona, C. E. (1980). The Revised UCLA Loneliness Scale: Concurrent and discriminant validity evidence. *Journal of Personality and Social Psychology, 39,* 472–480.

Schneider, C. J. (1982). The Michigan Screening Profile of Parenting. In R. H. Starr, Jr. (Ed.), *Child abuse prediction: Policy implications* (pp. 157–174). Cambridge, MA: Ballinger.

Shavelson, R. J., Hubner, J. J., & Stanton, G. C. (1976). Self-concept: Validation of construct interpretations. *Review of Educational Research, 46,* 407–441.

Shaw, M. E., & Wright, J. M. (1967). *Scales for the measurement of attitudes.* New York: McGraw-Hill.

Spielberger, C. D., Gorsuch, R., & Lushere, R. (1970). *Manual for the State-Trait Anxiety Inventory.* Palo Alto, CA: Consulting Psychologists Press.

Starr, R. H., Jr. (1988). Physical abuse of children. In V. B. Van Hasselt, R. L. Morrison, A. S. Bellack, & M. Hersen (Eds.), *Handbook of family violence* (pp. 119–155). New York: Plenum Press.

Stasiewicz, P. R., & Lisman, S. A. (1989). Effects of infant cries on alcohol consumption in college males at risk for child abuse. *Child Abuse & Neglect, 13,* 463–470.

Straus, M. A. (1969). *Family measurement techniques: Abstracts of published instruments, 1935–1965.* Minneapolis: University of Minnesota Press.

Straus, M. A. (1979). Measuring intrafamilial conflict and violence: The Conflict Tactics (CT) Scale. *Journal of Marriage and the Family, 41,* 75–88.

Straus, M. A., & Brown, B. W. (1978). *Family measurement techniques: Abstracts of published instruments, 1935–1974* (rev. ed.). Minneapolis: University of Minnesota Press.

Straus, M. A., & Gelles, R. J. (1990). *Physical violence in American families.* New Brunswick, NJ: Transaction.

Strube, M. J. (1989). Evidence for the type in Type A behavior: A taxometric analyses. *Journal of Personality and Social Psychology, 56,* 972–987.

Sweetland, R. C., & Keyser, D. J. (1986). *Tests: A comprehensive reference for assessments in psychology, education, and business.* Kansas City, KS: Test Corporation of America.

Touliatos, J., Perlmutter, B. F., & Straus, M. A. (1990). *Handbook of family measurement techniques.* Newbury Park, CA: Sage.

Turner, C. F., & Martin, E. (1984). *Surveying subjective phenomena* (Vol. 2). New York: Russell Sage Foundation.

Turner, S. M., & Hersen, M. (1985). The interviewing process. In M. Hersen & S. M. Turner (Eds.), *Diagnostic interviewing* (pp. 3–23). New York: Plenum Press.

Veit, C. T., & Ware, J. E., Jr. (1983). The structure of psychological distress and well-being in general populations. *Journal of Consulting and Clinical Psychology, 51,* 730–742.

Walker, C. E., Bonner, B. L., & Kaufman, K. L. (1988). *The physically and sexually abused child: Evaluation and treatment.* New York: Pergamon Press.

Wolfe, D. A. (1985). Child-abusing parents: An empirical review and analysis. *Psychological Bulletin, 97,* 462–482.

Wolfe, D. A. (1987). *Child abuse: Implications for child development and psychopathology.* Newbury Park, CA: Sage.

Wolfe, D. A., Fairbanks, J. A., Kelly, J. A., & Bradlyn, A. S. (1983). Child abusive parents' physiological responses to stressful and non-stressful behavior in children. *Behavioral Assessment, 5,* 363–371.

Wolfe, D. A., Sandler, J., & Kaufman, K. (1981). A competency-based parent training program for abusive parents. *Journal of Consulting and Clinical Psychology, 49,* 633–640.

Zuckerman, M., & Lubin, B. (1965). *Manual for Multiple Affect Adjective Check List.* San Diego: Educational and Industrial Testing Service.

9

Psychological Abuse and Childrearing Belief Systems

JOAN E. GRUSEC
GARY C. WALTERS
University of Toronto

In this chapter we discuss the view that psychological abuse is the core component of child maltreatment. Accordingly, we argue that the study of psychological abuse should take as its starting point what is known about the effects of adaptive and maladaptive parenting practices on child development. In the second half of the chapter we consider techniques for addressing and understanding parenting practices through the study of parent attitudes and parent belief systems.

THE NATURE OF PSYCHOLOGICAL ABUSE

Definitions of psychological abuse have ranged from broad to narrow. Garbarino, Guttman, and Seeley (1986) suggest psychological abuse falls into six domains: mental cruelty, sexual abuse and exploitation, emotional neglect, cultural bias or prejudice, institutional abuse, and living in dangerous environments. Besharov (1981), however, has argued that such a broad definition runs the risk of losing focus on the serious cases of psychological abuse and proposes targeting those cases where abuse is severe and has demonstrable effects on the child. Researchers have concentrated on the need for an operational definition of psychological abuse (Hart, Germain, & Brassard, 1987). Thus, McGee & Wolfe (in press) recommend defining maltreatment in terms of communications assessed by behavioral observations of parent–child interactions.

Conceptually, psychological abuse represents the core issue in the study of maltreatment. It is believed to be more prevalent than any of the other so-called types, it almost always accompanies other incidents of maltreatment, and its social consequences are more destructive of the developing child (see Garbarino & Vondra, 1987). As an illustration, consider the assumption that psychological maltreatment accompanies the more blatant forms of physical maltreatment, that is, that all forms of physical maltreatment may be thought of as involving a psychological component. It is not just the broken arm, the sexual encounter, or the physical neglect but what these events signify to the developing child and how they affect his or her social and emotional growth that should be a primary focus of research in child maltreatment. As Garbarino and Vondra (1987) have recently argued, "... it is the psychological consequences of an act that define that act as abusive — be it physical abuse (e.g., the meaning to a child of an injury inflicted by a parent in rage versus the same 'injury' inflicted by accident ...) or sexual abuse (since sexual acts have little or no intrinsic meaning apart from the social psychological connotations ...)." Psychological maltreatment "... is the critical aspect in the overwhelming majority of what appear as physical and sexual maltreatment cases" (p. 28).

Not only is psychological abuse an inherent part of acts of physical abuse but it can also occur independent of physically abusive acts; parents who physically abuse their children frequently also psychologically abuse them in other contexts as well. Data collected as part of an ongoing study by one of this chapter's authors indicate that when child protection workers were asked to classify their clients with respect to "type" of abuse, they listed psychological abuse as involved in 35 out of 38 cases originally called to the attention of their agency as physical, sexual, or neglect incidents (Walters, 1989).

There is also empirical evidence that at least one form of abuse (physical abuse) is associated with caregivers who differ markedly from each other in their style of parenting. Oldershaw, Walters, and Hall (1989) found that mothers screened by a child protection agency for "pure" physical abuse differed from a matched control group of nonabusive mothers on the behavioral and affective quality of their social interactions, including disciplinary encounters, with their children. Cluster analysis of these same behaviors revealed that abusive mothers in fact displayed three distinctly different styles of parenting: "distant," "intrusive," and "hostile." The distant mothers were characterized by their low involvement with, and apparent lack of interest in, their children. They displayed excessively flattened affect when interacting with their children, frequently ignored them, and exhibited low rates of both positive and negative interactive behaviors. In sharp contrast were the intrusive mothers who were constantly instructing their children to behave appropriately, and who expressed excessive disapproval throughout the interaction. These mothers, while relying heavily on power-assertive parenting techniques, also exhibited a variety of positively oriented displays of affection and approval. The hostile mothers directed subtle personal attacks against their children, ignoring them, denying them affection and approval, and displaying high levels of humiliating behaviors; they showed few positive behaviors and an extremely negative affective quality. The three subgroups also differed in the amount of affective involvement with their children, and the children of mothers in each subgroup also showed distinct patterns of behavior. Children of intrusive mothers exhibited more noncompliance and aggression than did children in the other groups, and those of hostile mothers displayed more bids for attention; there were no differences between children of distant mothers and those of control mothers.

These results accord with the findings of Egeland and Sroufe (1981) who have studied and described what may be similar subgroups (physically abusive, hostile/verbally abusive, neglectful, and psychologically unavailable) of mothers drawn from a large, high-risk population. In this case assignments to groups appear to have been based primarily on data obtained from personality tests, behavioral observations, and "each staff member's knowledge of the mother." Similarly, Lyons-Ruth, Connell, Zoll, and Stahl (1987), using in-home observations, were able to identify two groups of mothers of a high-risk infant population, which they termed "high hostile intrusive" and "low involvement."

The matter of classification of subjects is a major question that must be carefully considered in both designing and interpreting studies of child maltreatment. We must recognize that the classification of maltreatment, both between subject populations such as those responsible for physical abuse and neglect and within any given category, may be more a research convenience than a reality (see Aber & Cicchetti, 1984; Erickson, Egeland, & Pianta, 1989). The nature of abusive actions, as well as their frequency and patterning, no doubt vary considerably from child to child. As McGee and Wolfe (in press) have argued, there is a need in this area of research to precisely identify both the subtypes and patterns of maltreatment in individuals constituting our subject populations. How this is done by the researcher has important implications for the conclusions we draw about the consequences of abuse. What is clear is that we cannot assume a homogeneous subject population based on social service agency definitions or some other qualitative a priori classification scheme.

An Approach to the Study of Psychological Abuse

Our thinking about psychological abuse is based upon the extensive literature in developmental psychology concerning the general principles of adaptive and maladaptive parent–child relationships (Grusec & Lytton, 1988). Parental socialization practices can be arranged along a continuum that, for discussion purposes, can be called "good" to "bad," with abusive childrearing practices at the negative end of this continuum. The background literature in developmental psychology suggests that we can conceptualize parent–child relationships in terms of the following five categories of caregiver activities that can influence socialization practices.

1. *Harmful disciplinary practices.* To the extent that physical abuse occurs in disciplinary situations in which power-assertive interventions have escalated to dangerous levels, the connections of abuse to harmful disciplinary practices are obvious (Reid, 1986). But interest in the effects of discipline ought to go beyond this one focus. Some parents, for example, use excessive amounts of withdrawal of love and approval or threats of abandonment, that may have potentially negative outcomes for the child in terms of nonadaptive guilt (e.g., Hoffman, 1970). Others may use techniques that involve humiliation and attacks on the child's self-esteem (Oldershaw, Walters, & Hall, 1987, 1989). Parents who discipline in inappropriate ways or who are ineffective in their use of socialization techniques may well produce children who have not been adequately trained to comply with societal dictates. Those who rely on authoritarian and restrictive approaches to childrearing may produce children who are overly controlled and restricted in their behavior and who are unable to enjoy life within the bounds of reasonable conformity to the demands of others (Maccoby & Martin, 1983). Indeed, parental restrictiveness, particularly in association with the use of power assertion, is implicated in the development of submissiveness, dependency, lack of altruistic behavior, and lack of originality (Grusec & Lytton, 1988). The disciplinary practices described here clearly go well beyond the typical issues involved in physical abuse and neglect, and have an important place in studies of psychological abuse.

2. *Lack of responsivity, warmth, and acceptance.* These are parental characteristics that have been recognized as important in the development of children's attachment to their parents and, ultimately, of a whole range of social behaviors, including satisfactory peer relationships. The large literature concerned with the relationship between a history of abuse and the quality and security of children's attachment to their mothers (e.g., Crittenden & Ainsworth, 1989) is evidence of this awareness, as is research specifically concerned with the relationship between lack of empathy and a history of abuse (Bavolek, 1984). Insecure attachment, moreover, appears to be predictive of numerous other outcomes than physical abuse or neglect, including low self-esteem and inadequate social skills (Bretherton & Waters, 1985). Lack of parental acceptance and warmth has also been identified as a

contributor to a number of negative child outcomes, including aggression and maladjustment (Lytton, Watts, & Dunn, 1986; Siegelman, 1966).

3. *Exposure to deviant models.* The power of imitation to promote antisocial actions on the part of the child has been documented extensively by developmental researchers (Grusec & Lytton, 1988). Parents who themselves exhibit deviant behavior or who allow their children to be exposed to models of deviant behavior are setting the conditions for the acquisition of aberrant behavior by the child. Descriptive data gathered by one of us as part of an ongoing study indicates that 47 out of 50 cases of various types of child abuse (as classified by child protection services) involved exposure of the child to extremely deviant behavior (e.g., pornography, family violence and other forms of aggression, antisocial conduct, and acts of extreme humiliation) by parents or their acquaintances (Walters, 1989). Indeed, among child welfare workers who investigate instances of child abuse, such exposure is considered to be commonplace. A specific example in the area of family violence is wife battering; children of battered women are directly and negatively affected by exposure to such violence as revealed by measures of child behavior problems and social competence (e.g., Wolfe, Jaffe, Wilson & Zak, 1985).

4. *Extreme overprotection.* A form of deviant parenting that has received little attention is seen in parents who prevent their children from experiencing the effects of their behavior on the environment. The overprotective parent may produce children who are quite incapable of leading fulfilling lives and may, in extreme cases, set the conditions for certain types of psychopathology. The large literature on learned helplessness, and studies relating this phenomenon to depression, indicate that this should be an area of concern in the study of maltreatment. This literature is especially interesting in that independent and dependent variables influencing learned helplessness have been studied in a large number of experimental studies (e.g., Klein, 1987; Minor, Jackson, & Maier, 1984). However, we know little of the actual childrearing antecedents that may contribute to such an outcome.

5. *Exploitation.* The obvious example here is sexual exploitation, in which advantage is taken of the child's inability to refuse an unreasonable request on the part of a caregiver. Other kinds of exploitation that also carry the potential of psychological abuse include excessive demands for physical or psychological aid (e.g., the expectation on the part of a needy parent that the child's primary role is to provide love and comfort to the caregiver); in the extreme, such children are prevented from experiencing childhood, with the consequences of such long-term socialization experiences, where there is a reversal of family roles, not yet understood. A related example is the child who is required to do unreasonable amounts of household work and is thereby denied the time necessary to pursue childhood activities that are needed to promote good adjustment.

CHILDREARING ATTITUDE AND
PARENT BELIEF SYSTEM MEASURES

If one grants that an understanding of psychological abuse is fruitfully pursued through the study of parenting practices and behaviors of the sort just described, then the assessment of these practices becomes an important concern. One of the most frequently employed approaches to assessment has been the measurement of childrearing attitudes, on the assumption that these attitudes are a reflection of or are predictive of actual parenting behavior. In this part of the chapter we address this assumption and argue that it is problematic. We then describe some current and more refined approaches to the assessment of parenting attitudes and belief systems and their role in the production of parenting behavior.

PARENTING ATTITUDE MEASURES AND THEIR DEFICIENCIES

Tests designed to measure attitudes to parenting have been popular for a number of reasons. They are quick and easy to administer (much easier than observing actual behavior), produce easily quantifiable results, are seen to be free of the apparent contamination of situational pressures, and are also perceived to produce an aggregate measure that is a more reliable assessment of parental dispositions than are a few behavioral observations. In spite of these appealing features, however, the outcomes of studies employing parenting attitude measures have been rather disappointing.

In a recent review of parenting attitude measures Holden and Edwards (1989) demonstrated that they have serious limitations that no doubt help to account for their disappointing performance. These authors found more than 80 paper-and-pencil surveys (as opposed to interviews) of parenting attitudes, with 21 new instruments appearing in the first half of the 1980s; the popularity of these measures has not diminished in recent years. Holden and Edwards's review, however, indicates that the more recently developed instruments do not represent a marked improvement over what was available 10 or more years ago. Problems revolve primarily around three areas of concern: content, reliability and validity, and conceptual issues.

Content

Holden and Edwards note that parenting attitude questionnaires do not, in fact, measure only attitudes, that is, beliefs and their accompanying evaluations. They may measure beliefs alone, behavioral intentions, values alone, or self-perceptions (such as views about parenting ability and the parenting role)—aspects of parent cognition and affect that probably relate to behavior in different and as yet largely undetermined ways from attitudes. Also, items on parent attitude questionnaires are often worded in an ambiguous fashion (e.g., "I sometimes feel I am too involved with my child"), with resultant difficulties that are only enhanced by the common practice of phrasing items in the third person so as to make it unclear whether or not answers are to be in terms of the parent's own activities. All too often items are double-barreled (e.g., "I find that toddlers act like they are the most important people in the house and are always demanding things"), making it impossible for a parent to know which part of the statement to respond to. Confusion for the respondent also arises from the fact that some questionnaires include items that span the child's whole developmental progression, so that respondents are forced to remember what they did in the past or to predict what they will do in the future. Contextual information is deliberately omitted from items, which makes responding difficult for parents because their reaction to a child depends on the setting or context (e.g., whether or not the child and parent are in a public or private setting, whether or not the child is the parent's own, and so on).

Psychometric Issues: Reliability and Validity

Holden and Edwards note that there is adequate information about reliability on only half of the instruments they surveyed. Moreover, only 11% of the questionnaires they reviewed had been subjected to both test-retest and internal consistency reliability assessments, each of which provides important and distinctive information.

When reliability of measurement is an issue, of course, relations with outcome measures are underestimated, and so it becomes more difficult for the investigator to establish validity. In fact, the validity data for parent attitude measures are not very impressive. The strongest validity data consist of evidence that many instruments do differentiate clinical from control groups, although occasionally the direction of relationship has been the opposite of what researchers had predicted. The most important validity measure, however, has to do with prediction from responses on parenting attitude questionnaires to actual parent behavior. Here the findings are clearly disappointing, partly because few studies have attempted to measure concurrent validity. In a recent study of this issue, Kochanska, Kuczynski, and Radke-Yarrow (1989) attempted to link attitudes measured by the Child-Rearing Practices Report (Block, 1981) and mother–child interaction in a homelike setting. Their findings suggest that actual behavior may be more easily predicted from the measurement of parenting attitudes when the interpretation of that behavior does not depend on knowing the context in which it occurred.

Conceptual Issues

The assumed usefulness of parent attitude surveys lies in a number of assumptions that are not necessarily accurate. For one thing, the sorts of attitudes they assess can involve either automatic, unaware processing or intentional, controlled cognitions subject to the individual's awareness. The latter are available for conscious deliberation and might therefore be expected to have some effect on behavior. But the former are overlearned schematic representations of past experience that never come sufficiently into the individual's awareness to have an impact on actions (Schneider & Shiffrin, 1977). Holden and Edwards cite a large number of other untested assumptions, such as the following:

1. Attitudes may not even exist until they are elicited as newly constructed beliefs by the researcher's questions.
2. Attitudes may not be as unidimensional as has been suggested (e.g., accepting-rejecting, warm-hostile) but complex, depending on variables such as the number of competing thoughts a parent has about how to raise a child.
3. Although the measurement of attitudes is based on the assumption that they are global in their application, they are likely, in fact, to be mediated by a variety of contextual considerations such as short-term goals, whether or not others are present, and parental mood.
4. Attitudes may change over time; they may not correspond with behavior that is determined by other nonattitudinal elements of parental social cognition, such as subjective norms, behavioral intentions, and immediate context.
5. Finally, parenting attitude questionnaires fail to take into account one of the major characteristics of parent–child relationships, which has become compellingly clear—children affect parents as well as vice versa.

Holden and Edwards (1989) conclude that parenting attitude questionnaires are not particularly useful in their current form and that they should be retired from use. One alternative, of course, is to develop new measures that are less subject to the kinds of criticisms raised by Holden and Edwards. Another is to move away from global measures of parenting attitudes to more specific assessments of parent social cognition, a move that is becoming increasingly evident in the field and that appears to be a promising one. We turn now to a discussion of this new approach.

PARENTING BELIEF SYSTEMS: A NEW APPROACH

The recent major interest in parent cognition has been inspired largely by a swing from the unidirectional model of socialization, with virtually all its emphasis on how parents affect children, to a bidirectional model that recognizes the impact children have on their parents. This shift has oriented researchers and theoreticians to a greater focus on the effects of different socialization situations on the parent and, in the course of that focus, to a realization that parents are complex and responsive organisms worthy of study in their own right. In an era in which cognition is so central to psychological concerns it was only natural that parent cognition should become a central focus of investigatory activity.

The new approach to parent cognition is different, however, from that taken by those researchers who wish to relate parent childrearing attitudes to parent behavior. The traditional approach, as we have noted, focuses on global attitudes or general styles of parenting that are seen to determine a whole variety of parenting behaviors. Recent approaches are more concerned with specific thoughts or beliefs that pertain to a particular interaction between parent and child. For example, rather than focusing on the relationship between an attitude of acceptance or rejection on the part of the parent and the level of dependent behavior shown by a child, investigators within the new tradition would be more likely to consider the thoughts of a parent when the child was behaving in a dependent manner (e.g., "She's doing it because she's tired and frustrated"; "I can't stand this behavior"; "I know how to handle this problem") as those thoughts mediate the action of the parent (e.g., telling the child to solve the problem herself). In the new model, then, cognitions are seen as mediators between a child's specific behavior and the parent's specific response.

In addition to distinguishing between the global and specific nature of parent cognitions, these two approaches also distinguish between their contents. Traditionally, developmental researchers have focused on attitudes toward or styles of parenting, that is, whether parents are accepting or rejecting, responsive or unresponsive, controlling or permissive, democratic or authoritarian. The new interest has ranged more broadly, motivated at least in part by a concern with the naive or informal theories that parents bring with them to the childrearing situation. The new interest includes the goals that parents set for their children—what they want *from* them (e.g., economic assistance, affection, emotional gratification, an expression of themselves, status) as well as what they want *for* them (e.g., happiness, productivity). It ranges through parents' conceptions of the basic nature of children as good, bad, or neutral(and, therefore, of how much direction and control they need); their beliefs about the impact children will have on them and their own happiness and fulfillment; and their notions about stages through which children move and their developmental timetables as well as about the relative influences of heredity and environment on development. Attention has also been paid to the kinds of causal attributions parents make for various kinds of behavior, the ideas they have about their responsibilities as parents, and the beliefs they hold about the best methods for achieving the outcomes they desire for their children.

We believe that child maltreatment research would benefit greatly from consideration of these parent cognitions as they affect parenting behavior and as they change over time. To convey the flavor of the sort of cognitions that might be studied we briefly review four major areas of study in which investigators have linked parent thinking with parent affect and behavior and child outcome.

Causal Attributions

In an application of attribution theory to the understanding of parent–child relationships, Dix and Grusec (1985) argue that the appraisal parents make of the causes of specific child behaviors has an impact on their discipline interventions. If parents hold their children responsible for specific antisocial acts, believing that a child caused negative effects that were both foreseen and intended, they will be more likely to punish the behavior than if they believe it was unintentional. There are at least two reasons for this greater tendency to punish. First, Western legal and ethical systems dictate that punishment is appropriate only when wrongdoers are responsible for their transgression, and, second, a parent's belief that bad behavior was intentionally performed produces anger and an accompanying level of arousal that may lead the parent to be more punitive. When a parent believes, on the other hand, that a child lacks knowledge about the negative outcomes of his or her acts and therefore has not intentionally caused harm, the parent will be more likely to employ explanation and reasoning because these are techniques that impart knowledge to the child. As well, the parent will be less upset and so will be less inclined to respond strongly.

There is promising support for these proposals. Dix, Ruble, Grusec, and Nixon (1986) report that parents think misconduct is more intentional when it is performed by older children (who have more knowledge) than by younger children and that they are correspondingly more upset by it. Dix, Ruble, and Zambarano (1989) found that the more mothers believed their children knew a misdeed was wrong and the more responsibility they attributed to their children for the negative outcomes of that misdeed, the more upset they reported being, the more sternness and disapproval they said they would express, and the longer they thought their child should be punished.

If inaccurate belief systems in the form of inappropriate attributions for behavior lie at the base of at least some forms of psychological abuse, then we would expect that some psychologically abusive parents should have higher expectations for their children's knowledge of what is acceptable behavior. They would therefore see their children as more responsible for the effects of unacceptable behavior and, accordingly, would be less inclined to reason or explain and more inclined to punish frequently and at inappropriate times. The socialization practices of these parents would thereby be ineffective in teaching their children appropriate behavior, as well as run the danger of becoming physically or emotionally abusive. A high level of anger aroused by attributions of intentionality and spitefulness could make parents increasingly sensitive to even small deviations from acceptable behavior and thus cause them to react to events that would, under other circumstances, simply be ignored; such parents would be characterized as intrusive in their style of parenting. In fact, when asked to respond to stories depicting children's misbehavior, parents who have been identified as physically abusive are more likely to attribute malevolent intention to the children (Bauer & Twentyman, 1985). (Cognitive dysfunctions in abusive mothers, incidentally, do *not* appear to extend to a general belief that developmental milestones, such as being able to play quietly for long periods of time, should be reached earlier than they are [Azar, Robinson, Hekimian, & Twentyman, 1984].)

Goals for Childrearing

When they attempt to modify child behavior, parents can have either short-term or long-term goals in mind. In the first case the goal is immediate compliance, whereas in the second it is internalization of parental values and standards. A parent confronted with battling siblings, for example, may choose either to terminate the battle or to attempt to ensure that future battles are not likely to occur, even in the absence of parental surveillance. These differing goals elicit differing parenting strategies as demonstrated by Kuczynski (1984). He found that mothers who want their children to comply when they are absent interact in a more nurturant manner, reason more, make more statements about their child's character, and converse more frequently with their child than those who are not attempting to elicit long-term compliance. Trickett and Kuczynski (1986) report a difference in the discipline styles of abusive and nonabusive mothers, which they attribute to differences in the goals set by these two groups. They discovered that nonabusive parents were likely to modify their discipline techniques according to the nature of the misdeed with which they were dealing. Thus, a child's high-arousal transgression, where the goal of discipline presumably is immediate suppression, was reacted to with punishment, while violations of social rules, where long-term compliance is more likely the goal, elicited parental reasoning, and moral violations elicited a combination of reasoning and punishment. Identified physically abusive mothers, on the other hand, responded to all these classes of misdeeds with punishment, an indication to Trickett and Kuczynski that their goals in all behavioral domains were short-term with a focus simply on immediate compliance rather than internalization.

Expectations about Parenting Efficacy

The major work in the area of parental expectations of efficacy has been carried out by Daphne Bugental (e.g., Bugental, Mantyla, & Lewis, 1989). In her research Bugental has identified two groups of mothers: those who believe they have the ability to control children's behavior and those who believe the control resides in the child and that they themselves have little impact on how the child behaves. To demonstrate how these beliefs influence their social interactions with children Bugental observes mothers as they spend time with children (not their own) who are relatively unresponsive to adults. She reports that mothers who have low expectations concerning their own parenting efficacy behave differently from those with high expectations. The former display a condescending and unconvincing pattern of positive affect toward the child, a pattern marked by inappropriate voice level, smiles without eye involvement, smiles accompanied by eyebrow flashes or a worried brow or frown, head tilted to one side, and head brought into a lower and closer position relative to the chest than normal. Such a pattern of behavior, which Bugental suggests reflects a "leakage" of feelings of powerlessness, is confusing to the child because it sends conflicting messages—reassurance on the one hand and a suggestion that the child lacks competence on the other. This conflicting message appears to maintain the child's lack of responsiveness and noncompliance by slowing responses and increasing avoidant behavior. High expectation mothers, on the other hand, are able to encourage responsiveness by their more appropriate and less confusing behavior. The two groups of mothers do not differ in their reactions to responsive children, an indication of the important role played by the child in social interaction.

In an extension of this work to child maltreatment Bugental, Blue, and Cruzcosa (1989) report that mothers with low perceptions of parenting efficacy are more likely to use abusive discipline such as kicking, biting, and beating up, as well as coercive discipline such as spanking, pushing, and slapping. Bugental and associates also found that children who are at risk for abusive or coercive caregiving, that is, who have a history of abuse or who are rated as difficult by their mothers, are also more inclined to elicit negative affect from strangers who are low in perceived parenting efficacy than are children not at risk for child abuse. This differential pattern of reaction is not evident in the case of women who are high in feelings of efficacy. Bugental suggests that a mother's attributions of high parenting efficacy act as a buffer against the environment for her while attributions of low self-efficacy make a parent more reactive to the characteristics of the child (but not more responsive, i.e., not more attuned to the needs of the child). Bugental (1989) also reports that low power mothers more easily retrieve problem-focused thoughts such as "Is she doing this on purpose?" whereas high power mothers are more inclined to such cognitions as "Maybe he needs reassurance," a suggestion that low power mothers structure events in a way that makes them more likely to perceive problems in relationships.

Agreement between Parent and Child Concerning Domains of Authority

Eliot Turiel and his colleagues (e.g., Nucci, 1981; Turiel, 1983; Smetana, 1981) have demonstrated that children distinguish among three different domains of behavioral transgression. Specifically, children think differently than adults about (1) moral transgressions—that is, misdeeds such as hurting and stealing that have an intrinsic effect on the welfare and rights of others; (2) violations of social conventions—that is, misdeeds such as forms of address and modes of eating that violate rules designed to ensure fluid social interaction and maintain social order; and (3) personal issues—that is, choice of friends and recreational activities that have consequences that pertain only to the children themselves. By and large, parents and children tend to agree that parents have authority to legislate child behavior in the moral and social convention domains but not in the area of personal issues (Smetana, 1988). The problem arises if a parent labels an activity as a social convention or a moral issue when the child believes it to be a personal issue. Indeed, Smetana suggests that much of adolescent conflict is a result of the fact that parents see certain events, such as sleeping late in the morning or watching too much TV, as violations of social conventions and their adolescent offspring see them as personal issues and therefore beyond the realm of parental dictate. Smetana notes as well, however, that even when parents and adolescents disagree concerning who should have final authority on an issue, there is less feeling of conflict if they reason in the same way about the issue and approve of each other's style of reasoning.

Although these ideas have not been extended specifically to the area of child maltreatment they certainly have implications for further understanding of psychological abuse. Thus, parents and children in conflict about the degree to which parental intervention is reasonable will set the stage for maladaptive social interactions and harmful parent intrusion.

IMPLICATIONS FOR RESEARCH

Given the promising start that has been made by investigators who are studying both normal and abusive parenting, we strongly urge that studies of the psychological dimensions of maltreatment include evaluations of parent cognitions. There is good reason to believe that cognitions mediate parent affect and behavior and, in that capacity, have a role to play in determining the psychological adjustment or maladjustment of the child. To the extent that this is true, psychological abuse presumably could ultimately be avoided or stopped through the appropriate modification of parent thinking.

SUMMARY

We have argued that child maltreatment should be conceptualized in terms of its psychological dimensions. This was done through a consideration of the nature of psychological abuse, an emphasis on the need to conceptualize parenting behavior along a continuum, a discussion of the inadequacies of traditional ways of measuring this continuum, and a reconceptualization of parenting maltreatment in terms of specific parent belief systems. Through such a reconceptualization of maltreatment we should be able to evaluate more thoroughly the effects on child development of less than optimal discipline practices, rejection and restrictiveness, the provision of deviant models, extreme overprotection, and exploitation. In focusing on parents we should not, however, lose sight of the role child characteristics play in determining parental behavior, affect, and cognition. For example, many children are seemingly invulnerable to the effects of maltreatment. We need to examine the characteristics underlying this invulnerability (see Starr, MacLean, & Keating, Chapter 1, this volume).

REFERENCES

Aber, J. L., & Cicchetti, D. (1984). The social-emotional development of maltreated children: An empirical and theoretical analysis. In H. Fitzgerald, B. Lester, & M. Yogman (Eds.), *Theory and research in behavioral pediatrics* (pp. 147–199). New York: Plenum.

Azar, S. T., Robinson, D. R., Hekimian, E, & Twentyman, C. T. (1984). Unrealistic expectations and problem-solving ability in maltreating and comparison mothers. *Journal of Consulting and Clinical Psychology, 52,* 687–691.

Bauer, W. D., & Twentyman, C. T. (1985). Abusing, neglectful, and comparison mothers' responses to child-related and non-child-related stressors. *Journal of Consulting and Clinical Psychology, 53,* 335–343.

Bavolek, S. J. (1984). *Handbook for the Adult–Adolescent Parenting Inventory.* Eau Claire, WI: Family Development Resources.

Besharov, D. J. (1981). Toward better research on child abuse and neglect: Making definitional issues an explicit methodological concern. *Child Abuse & Neglect, 5,* 383–390.

Block, J. H. (1981). *The child-rearing practices report (CRPR): A set of Q items for the description of parental socialization attitudes and values.* Unpublished manuscript, University of California, Institute of Human Development, Berkeley.

Bretherton, I., & Waters, E. (Eds.). (1985). Growing points of attachment theory and research. *Monographs of the Society for Research in Child Development, 50* (Nos. 1–2, Serial No. 209).

Bugental, D. (1989, April). *Caregiver cognitions as moderators of affect in abusive families.* Paper presented at the Biennial Meeting of the Society for Research in Child Development, Kansas City, MO.

Bugental, D., Blue, J., & Cruzcosa, M. (1989). Perceived control over caregiving outcomes: Implications for child abuse. *Developmental Psychology, 25,* 532–539.

Bugental, D. B., Mantyla, S. M., & Lewis, J. (1989). Parental attributions as moderators of affective communication to children at risk for physical abuse. In D. Cicchetti & V. Carlson (Eds.), *Child maltreatment: Theory and research on the causes and consequences of child abuse and neglect* (pp.254–279). New York: Cambridge University Press.

Dix, T. H., & Grusec, J. E. (1985). Parent attribution processes in child socialization. In I. Sigel (Ed.), *Parent belief systems: Their psychological consequences for children* (pp. 201–233). Hillsdale, NJ: Erlbaum.

Dix, T., Ruble, D. N., Grusec, J. E., & Nixon, S. (1986). Social cognition in parents: Inferential and affective reactions to children of three age levels. *Child Development, 57,* 879–894.

Dix, T., Ruble, D., & Zambarano, R. J. (1989). Mothers' implicit theories of discipline: Child effects, parent effects, and the attribution process. *Child Development, 60,* 1373–1391.

Egeland, B., & Sroufe, L. A. (1981). Developmental sequelae of maltreatment in infancy. *New Directions for Child Development, 11,* 77–91.

Erickson, M. F., Egeland, B., & Pianta, R. (1989). The effects of maltreatment on young children. In D. Cicchetti & V. Carlson (Eds.), *Child maltreatment: Theory and research on the causes and consequences of child abuse and neglect* (pp. 647–684). New York: Cambridge University Press.

Garbarino, J., Guttman, E., & Seeley, J. (1986). *The psychologically battered child: Strategies for identification, assessment and intervention.* San Francisco: Jossey-Bass.

Garbarino, J., & Vondra, J. (1987). Psychological maltreatment: Issues and perspectives. In M. Brassard, R. Germain, & S. Hart (Eds.), *Psychological maltreatment of children and youth* (pp. 25–44). New York: Pergamon Press.

Grusec, J. E., & Lytton, H. (1988). *Social development: History, theory, and research.* New York: Springer-Verlag.

Hart, S., Germain, R., & Brassard, M. (1987). The challenge: To better understand and combat psychological maltreatment of children and youth. In M.

Brassard, R. Germain, & S. Hart (Eds.), *Psychological maltreatment of children and youth* (pp. 3–24). New York: Pergamon Press.

Hoffman, M. L. (1970). Conscience, personality, and socialization techniques. *Human Development, 13*, 90–126.

Holden, G., & Edwards, L. (1989). Parental attitudes toward child rearing: Instruments, issues, and implications. *Psychological Bulletin, 106*, 29–58.

Klein, S. B. (1987). *Learning: Principles and applications.* New York: McGraw-Hill.

Kochanska, G., Kuczynski, L., & Radke-Yarrow, M. (1989). Correspondence between mothers' self-reported and observed child-rearing practices. *Child Development, 60*, 56–63.

Kuczynski, L. (1984). Socialization goals and mother–child interaction: Strategies for long-term and short-term compliance. *Developmental Psychology, 20*, 1061–1073.

Lyons-Ruth, K., Connell, D. B., Zoll, D., & Stahl, J. (1987). Infants at social risk: Relations among infant maltreatment, maternal behavior, and infant attachment behavior. *Developmental Psychology, 23*, 223–232.

Lytton, H., Watts, D., & Dunn, B. E. (1986). Stability and predictability of cognitive and social characteristics from age 2 to age 9. *Genetic, Social and General Psychology Monographs, 112*, 363–398.

Maccoby, E. E., & Martin, J. A. (1983). Socialization in the context of the family: Parent–child interaction. In E.M. Hetherington (Ed.), *Handbook of child psychology: Vol. 4. Socialization, personality and social development* (pp. 1–102). New York: Wiley.

McGee, R. A. & Wolfe, D. A. (in press). Psychological maltreatment: Toward an operational definition. *Developmental Psychopathology.*

Minor, T. R., Jackson, R. L., & Maier, S. F. (1984). Effects of task irrelevant cues and reinforcement delay on choice escape learning following inescapable shock: Evidence for a deficit in selective attention. *Journal of Experimental Psychology: Animal Behavior Processes, 10*, 543–566.

Nucci, L. (1981). The development of personal concepts: A domain distinct from moral or societal concepts. *Child Development, 52*, 114–121.

Oldershaw, L., Walters, G. C., & Hall, D. K. (1987). Control strategies and noncompliance in abusive mother–child dyads: An observational study. *Child Development, 57*, 722–732.

Oldershaw, L., Walters, G. C., & Hall, D. K. (1989). A behavioral approach to the classification of different types of physically abusive mothers. *Merrill-Palmer Quarterly, 35*, 255–279.

Reid, J. B. (1986). Social-interactional patterns in families of abused and nonabused children. In M. Zahn-Waxler, M. Radke-Yarrow, & M. Cummings (Eds,), *Biosocial origins of altruism and aggression* (pp. 238–255). Cambridge: Cambridge University Press.

Schneider, W., & Shiffrin, R. M. (1977). Controlled and automatic human information processing: I. Detection, search, and attention. *Psychological Review, 84*, 1–66.

Siegelman, M. (1966). Loving and punishing parental behavior and introversion tendencies in sons. *Child Development, 37*, 985–992.

Smetana, J. G. (1981). Preschool children's conceptions of moral and social rules. *Child Development, 52,* 1333–1336.

Smetana, J. G. 1988. Concepts of self and social convention: Adolescents' and parents' reasoning about hypothetical and actual family conflicts. In M. R. Gunnar (Ed.), *Minnesota symposium on child psychology* (Vol. 21, pp. 79–122). Hillsdale, NJ: Erlbaum.

Trickett, P. K., & Kuczynski, L. (1986). Children's misbehavior and parental discipline in abusive and non-abusive families. *Developmental Psychology, 22,* 115–123.

Turiel, E. (1983). *The development of social knowledge: Morality and convention.* Cambridge: Cambridge University Press.

Walters, G. C. (1989). *Parenting behavior and emotional status of physically abusive mothers.* Unpublished manuscript, University of Toronto, Toronto.

Wolfe, D. A., Jaffe, P., Wilson, S. K., & Zak, L. (1985). Children of battered women: The relation of child behavior to family violence and maternal stress. *Journal of Consulting and Clinical Psychology, 53,* 657–665.

10

Measurement of Parent–Child Interaction in Studies of Child Maltreatment

ERIC J. MASH
University of Calgary

By definition, almost every form of child maltreatment represents a serious disturbance in the parent–child relationship (Giovannoni, 1989). Furthermore, it has been assumed that child maltreatment occurs along with other kinds of disturbances in the parent–child interaction, with maltreatment being just one of several manifestations of a more general pattern of dysfunctional parenting and psychosocial maladjustment (Rutter, 1989). While many of these other disturbances in parenting would not be classified as abusive according to legal definitions, they are nevertheless part of the problem as precursors, correlates, and/or outcomes of maltreatment. The demarcation of clear boundaries between maltreatment and these other forms of disturbed parent–child interchange is often arbitrary and subject to disagreement, particularly in cases of psychological maltreatment (McGee & Wolfe, in press). Nevertheless, these seemingly less sinister disturbances in the parent–child interaction are likely to be more frequent, more continuous, more subtle, and, perhaps, more damaging in their cumulative impact on the child and family than those interactions characterized, specifically, as abusive (Lyons-Ruth, Connell, Zoll, & Stahl, 1987).

For conceptual, pragmatic, and ethical reasons, the preponderance of efforts to describe and measure parent–child interactions in maltreating families has focused on these "other" interactional disturbances. This work has attempted to: (1) identify unique features of the parent–child interaction that reliably discriminate between populations in which maltreatment does and does not occur; (2) describe the features of parent–child interaction characteristic of differing types of maltreating groups; (3) understand the parent–child-environment conditions that contribute to disturbances in the parent–child interaction; (4) establish the causal links between general disturbances in the parent–child interaction and specific abusive interchanges; (5) map out the relationships among perturbations in the parent–child interaction and both current and future negative and positive psychosocial outcomes for the child, parent, and family; (6) develop early intervention programs for enhancing the quality of the parent–child relationship; and (7) evaluate the as yet undetermined benefits of involving parents in such programs (e.g., White, Taylor, & Moss, 1989).

Longitudinal research is vital to all of the aforementioned pursuits, since the early identification, understanding, and remediation of less extreme disturbances in the parent–child interaction that may precede the onset of abuse and subsequent developmental disruptions are essential if we are to judge their seriousness accurately and to institute effective prevention programs. For this reason, the current chapter will emphasize the development and utilization of reliable, valid, and meaningful measures of parent–child interaction in the context of longitudinal research.

Unfortunately, research into the parent–child interactions of families in which maltreatment occurs is difficult to conduct and, as a result, studies have yielded inconsistent and uninterpretable findings (Cicchetti & Todd-Manly, 1990; Mash & Wolfe, 1991; Plotkin, Azar, Twentyman, & Perri, 1981). For many dimensions, it has proven extremely difficult to identify interactional disruptions that are *unique* to maltreating families (Azar, 1986) or that reliably distinguish between abusive and nonabusive groups (e.g., Dowdney, Skuse, Rutter, Quinton, & Mrazek, 1985; Starr, 1987). This is particularly so when comparisons are made between families that are well matched with respect to important demographics. It is not yet known whether the primary interactional risks to the child stem from a lack of affectionate care, actively hostile, cruel, or punitive parenting; the general effects of social impoverishment or, as is likely, from some combination of all of these factors (Rutter, 1989).

The relationships between different forms of maltreatment and distinct types of parent–child interaction are just beginning to be uncovered (e.g., Crittenden, 1988c), a state of affairs due, in part, to the heterogeneity that has characterized most maltreatment samples. Such heterogeneity is evident not only in samples that mix cases of physical abuse and neglect, but also in samples where within-category differences in age of onset, frequency, severity, and chronicity of abuse are not considered. And finally, with few exceptions, it has proven extremely difficult to establish direct links between specific patterns of parent–child interaction and specific developmental outcomes for maltreated children and/or their parents.

To date, well-controlled research into the parent–child interactions of maltreating families is sparse, and particularly so for forms of maltreatment other than physical abuse. Many studies have used parent–child assessment instruments and procedures that were initially developed for general populations, and the use of these conventional procedures with populations whose life course may include poor quality of caregiving, marital strife, family disruptions, social isolation, environmental risks, emotional instability, ongoing involvement with social agencies, and frequent health problems is of questionable validity (Cicchetti & Wagner, 1990). On occasion, the uncritical application of conventional indices of parent–child interaction seems only to confirm the obvious (e.g., that physically abusive parents may use harsher forms of discipline than nonabusive parents). In addition, the full range of parent–child interactional outcomes that are possible in maltreatment samples may not be encompassed by conventional parent–child assessment protocols (Crittenden, 1988c). For example, findings from studies using the Ainsworth Strange Situation (StS) with maltreatment populations have necessitated the development of new attachment classifications to describe patterns of behavior that were not observed in the original normative samples (e.g., Carlson, Cicchetti, Barnett, & Braunwald, 1989a, 1989b; Main & Solomon, 1986, in press).

In general, many of the instruments used to study parent–child interaction in maltreatment populations have been: investigator- and/or study-specific; used infrequently; inconsistently applied from study to study; developed via guesswork or in an ad hoc fashion; lacking in consistent links between the instrument and its underlying theoretical model; characterized by poorly operationalized constructs of parent–child interaction; narrow in their sampling of developmental domains and stage-salient interactional tasks; applied to very small samples; and of unknown or inadequate reliability and validity.

It is also somewhat ironic that the richness and complexity of our theoretical formulations concerning parent–child relationships in maltreatment populations (e.g., Belsky & Vondra, 1989; Carlson et al., 1989b; Crittenden & Ainsworth, 1989) seem to have far exceeded the measurement operations that we have used to study such relationships. To date, even our best longitudinal investigations into the roots and consequences of child maltreatment have used measures of parent–child interaction that seem quite primitive in relation to the rather sophisticated developmental models that have been proposed as the basis for these studies.

On a more optimistic note, this state of affairs is gradually changing for the better. As will be discussed, there are now several well-developed and psychometrically adequate parent–child and family assessment instruments that are available for use in studies on maltreatment. However, many of these instruments have not yet been used in a longitudinal framework with high-risk families, and their psychometric properties over longer time intervals and with high-risk groups are unknown. Consequently, there is much work that needs to be done.

This chapter addresses a number of representative issues and procedures associated with the measurement of parent–child interaction in the context of maltreatment. Given the enormity of the literature on parent–child interactions (see Lytton, 1980, and Maccoby & Martin, 1983, for reviews), I can only highlight several broad conceptual and methodological issues that seem especially relevant to the selection of specific measurement procedures for use in longitudinal research on child maltreatment. To make this task more manageable, the discussion centers on infants and young children and on forms of maltreatment that usually involve parents. I discuss some areas in detail (e.g., measures of attachment quality, contexts for assessment) in order to illustrate some general points that apply equally to other important areas of parent–child interaction that space restrictions do not permit me to discuss (e.g., measures of communication). On the other hand, I need to discuss measures of parent–child interaction that have not been used very often in studies of maltreatment, but probably should be. At the outset, I would note that both common sense and research findings preclude the recommendation of a standard battery of parent–child interaction measures to be used in research on maltreatment, even though certain general principles may be applied to govern one's choice of measures. The appropriateness of any measure(s) will be a function of a complex set of interacting conditions, not the least of which is the purpose of one's investigation (e.g., to assess the impact of a specific type of intervention, to examine intergenerational continuities, to identify developmental outcomes associated with differing types of maltreatment).

A FRAMEWORK FOR SELECTING MEASURES
OF PARENT–CHILD INTERACTION

A comprehensive inventory prepared by the Social Science Research Council in 1984 indicated that almost all of 116 major longitudinal research investigations on childhood and adolescence included multiple measures of parent–child interaction (Verdonik & Sherrod, 1984). Even the most cursory review of this important inventory leaves one with the feeling that the actions and events surrounding parent–child interaction appear limitless, as do the number and variety of methods that have been used to assess them. This complexity seems especially apparent in longitudinal investigations that attempt to identify early disturbances in the parent–child interaction, since such studies often require the use of sophisticated measurement instruments that are sensitive to the subtle variations, adjustments, and readjustments in parent–child interaction and family relationships that are known to occur over the first few years of life.

The growing sophistication of current theories of development adds to the inherent complexity of studying parent–child relationships. Transactional and dynamic-systems models, which emphasize the child's social system as a primary mediator for all aspects of development, necessitate the use of multiple measures that assess the relationships among the social, emotional, cognitive, perceptual, linguistic, and biological domains of parent–child interaction (Cicchetti & Rizley, 1981; Fogel, in press; Hartup, 1986; Hinde & Stevenson-Hinde, 1988; Sroufe & Fleeson, 1986). The multilevel contextual constructs that are characteristic of an ecological orientation highlight the importance of evaluating parent–child interactions across a variety of settings, data sources, and informants (Belsky & Vondra, 1989; Bronfenbrenner, 1986).

Given these views, it should be evident that assessments of parent–child interaction in studies of maltreatment could potentially encompass an enormous number of events, many of which may seem somewhat distal or remote from the interaction. In light of this, it should also be evident that both conceptually derived and empirically validated decision rules are needed for determining what aspects of parent–child interaction are most important, how they should be measured, and how information is to be aggregated across domains, methods, and sources. Without such decision rules, researchers and the families they study are likely to be overwhelmed and/or needlessly burdened by the inefficiencies and excessive demands that are known to be associated with the "blind use of instruments" or "shotgun approaches," namely, the gathering of data on *all* possible aspects of the parent–child interaction. Apart from the fact that such approaches are likely to exceed most researchers' capabilities and resources, the simultaneous assessment of multiple forms and levels of parent–child interaction can create quite complicated reactive effects that could diminish the interpretability and external validity of the research findings (Lorion, 1987).

Unfortunately, decision rules concerning which elements of the parent–child interaction in maltreatment populations are most important to assess and how they should be measured are not yet available, and the theoretical models and empirical bases needed to generate such rules are just beginning to emerge. Nevertheless, it is believed that sensible decisions regarding the assessment of parent–child interaction in any study of maltreatment will require the consideration of a number of specifiable parameters and their interrelationships. These general parameters are depicted in Figure 10.1, and include: (1) one's conceptual framework and underlying assumptions regarding parenting, normal development, and the various forms of maltreatment; (2) the broader environmental and cultural conditions in which parent–child interaction is embedded; (3) the unit(s) of interaction or family subsystem(s) of interest; (4) the relevant contexts and subcontexts in which parent–child interaction occurs; (5) the developmental periods during which parent–child relationships are to be assessed, and the stage-salient tasks within these periods that are viewed as most critical to the child's current and future adaptive functioning; (6) the interactional domain(s) of interest as reflected in sets of major interactional constructs (e.g., affect, control), the content of interaction (e.g., cognitive complexity, language, affective communication), the structural organization of interaction (e.g., reciprocity, flexibility), and the functions of interaction (e.g., regulation of distress, avoidance); (7) the methods for assessing parent–child interaction, including choices concerning specific procedures (e.g., direct observation or questionnaires), level of analysis (e.g., molecular versus molar events), and sources of information (e.g., parent, trained observers, clinician); and (8) one's research goals, purposes, and resources.

PARENT–CHILD INTERACTION AND TYPES OF MALTREATMENT

Our understanding of the various forms of maltreatment and their effects is an important precondition for the selection of meaningful dimensions of parent–child interaction to measure. Across the broad categories of maltreatment, different dimensions of parent–child interaction may vary in their relative importance. For example, measures that are sensitive to issues of denial, defensiveness, or the use of avoidant behavioral and emotional coping strategies may be especially appropriate in the area of sexual maltreatment (e.g., Cole & Woolger, in press); measures sensitive to the use of power in relationships may be especially important in assessments of physical abuse (e.g., Crittenden, 1988b); and measures sensitive to the cognitive/linguistic elements of parent–child interaction may be crucial for studies on neglect. There is a need for the development of measures of parent–child interaction that are tailored to the differing patterns of maltreatment. As is true in the area of maltreatment more generally, there has been a disproportionate emphasis on the development of measures of parent–child interaction in physically abusive families, even though parent–child disturbances are characteristic of all types of maltreatment. For

CONCEPTUAL FRAMEWORK

Concepts of Normal Development   Concepts of Maltreatment

Systems, Ecological, Dynamic   Physical Abuse
Parenting   Neglect
Children's Development   Psychological Maltreatment
Parent–Child and Family Relations   Sexual Maltreatment

ENVIRONMENTAL CONDITIONS

Social Support   Stress   Cultural Milieu

INTERACTION UNIT	INTERACTION CONTEXTS & SUBCONTEXTS	DEVELOPMENTAL PERIOD
FAMILY	Home	Prenatal
Mother, Child, Father	Laboratory Clinic	Infancy
Mother–Child	Day-care Center	Preschool
Father–Child	School	Childhood
Siblings	Summer Camp	Adolescence
Parent–Siblings		Adulthood
Marital		

INTERACTIONAL DOMAINS

Major Constructs

Caregiving, Affect, Control, Communication, Systems Properties

Interactional Content	Interactional Structure	Interactional Function
Cognitive Linguistic	Mutuality, Reciprocity	Avoidance
Social	Organization	Protection of Self-Esteem
Emotional	Flexibility	Regulation and Coping
Health/Lifestyle	Contingency	

METHODS OF ASSESSMENT

Procedures	Level of Analysis	Informant/Data Source
Direct Observation	Molecular vs. Molar	Parent
Interview	Quantitative vs. Qualitative	Child
Questionnaire		Observer, Rater
Ratings		Clinician

RESEARCH GOALS, PURPOSES, & RESOURCES

FIGURE 10.1. A general framework for selecting measures of parent–child interaction for use in the longitudinal study of child maltreatment.

example, while research has suggested that dysfunctional parent–child relations may occur in parents who were victims of sexual maltreatment during their own childhood, there are few observational studies of parent–child interactions in such groups (Cole & Woolger, 1989). The need for maltreatment-group-specific measures of parent–child interaction is also suggested by the different age trends associated with different forms of maltreatment (e.g., Sedlak, 1989).

There is also a need to differentiate subtypes within each of the broader maltreatment categories, although empirical efforts of this nature are sparse.

Using cluster analytic techniques, Oldershaw, Walters, and Hall (1989) identified Emotionally Distant, Hostile, and Intrusive patterns of parent–child interaction. Crittenden (1981, 1985) presented a similar classification for subgrouping maltreating parents, and reported differences in the parent–child interactions of abusive versus neglectful mothers. It should be noted that these types of subclassifications are based heavily on maternal behaviors rather than on features of the interaction. They are also categorical in their emphasis on characterizing parents as belonging to one type versus another. It should be remembered, however, that most parents are hybrids in their styles of interaction, altering these styles in relation to contextual information (Holden & Ritchie, 1987). Parents may only fall into global categorizations when we use general rather than specific measures and situations. In our efforts to develop subtypes we might wish to consider a more dimensional approach in which individual parent–child or family interactions can be described on several different dimensions (e.g., control, affect), with subtypes based on the patterning or profile of these dimensions.

Based on her data and clinical observations of several hundred maltreating/low functioning families, Crittenden (1988b) has recently presented such a multidimensional approach to sub-grouping differing types of maltreating families. The *rationally* derived subgroupings were based on a constellation of factors that included parental skills, family structure, parent's childhood experience, parental expectations, network support, parental coping strategies, children's behavioral characteristics and coping styles, and prognosis. On the basis of such a scheme, families were described as abusing, neglecting, abusing and neglecting, marginally maltreating (crisis-driven), and adequate. Such subgroupings may change over time. For example, Crittenden (1988b) has described how family transitions related to increasing family size may lead abusing parents to become neglecting, or neglecting parents to become abusing.

Expanded family subtypes of the kind proposed by Crittenden (1988b) may be necessary for longitudinal studies of high-risk groups, since many of the other systems for categorizing maltreatment groups are often derived after the fact of maltreatment. Studying the emergence of differences in parent–child interactions for subtypes of family risk based on differences in family background, family structure, individual and interpersonal resources, prior parenting experience, and attitudes and beliefs seems a worthwhile research direction.

INTERACTIONAL DOMAINS

In describing measures of parent–child interaction, it must be recognized that such relationships are multidimensional, encompassing many different aspects of child, parent, parent–child, and family functioning (NCCIP, 1987). Parental characteristics such as general health, socio-emotional adjustment (e.g., psychopathology, moods, style of dealing with others), cognitive functioning (e.g., judgment, problem solving ability, capacity to organize thoughts), life-course development (e.g., work, school), and functioning as a parent (e.g., physical caregiving, parent's attitude about himself or herself as a parent, psychological availability, sensitivity to child's cues and signals, appropriate multisensory communication, and effectiveness as a teacher) are all embedded in the parent–child relationship. So, too, are child characteristics such as physical health, temperament (e.g., responsiveness-engageability, general adaptability, and coping), physical appearance, dominant mood, motor development and activity, social and emotional functioning, cognitive functioning, language, and play. A variety of parent–child relationship dimensions have also been shown to exert important influences on development (e.g., dominant affective tone, intensity of engagement, frequency of interaction, modes of communication, attachment relationships, and play interactions).

Measures of the parent–child relationship in maltreatment samples have typically encompassed several of these areas. Because functioning in different aspects of the parent–child relationship may not show uniformity (e.g., a parent may provide adequate physical care, but show incompetence as a playmate) or because different areas of functioning may be related to different developmental outcomes for both child and parent (Crittenden, 1988c), the assessment of multiple dimensions has become the norm for most studies of parent–child interaction in maltreatment samples.

Major Constructs

The measurement emphasis given to any particular area will, of course, depend on one's theoretical model, the objectives of a particular study, and the current and future areas of functioning that are of interest (e.g., behavioral, cognitive, affective). However, in light of the inordinately large number of potentially relevant variables, there is a need to specify a smaller set of interrelated constructs that seem most relevant to understanding maltreatment family relationships across a variety of different content areas. Jacob and Tennenbaum (1988) have delineated four such common sets of constructs in the study of family psychopathology more generally. These constructs, equally relevant to maltreating families, are: affect, control, communication, and family systems properties. Similarly, Epstein, Rakoff, and Sigal (1968) have specified such constructs as task accomplishment, role performance, communication, affective expression, involvement, control, and values and norms. While the number, clarity, and independence of these various constructs are still being worked out, they do serve as a convenient way of organizing some of the more specific measures of parent–child and family interaction that have been used in studies on maltreatment.

Theoretically, each of the aforementioned sets of constructs could be evaluated for individuals, family dyads, triads, or the entire family. However, in practice, certain constructs have received greater attention in relation to particular family units (e.g., control at the level of the parent–child versus sibling dyad). Also, each of these sets of constructs could be evaluated using any of the differing procedures (e.g., observations, ratings, self-report) or data sources (e.g., parent, child). Again, however, certain procedures have been more commonly used to evaluate some constructs than others (e.g., observation to measure control). Of course, the convergence of different measures of the same construct taken at the same point in time will increase our confidence in the validity of that construct for the study of parent–child relationships.

What has been, and continues to be, one of the most pressing issues for researchers concerns the equivalency of similar sets of constructs across developmental periods. Since the specific manifestations of a broader construct (e.g., affective expression) will change with development, it becomes necessary to define and measure topographically dissimilar expressions that are, nevertheless, considered to be indicative of the same underlying construct (e.g., attachment at 12 months versus attachment at 6 years). Therefore, our measures must be sensitive to continuities or discontinuities in the underlying organizational processes, rather than attempt to achieve isomorphic correspondence over time. However, since we do not yet fully understand the dynamics of the underlying processes that are involved in maltreating parent–child relationships, many unresolved issues remain. For example, are we to define underlying processes in relation to the functions they serve or in some other fashion? Unfortunately, we are often in the position of modifying our views of various parent–child constructs at the same time that we are attempting to develop measures to assess these constructs.

In light of the large number of measures that have been used to describe affect, control, communication, and systems properties in maltreatment populations, the discussion that follows focuses on the assessment of affective dimensions—and particularly the assessment of attachment relationships—as an example.

Interactional Content

Affective Dimensions

Affective dimensions have played a central role in maltreatment theory and research. The primacy of early affective attachments as determinants of relationship satisfaction, ability to cope with interactional distress, and a variety of important developmental outcomes has resulted in a great deal of attention directed at the assessment of attachments in maltreatment samples.

Attachment Relationships

Ainsworth Strange Situation. The Ainsworth Strange Situation (StS) assessment of attachment may qualify as the most frequently used measure of the parent-infant relationship in longitudinal studies with high-risk infants (e.g., Carlson et al. 1989a, 1989b). Infants' responses in the StS are generally viewed as a reflection of the history of the parent–child interaction in the home. As such they represent an indirect measure of the parent–child interaction and presumably of the overall quality of the relationship. Secure attachments are associated with parent–child interactions characterized by relatedness and synchrony, resiliency to stress, adaptive coping with interactional disruptions, the use of the parent–child relationship as a distress regulating system, and appropriate affective interchanges.

Recent studies with maltreated infants have supported the link between insensitive caregiving and the development of insecure attachments (see Crittenden & Ainsworth, 1989, and Spieker & Booth, 1988, for reviews). A number of studies have identified patterns of insecure attachment in maltreated infants and toddlers (e.g., Carlson et al., 1989a; Crittenden, 1985, 1988a; Egeland & Sroufe, 1981; Gaensbauer & Harmon, 1982; Lamb, Gaensbauer, Malkin, & Schultz, 1985; Lyons-Ruth and associates 1987; Schneider-Rosen, Braunwald, Carlson, & Cicchetti, 1985). However, findings from some of these studies were somewhat perplexing in that many maltreated infants did not show an insecure attachment, a finding inconsistent with attachment theory. This led some investigators to qualify their findings, and others to develop new categories to describe the peculiarities in attachment that they observed. New categories have included the Avoidant/Resistant (A/C) classification of Crittenden (1985, 1988a), the Unstable/Avoidant category of Lyons-Ruth and associates (1987), and Main and Solomon's (1986, in press; Carlson et al. 1989a; O'Conner, Sigman, & Brill, 1987; Spieker & Booth, 1988) Disorganized/ Disoriented (Type D) classification. Carlson and associates (1989a, 1989b) reported that 82% of their sample of maltreated infants could be categorized as Disorganized/Disoriented. These infants showed no coherent strategy in the manner in which they dealt with the stress of separation and reunion.

While a detailed review and critique of the StS assessment of attachment is beyond the scope of this chapter, a few points are highlighted in the following paragraphs. For critical reviews of the StS as an assessment technique the interested reader is directed to Lamb, Thompson, Gardner, and Charnov (1985) and Teti and Nakagawa (in press).

1. The StS is noteworthy for its frequency of use across different investigators, laboratories, and populations. Relatively speaking, it is one of the more standardized measures of parent–child interaction, although it is by no means exempt from the frequent investigator-specific adaptations in setting and coding procedures (e.g., rater versus multivariate classifications of attachment; Connell, 1986) that have characterized most measures of parent–child interaction. Although the cumulative evidence regarding the relative strength of the associations is still inconclusive (e.g., Goldsmith & Alansky, 1987), variations in attachment quality as assessed in the StS have been found to be either positively or inversely related to variations in one or more of the following dimensions of maternal behavior: support and acceptance, sensitivity, accessibility, responsiveness to crying, timing of feeding, active encouragement of learning, competence, overinvolvement, indulgence, rejection, hostility, and discouragement of independence. These maternal dimensions have been assessed using a variety of methods including Ainsworth ratings, face-to-face interactions, and home and play observations (e.g., Goldsmith & Alansky, 1987; Solomon, George, & Ivans, 1987).

Purportedly, attachment quality has also been predictive of the child's later functioning in areas such as self-development, self-regulation, cognitive competence and problem solving, linguistic competence, sociability with adults and peers, ego resiliency/ego control, adaptation to school, and behavioral adjustment, although as was the case for attachment quality and maternal behavior, the findings have been infrequently replicated and inconsistent with respect to the magnitude of these associations (Ainsworth, Blehar, Waters, & Wall, 1978; Fagot & Kavanagh, 1990; Sroufe, 1988). Nevertheless, in the context of the purposes and resources of a particular investigation, the cumulative weight of the aforementioned findings would support the use of the StS assessment in studies of high-risk infants and young children.

2. The coding scheme developed by Main and Solomon (1986, in press), which includes the Disorganized/Disoriented category, seems especially sensitive to the problems of high-risk infants and, as such, appears to be the preferred coding strategy in studies of maltreatment.

3. The validity of the Ainsworth StS as a minimally stressful procedure for infants older than 24 months has been questioned, and different situations may be required with older children. However, the disorganization and immaturity characteristic of the attachments of maltreated youngsters has led some to suggest that the Ainsworth procedures may be stressful for maltreated children up to the age of 30-32 months (Crittenden, 1988c).

4. Until recently, laboratory assessments of attachment have not been available for toddlers and older children (Cicchetti, Cummings, Green-

berg, & Marvin, in press). However, the revised separation and reunion assessments for 3- and 6-year-olds, developed by Main, Cassidy, and colleagues (e.g., Cassidy, Marvin, & Colleagues, 1987; Main & Cassidy, 1988) provide researchers with some promising new approaches to the assessment of attachment quality beyond infancy.

5. These laboratory procedures for older children are new, and will require further psychometric development. In particular, Main and Cassidy (1988) report low reliability for the D categorization and have adopted a rating scale for describing disorganized/disoriented infant behavior, while reserving the use of the Type D categorization for more extreme scores. A comparable rating scale for child controlling behavior is also being developed (the classification for 6-year-olds that replaces the Type D category for infants is Insecure/Controlling).

6. Main and Cassidy (1988) note that assessments of attachment with older children should be based on more than a single reunion observation and that more than one type of method should be used. In particular, they recommend that measures of the child's representation of relationships with parents, such as family drawings and responses to family photographs, be used in addition to the behaviorally based reunion procedures. While such a multimethod approach to the assessment of attachment is needed, it should be recognized that laboratory separation and reunion assessments are both labor- and time-intensive. This is especially so for older children, for whom longer separations may be required to produce interactional stress and for whom the ways in which attachment relationships are expressed become increasingly complex.

So, while the revised StS may have some validity with older children, its utility and efficiency relative to alternative approaches are yet to be demonstrated. Main and Cassidy's (1988; Kaplan & Main, 1985; Main, Kaplan, & Cassidy, 1985) recommendation to use additional measures of attachment requires further investigation, but family drawings and responses to photographs have not proven to be the most reliable or valid methods of assessing children's functioning in other areas (Mash & Terdal, 1988). Moreover, the use of such representational procedures with children from low-functioning families who may show cognitive or linguistic deficits may serve to attenuate reliability and validity. While it is highly recommended that a multimethod approach to the assessment of parent–child relational quality be adopted, it is not yet clear what specific methods should be used. Further convergent validation studies are needed.

7. Attachment classifications appear to be stable for children from 12 to 20 months and predictable from infancy to early childhood in most unstressed middle-class families. However, such stability may not characterize maltreatment samples who are experiencing high levels of stress (Egeland & Farber, 1984; Main & Cassidy, 1988; Schneider-Rosen et al.,

1985). Associations between StS behavior and other child characteristics may be less reliable when there is discontinuity in caregiving conditions (Lamb, 1987). Given the variations in attachment classifications that may be associated with major life stressors and changes, more frequent assessments of the reorganizations in attachment relationships over time seem especially relevant for longitudinal studies with maltreatment samples. The assessment of such reorganizations in relation to life changes, as well as the interaction of such changes with other important variables such as the sex of the child and parent, seems important. For example, Carlson and associates (1989b) reported that boys were more likely than girls to be classified as Type D when the husband was absent from the home, whereas girls were more likely to be classified as Type D when the husband was present.

8. Research into the stability of behaviors during StS assessments has found the emotional dimensions of interactive behavior (e.g., distress to stranger) generally to be more stable over time and situations than the social interactive dimensions (e.g., proximity/contact, avoidance, unsociability), although the idiosyncratic patterning of emotional responses does tend to increase with age (Connell & Thompson, 1986). Such findings have important implications for the design of longitudinal studies in terms of both the frequency of assessments and the contexts in which different dimensions of parent–child interaction are to be evaluated.

Main and Cassidy (1988) make the important point that it is the *predictability* rather than the stability of attachment relationships from infancy through childhood that must be understood. Changes in attachment quality that can be shown to reflect progressive adaptations to family circumstances are important in their own right. For example, the shift from a Disorganized/ Disoriented pattern at 12 months to an Insecure/Controlling pattern at 6 years has been hypothesized to represent a predictable adaptation to an insecure, disorganized, and at times frightened/frightening parenting environment, that is, it is posited that as the child matures he or she develops the capacity to organize the parent through direct control of the parent's mood or behavior (Main & Cassidy, 1988).

9. Thus far, studies have been inconsistent in identifying specific attachment classifications that are associated with specific maltreatment subgroups, or even in showing that the insecure attachments observed in maltreatment samples are specific to maltreatment. For example, O'Conner and associates (1987) reported that the Type D classification was also common in infants of mothers exhibiting excessive alcohol consumption. The inconsistencies in findings related to maltreatment subgroup specificity are, in part, a reflection of small and heterogeneous samples, a lack of adequate control groups, the unequal representation of maltreatment subgroups in research studies to date, the restricted age range in which assessments of attachment have been conducted (e.g., mostly with in-

fants), and the rather unidimensional methodological approach (StS) that has dominated the assessment of attachment quality. Research that attempts to rectify some of these difficulties may well reveal stronger relationships between maltreatment subtype and attachment quality than has previously been the case.

10. As an indirect measure of parent–child interaction, attachment classifications have been shown to be one useful index of the quality of the parent–child relationship. However, research findings have suggested that observed patterns of parent–child interaction may be an even more sensitive measure of this relationship, since findings regarding differences in interactional patterns between typical and atypical populations are more consistent than those for attachment classifications (Field, 1987). Therefore, the development and utilization of assessments of relationship quality that are designed to evaluate parent–child interactional behaviors across a wider range of ecological contexts (both stressful and nonstressful) more meaningful than the StS is recommended.

11. Related to the previous point is the finding that global early intervention programs seem to have had greater success in altering parent–child interaction patterns than in altering attachment classifications (Field, 1987). On the surface, such findings would contraindicate the use of attachment classifications as an outcome measure in studies designed to bring about changes in interactional patterns in maltreatment populations. However, it is also the case that interventions that focus more specifically on attachment-related issues (e.g., Lieberman, Weston, & Pawl, 1989) may be more effective in altering attachment classifications than are global early intervention programs. Moreover, researchers' accounts of changes from insecure to secure attachment classifications that have accompanied improvements in life circumstances in maltreatment populations (e.g., Pianta, Egeland, & Erickson, 1989) would suggest that directed systematic efforts to produce changes in attachment might prove to be successful.

Attachment Behavior Q-Set. A procedure for assessing attachment in the home has been developed by Waters (Waters, 1987; Waters & Deane, 1985). Although not widely used with maltreatment samples to date, the Attachment Behavior Q-Set will be mentioned briefly here because it evaluates behavior in the home, can be used with preschool children, and illustrates an alternative method for assessing parent–child interaction (Q sort) not only in the area of attachment but in other areas as well (e.g., Pederson et al., 1989).

The Attachment Q-Set consists of 90 items that are sorted by a trained observer or by the caregiver into nine piles based on how like or unlike a given descriptor is of the child during the previous week. Waters (1987) reports that the procedure takes middle-class parents approximately 45 minutes to complete. When parents are the informants, they are asked to become familiar with the cards prior to sorting and to observe their child for about a week with these cards in mind. Attachment scores are obtained by correlating the sort for a given child with a criterion sort done by attachment experts. It should be noted that the use of such scores may be somewhat problematic in longitudinal studies, where the proto- types of "experts" have been known to change over time (Main & Solomon, 1986).

The Attachment Behavior Q-Set is a promising research instrument. Evidence for its validity comes from a number of reports of correspondence between Q-Set scores and StS attachment classifications. Its use with lower functioning parents will need to be explored since the written instructions, as described in the manual (p. 6), may be too abstract and complex for low functioning parents (e.g., "Keep the ten that are very most unlike your child in Pile 1, and move the rest toward the middle to Pile 2. If you have fewer than ten cards in Pile 1, add in the cards from Pile 2 and pick the ten most unlike your child. Put any leftover cards in Pile 2."). It has been sug- gested that subsets of the Q-Set items might be used for certain purposes (Teti & Nakagawa, in press), although the reliability and validity of such altered measures will need to be evaluated. The Q-Set also contains a vari- ety of different types of items (e.g., child's facial expressions are strong and clear when he is playing with something; when he is in a happy mood, he stays that way all day) and likely taps several different dimensions of the parent–child relationship in addition to attachment.

Older Children's Ratings of Relationship Quality. Recently, attach- ment relationships have been assessed in older children through the use of rating scales based on the construct of *relatedness.* In a study by Lynch and Wellborn (1989) of 6- to 11-year-old maltreated children, relation- ship quality was assessed along two continuous dimensions believed to tap the child's internal models of attachment. These dimensions—*emotional quality* (e.g., when I'm with my mother I feel . . . happy, safe, scared) and *psychological proximity seeking* (e.g., I wish my mother knew me bet- ter)—were derived from a 17-item self-report questionnaire, and the pur- ported inverse relationship between these dimensions was presumed to reflect the child's representation of the *organization* of the relationship (i.e., lower emotional quality should be associated with a greater need for proximity). Although maltreated children did not differ from controls on these dimensions, they did show a pattern of relatedness characterized as "disorganized" (i.e., high positive affect with wanting to be closer).

Other patterns of relatedness, described by Cicchetti and his cowork- ers on the Rochester Project (see Lynch & Wellborn, 1989), have included *optimal* (i.e., high positive emotion and satisfaction with current levels of proximity), *enmeshed* (i.e., extreme positive and no need to be closer), *deprived* (i.e., low emotion and desire to be closer), and *disengaged* (i.e., low emotion and no desire to be closer) categories. These efforts to understand attachment in older children, and to identify individual patterns is an interesting new approach to the assessment of parent–child relationships that is theoretically well-grounded. However, the approach is in its developmental stages, and the reliability and validity of these procedures and categories await further empirical examination. The facts that these measures are based on children's self-reports, have not yet been cross-validated, and do not discriminate between maltreated and control children at a global level are all areas of concern.

Adult Attachment Interview. George, Kaplan, and Main (1984) and Main and Goldwyn (in press) have developed an interview for the assessment of attachment organization in later life and have described a tripartite classification for describing adult representations of their own early childrearing environments: *secure* (i.e., at ease in integrating experiences into a coherent model and in recalling positive attachment experiences), *dismissing* (i.e., devalues and has difficulty recalling specific attachment experiences), and *preoccupied* (i.e., has difficulty integrating attachment experiences into a coherent model). The interview asks respondents to recall specific memories of their childhood as well as to conceptualize relationship influences. Interview classifications have been cross-validated with ratings of interview responses (e.g., rejection, role-reversal, loved versus unloved, idealization of the parent, persistence of not remembering, and coherence of interview; Kobak & Sceery, 1988). Also, Dozier, Bast, and Meston (1989) reported that adults who were categorized as "dismissing" during the Adult Attachment Interview showed higher levels of autonomic nervous system reactivity than those categorized as "secure." Q-sort methodologies have also been developed for adult attachment classifications. These involve the comparison of individual ratings with a Q-sort prototype for each classification (Kobak, 1988). Main and Goldwyn (1984) have reported a significant association between representations held by parents of their own attachment experiences and the quality of their infants' attachments to them.

Measures of adult attachment are useful in identifying continuities in the representation of relationships across generations and exploring relationships between such representations and current parent–child interactions. While these measures of adult perceptions may have predictive validity in their own right, they should not be viewed as accurate representations of childhood experiences. This point is brought home by findings from recent studies that have found a strong heritability factor in adult recollections of their early family experiences, particularly in relation to perceptions of the affective (e.g., warmth) versus control dimensions of such experiences (Plomin, McClearn, Pedersen, Nesselroade, & Bergeman, 1988).

Measures of Emotional Expression

Concepts related to emotionality, physiological arousal, and reactivity have been central in many discussions of maltreatment (e.g., Vasta, 1982; Wolfe, 1987). In the case of physical abuse, it has been proposed that constitutional factors and/or socialization history may cause some parents to overreact even to mild forms of negative child behavior (e.g., whining) or to show undifferentiated patterns of physiological reactivity in response to negative (e.g., crying) versus positive (e.g., smiling) child behaviors (e.g., Disbrow, Doerr, & Caulfield, 1977; Frodi & Lamb, 1980; Wolfe, Fairbank, Kelly, & Bradlyn, 1983). The potential importance of measures of arousal and emotionality for understanding parent–child relationships is suggested by findings from a number of recent studies. Donovan and Leavitt (1989), for example, reported a relationship between maternal patterns of physiological arousal in response to infant cries at 5 months (e.g., heart rate acceleration characteristic of aversive conditioning) and 16-month attachment quality as assessed in the Ainsworth StS.

While patterns of anger and overarousal have received the most attention in research on maltreatment, it would seem that emotional hyposensitivity and underarousal may be equally relevant in light of the depressed and/or apathetic moods that characterize many maltreating parents and maltreated children (e.g., Cummings & Cicchetti, in press) and disturbances in patterns of sexual arousal may play an important role in sexual maltreatment. The need for obtaining measures of a range of more subtle emotional responses seems especially apparent in cases of psychological maltreatment.

These brief comments suggest the importance of assessing the more affective features of parent–child interaction. To date, the few studies that have assessed emotional expression in maltreating parent–child interactions have used laboratory-based measures of mothers' autonomic arousal in response to somewhat contrived child stimuli, global rating scales describing the overall emotional tone of the interaction (e.g., positive, negative, neutral), or ratings of more specific emotions (e.g., covert hostility). While such measures are useful for some purposes, two points regarding the assessment of emotional expression seem especially relevant.

First, there is a need to expand the measurement procedures used to assess emotional expression in parent–child interaction (Wolfe & Bourdeau, 1987). In addition to the use of "on or under the skin" measures of arousal, such as those assessing heart rate, skin conductance, respiration, or muscle tension, other sensitive but rarely used indicators of emotion include the following: (1) *voice quality*, as assessed by judgment analysis or the acoustical analysis of specific prosodic features such as mean, contour, or variability in fundamental frequencies (e.g., Bugental, Mantyla, & Lewis, 1989; Scherer, 1986); (2) nonverbal *facial displays*, as assessed by judgment analysis or through the use of complex coding systems such as Ekman and Friesen's (1978) Facial Action Coding System (FACS) or Izard's (1983) Maximally Discriminative Facial Movement Coding System (MAX); (3) *visual responsiveness*, as assessed by measures of attentional focus (e.g., central versus peripheral), gaze, or eye contact (e.g., Kleinke, 1986; Messer & Vietze, 1988); (4) *body orientation* as assessed through judgmental analysis or coding of body positioning, posture, and distancing; and (5) *aggregate measures of affect* that utilize two or more of the preceding indicators. For example, procedures such as Tronick, Cohn, and colleagues' (e.g., Cohn & Tronick, 1987) revised Monadic Phases Coding System combine information about gaze, facial and vocal affective expressions, posture, and type of activity.

Second, there is a need to examine, in both laboratory and naturalistic situations, the emotional reactions of both parent and child, concomitant with their behaviors, in the context of ongoing social interactions as they unfold over time (Cohn & Tronick, 1988a). This would permit a sequential analysis of emotional states in relation to particular behavioral or emotional expressions on the part of parent, child, or other family members. The identification of the behavioral or emotional antecedents or consequences of harsh discipline is only one of many interesting research issues that might be explored. The use of these types of assessments in parent–child interaction research is in its beginning stages and is likely to be facilitated by the utilization of telemetric recording procedures.

The preceding recommendations represent a formidable challenge. In addition to the sophisticated resources that may be required to carry out these assessments of emotion and the practical difficulties involved, many of the specified measures are of unknown reliability and validity in the context of ongoing parent–child interactions, especially over the extended time frames typical of longitudinal research. Therefore, psychometric validation and cross-validation studies will be needed (e.g., Cohn & Tronick, 1988b; Matias, Cohn, & Ross, 1989). Nevertheless, the central role ascribed to affective processes in most forms of maltreatment would support the substantial efforts that will be required to develop and employ more sensitive measures of the emotional features of parent–child interaction than has been the case in studies to date.

Control

Considerations of interpersonal influences in the parent–child dyad have emphasized the behaviors, strategies, techniques, and styles of parenting behavior by which parents attempt to teach, shape, or control the behavior of their children. Studies have shown that by 2 years of age, 50% to 60% of mothers' behaviors are intended to exert a control function

(Schaffer, 1984), and it has been estimated that during the first 10 years of their life children experience pressure from their parents to change their behavior on the average of every 6 to 7 minutes throughout their waking day (Hoffman, 1983). While bidirectional influences in the parent–child interaction are acknowledged, most measures of control have focused on parental rather than child behavior.

One example of a multicategory code system that was developed specifically to look at the control strategies of abusive parents in attempting to gain compliance from their children was developed by Oldershaw, Walters, and Hall (1986). Positively oriented (e.g., reasoning, bargaining, cooperation, modeling, approval, positive physical behaviors, laughing), negatively-oriented (e.g., threats, negative physical behaviors, humiliation, disapproval, negative demands, ignoring) and neutral (e.g., commands) control strategies were included. With this coding procedure, it was found that abusive mothers used more negative control strategies, were more directive, and showed less positive affect as compared with controls.

Interactional Structure

Fundamental to measures of interactional structure are notions that the parent–child interactional system is dynamically self-organizing and that this dynamic self-organization creates interactional regularities or patterns (Fogel, in press). A great deal of research has shown that the timing and patterning of social influence is critical in determining developmental outcomes, and in some cases may be more important than the content of interaction. It is these *patterns* of interaction that measures of structure attempt to assess. In the context of maltreatment, structural measures of parent–child interaction have included such overlapping constructs such as consistency, flexibility, adaptability, reciprocity, bidirectional influence, mutuality, predictability, organization, contingency, affect matching, and indiscriminate responding.

There has been little uniformity in how these constructs have been assessed. Frequently, the dimensions have been descriptively defined and a unidimensional rating scale employed. Multicategory behavioral observation codes have derived measures based on sequential analysis in order to describe some of these structural features of interaction. For example, a mother's probability of responding negatively given her child's demanding behavior taken together with the probability that she will respond negatively in general provides some information about relational contingencies. However, there are few standardized transformation rules by which such measures of interactional structure can be derived across code systems. Sequential analyses have suggested that interactions in maltreatment families may be characterized by inconsistency, a lack of mutuality, disorganization, inflexibility, and indiscriminate responding. For example, Old-ershaw and associates (1986) found that abusive mothers were more inconsistent and inflexible in their use of discipline than controls.

Whole family measures have also looked at structural features of the larger family unit in terms of such constructs as organization and adapt-ability, alliances, and permeability of boundaries. Measures of family structure have been derived using questionnaires, rating scales, and obser-vations of family interactions during standard discussion tasks. (For a comprehensive review of these measures the reader is referred to Grote-vant and Carlson, 1989, Jacob and Tennenbaum, 1988, and Touliatos, Perlmutter, and Straus, 1990.)

It should be recognized that structural changes in the organization of the interaction are likely to occur with development and that such struc-tural elements as bidirectionality of effects and periodicity may vary with the child's age (e.g., Cohn & Tronick, 1988a). However, information con-cerning normative developmental reorganizations in interactional struc-ture is sparse, although it is acknowledged that variability is an inherent part of organization and that parent–child interactions are likely to show asymmetries as a function of both developmental and situational varia-tions. For example, interactions during the first year of life may be gov-erned more by the timing of events (e.g., when and how frequently events are performed) in contrast to later interactions that may depend a great deal more upon content (Fogel, 1988).

Fogel (1988) has made the point that if we wish to examine reorgani-zation and change, looking at discrete events rather than scaled events with no known validity is a preferred approach. He argues that investiga-tor-imposed scaling may not have the functional significance for the infant or mother that discrete behaviors do. Until we have a better understand-ing of the dynamic processes involved in mutual social adaptation, we must be careful that the summary measures that we use do not distort these processes.

Interactional Function

At a general level, the parent–child relationship serves a number of differ-ent but interrelated functions. It provides a context for many different areas of socialization (e.g., communication, emotion regulation, self-devel-opment), constitutes a resource that enables the child to function more independently in the world at large, and serves as a model for future rela-tionships (Hartup, 1986). Many measures of the parent–child relationship reflect interactional functions. For example, the quality of attachment is presumed to be an indirect measure of the distress-regulating function of the relationship. Some behavioral patterns may best be understood in relation to their function of avoiding unwanted demands, protecting self-esteem, or maintaining authority or intergenerational boundaries. Our conceptual models for describing interactional functions are quite limited, and our measurement operations are perhaps weakest in this area. From a longitudinal perspective, however, it is important to remember that dissimilar events may serve similar functions. If we can effectively and systematically delineate functions of the parent–child relationship we may be in a better position to describe developmental continuities and discontinuities. Crittenden (1988c) has described her efforts to develop interaction categories involving functionally equivalent behaviors. Thus far, such efforts have been based on theory or the face validity of certain combinations of behavior, rather than on efforts to define functions empirically. It may be that functional equivalence may be measured in terms of statistical associations and similarities in predicting particular events or outcomes.

INTERACTION UNIT

Conceptual approaches to the study of parent–child interaction have increasingly recognized that the relationship between child and parent can best be understood through the simultaneous consideration of other family members (e.g., Parke & Tinsley, 1987). The units of assessment for understanding family influences over time in maltreatment samples should appropriately involve individuals, relationships between two or more family members, the entire family, and/or the links between the family and extrafamilial environment. However, as has been the case in developmental research more generally, most studies of parent–child interaction in maltreatment samples have measured the mother–child relationship in isolation from other family members. Whole family, sibling, and father–child relationships have received far less attention.

Whole Family Measures

Consistent with recent family systems and family adaptation models (e.g., Kreppner, 1989a, 1989b), there has been a growing interest in assessment measures concerned with whole family functioning and/or with the functioning of multiple family relationships. This interest is reflected in the recent appearance of a number of excellent volumes that catalog and describe such measures in great detail (e.g., Grotevant & Carlson, 1989; Jacob & Tennenbaum, 1988; Touliatos et al., 1989). There is undoubtedly a need to include a greater number of "whole family" variables in studies on maltreatment, even though such basic issues as conceptualizing family structure may be difficult when one considers the elusive and transient composition that characterizes so many maltreating families (Cicchetti & Todd-Manly, 1990). However, it would make little sense to evaluate mother–child interaction in cases where, for example, the mother has not interacted with her child for some time and the grandmother has custody.

In populations in which family composition is often so fluid, the appropriateness of using family measures in longitudinal research might be questioned. However, it may be that measures reflecting whole system variables could prove to be more stable estimates of family functioning in unstable family situations than measures focusing on the characteristics associated with specific family subsystems. It is possible that some of the more global dimensions of family structure and functioning (e.g., patterns of dominance and submission, alliances, intergenerational boundaries) may endure, even though the individual "players" may change over time. Consequently, whole family measures may be especially well suited to longitudinal research on maltreatment. In considering such use, a few points seem relevant. First, few of the available family measures have been developed or used with low functioning and/or maltreating families, and therefore their coverage and psychometric properties when used with these populations are not known. Second, until recently, the use of family measures in longitudinal research has been infrequent, and the stability of these family measures over longer time periods encompassing important family transitions has not been extensively investigated. Third, many of the whole family constructs (e.g., defensive communication) and methods (e.g., family discussions) have been applied more frequently with families of older children and adolescents. Their use with families of infants and young children needs to be explored further. Certain types of family constructs may be salient for certain stages of family development, whereas others may be relevant across all stages.

A related point is the need to consider family development in maltreatment populations as a dynamic context for the evaluation of parent–child interaction. While an organizational systems model has been proposed for understanding individual children's adjustment, the progressive reorganizations of parent–child or family interaction that are associated with both normative family transitions (e.g., birth of a child) and specific adaptations that characterize maltreating families (e.g., temporary removal of the child from the home, or the report of abusive episodes) have received little attention. There is a need to explore the interplay between individual, dyadic, and family development.

Sibling Relationships

Of all family relationships, those between siblings have received the least attention, and there are few well-developed measures for describing sibling relationships, especially those of older children and adolescents. Given the disturbances in parent–child interaction that are known to occur in maltreatment populations, an examination of the possible unique roles, both positive and negative, that sibling relationships might play in maltreatment populations seems important (e.g., Pepler & Moore, 1989). Such roles may include serving as an attachment figure (Teti & Ablard, in press), informal support system, or caregiver. Studies of siblings provide an opportunity to consider nonshared family influences in maltreatment populations in relation to differential parental treatment, family structure, or extrafamilial networks. Moreover, systematic and direct comparisons of maltreating parents' interactions with their different children over time would help to better understand why some children in the same family are more likely to be targeted for maltreatment than others.

Father–Child Interactions

A number of investigators have noted that fathers have been understudied in maltreatment research (e.g., Cicchetti & Todd-Manly, 1990; Wolfe, 1987). Undoubtedly, this is related to reports in some maltreatment samples that as many as 70% to 80% of the families studied did not have a father or father figure in the home (e.g., Cicchetti & Todd-Manly, 1990), as well as to the more general difficulties associated with engaging fathers in developmental research. Nevertheless, efforts to understand father–child relationships in maltreatment situations where fathers are present, or the role that a changing and unstable father figure may play in relation to mother–child interaction and developmental outcomes more generally, are important avenues of research that need to be pursued in spite of the attendant difficulties.

INTERACTION CONTEXT AND SUBCONTEXTS

The context in which parent–child interaction is observed defines the nature of the interaction. Not only do different settings evoke different interactional organizations but the meanings of topographically similar interactions may differ as a function of where or when they occur. Since interaction and the social and physical context are fully interdependent, it is not surprising that certain dimensions of parent–child interaction may differ tremendously with even minor variations in the assessment setting (e.g., room size, play materials, presentation of instructions, arrangement of furniture, time of day). The recognized influence of context is likely to depend on the interactional domain of interest. For example, studies have reported that social dimensions of parent–child interaction show greater context-boundedness than the emotional dimensions of parent–child interaction (e.g., Connell & Thompson, 1986). Other reports have found maternal cognitive demands in a teaching task to be predictive of children's later cognitive competence, whereas measures of the affective tone of these interactions were not (Seifer, Sameroff, Baldwin, & Baldwin, 1989).

Settings may vary with respect to their physical location, demand characteristics, perceived meanings, the extent to which they evoke particular interactional repertoires, and the way in which they interact with other important individual, population, or environmental characteristics. It is essential that some consideration be given to all of these factors in selecting the contexts in which parent–child interactions will be measured. In spite of the importance of situational parameters for the study of parent–child interaction in maltreatment populations, very little systematic attention has been given to the development of standardized, reliable, and well-validated assessment contexts. With few exceptions, such as the Ainsworth StS, studies have varied widely in the conditions surrounding the assessment of parent–child interaction. Even where different studies have employed seemingly similar contexts, for example, unstructured play, there has been enormous variability in such things as the play materials, the instructions given to parents and/or children, and the length of the play period.

Direct assessments of parent–child interaction in maltreatment populations have taken place in the home, research laboratory, and clinic. An ongoing issue in research on parent–child interaction has been concern over the use of naturalistic versus laboratory/clinic assessments. While the pendulum of research opinion on this issue continues to swing back and forth, most investigators acknowledge that both types of assessment are important. It is also quite clear that no single assessment context provides a "truer" index of the overall parent–child interaction than another. The degree and type of structure that an investigator imposes on the interaction situation is crucial. For example, home observations requiring that the TV be turned off and that no phone calls be made and laboratory assessments that instruct parents to respond "normally" but to limit the interactions they initiate with their child (e.g., Ainsworth StS) may be equally "unnatural." Nevertheless both may provide important information about the parent–child interaction and have much predictive validity.

The major criterion for estimating the value of any assessment context should be its ability to generate parent–child interactions that are relevant for answering particular questions in light of available resources. Often, it is difficult to determine this in advance. However, it makes little sense to study private, infrequently occurring, high intensity events by sitting around for hours or days waiting for something to happen when it may be possible to induce these events by imposing structure on the situation through instructions. Structured interaction situations (Hughes & Haynes, 1978), whether in the home or laboratory, are known to be especially useful for studying infrequently occurring events, providing a high degree of control over the assessment situation, and creating a standard setting across different sets of interactants or the same set of interactants at different times. Since maltreatment populations are characterized by behaviors that are infrequent or private, by unstable home situations, and by variability both across families and within families over time, it would seem that structured interaction situations offer special promise in longitudinal studies on maltreatment.

While structured interaction situations have been used extensively in studies of maltreatment, with few exceptions (e.g., Ainsworth StS), the conceptual rationale underlying the specific type(s) of structured assessment situation(s) used has been implied (e.g., interaction was observed in "appropriate situations") but not clearly articulated. Home and laboratory observations of mother–child interaction during play, feeding, and face-to-face contact have been especially frequent with infants. Although these kinds of situations have been viewed as a window on the mother's behavior (e.g., caregiving, involvement, emotional intensity), the child's behavior (e.g, engagement, sociability, emotional reactions), and the dyad's behavior (e.g, synchrony, reciprocity), the emphasis with research involving infants has often been on describing parenting behavior.

Observation of unstructured play in a laboratory or clinic playroom has probably been the most frequently used situation with children from 24 months to 4 or 5 years. Other commonly used situations in this age range have involved tasks that focus on the mother as a teacher and those requiring cooperation or compliance (e.g., cleaning up). Home observations of preschool- and school-age children have either been "unstructured" (e.g., Bousha & Twentyman, 1984; Reid, Taplin, & Lorber, 1981) or have included structured skill games, discussions, or tasks calling for cooperative behavior or physical contact (e.g., Burgess and Conger, 1978). Commonly assessed dimensions in task situations have included child behaviors such as compliance, self-control, and positive and negative affect, and maternal behaviors such as involvement in child compliance, investment in teaching, and positive and negative affect (e.g., Feshbach, 1989). There are also numerous structured tasks that have been developed for the observation of interactions between parents and older children and adolescents (see Foster & Robin, 1988). However, observation of parent–child interaction in older samples of maltreated youngsters has been infrequent, presumably related to the assumption of heightened reactivity to observation and to the increased role of representational influences on the parent–child interactions of older children and adolescents (e.g., child's and parent's perceptions of the interaction).

In maltreatment populations, parenting as observed in unhurried circumstances is often better than that found over longer time spans during which parents must cope with competing demands and other life stressors (Dowdney et al., 1985; Mash, Johnston, & Kovitz, 1983). Hence, a number of studies have structured assessments of parent–child interactions so that progressively greater time or performance demands are placed on the parent or child. With infants, "stressful" situations have included physical examinations, inoculations, separations, or waiting room procedures. With older children, tasks requiring children to clean up toys (Mash et al., 1983), sort, fold, and hang up clothes (Volkin, 1987), complete tasks within a specified time frame, or engage in less preferred activities (e.g., schoolwork) are all designed to place stress on the parent–child interaction. Most investigators would agree that there is a need to assess interaction in a wide range of ecologically valid, stressful and nonstressful interaction situations (e.g., Field, 1987; Wolfe & Bourdeau, 1987) and that different types of situations are likely to provide insights into different aspects of the parent–child relationship (Crittenden, 1988c).

Parent–child assessment situations have varied a great deal with regard to the length of time over which interaction is rated/observed. For example, ratings of a dimension such as sensitivity have been made following observation periods ranging from 1 minute to 60 hours. Crittenden's (1988c) codings, using the third revision of the CARE-Index, are based on 3-minute observations of mother–infant interaction during semistructured play. Aragona and Eyberg (1981) used a 5-minute mother-directed and a 5-minute child-directed interaction task. Kavanagh, Youngblade, Reid, and Fagot (1988) used a 10-minute play and an approximately 2-minute clean-up task. Mash et al. (1983) employed a 15-minute play and a 15-minute task situation. Oldershaw et al. (1986) used a 40-minute clinic observation session that included a snack period, unstructured play, and a clean-up task. The frequently used Ainsworth StS involves 22-24 minutes of observation, of which mother and infant are actually together for 12 minutes (Ainsworth et al., 1978). Cicchetti (1989) reported using 20 minutes of unstructured free play and 30 minutes of structured interaction.

Observational studies in the home have tended to use longer observation/rating periods, ranging from a single 40-minute observation (Lyons-Ruth, Connell, & Zoll, 1989) to 90 minutes a day for three consecutive days (Bousha & Twentyman, 1984) to 60 minutes a day for four days (Burgess & Conger, 1978) to 45-60 minutes a day for six days over a period of 11-24 days (Lahey, Conger, Atkeson, & Treiber, 1984; Reid, Kavanagh, & Baldwin, 1987).

These examples are presented to highlight the fact that, in many cases, the designation of the length of the assessment situation in studies of parent–child interaction in maltreatment samples has been arbitrary, often based on precedent or pragmatics rather than upon reliability or validity considerations. In many observational studies the time frame over which interaction was assessed was very likely too brief to have produced stable measures of either parent or child behaviors, and certainly not of interactional sequences. Wachs (1987), for example, has found that specific indices of parent behavior (e.g., vocalization, physical contact, responsivity, level of involvement) derived from single observations of less than 45 minutes are not likely to be very stable, even over a time span as short as three weeks. However, when data are aggregated across observation sessions the stability of measures increases.

There are no steadfast rules for determining what constitutes an adequate sample of parent–child interaction, since the adequacy of the sample will depend on many factors, including the complexity of the coding system (e.g., number of categories), domain of parent–child interaction being studied, and time frame of interest. Presumably, the more structured or focused the situation, the briefer the time frame needed to sample the domains of interest. Also, the more global the ratings of parent–child interaction, the less time is likely to be needed. It is incumbent on each investigator to demonstrate that the measures being reported are reliable and representative of the parent–child interactions being sampled, in the context of the research issues being studied. From a longitudinal perspective it would seem that measures that aggregate behavior across multiple assessment sessions within short time frames would be important for obtaining reliable estimates of the constructs of interest.

While the contexts for the assessment of parent–child interaction have tended to include age-relevant and stage-salient tasks, the selection of such contexts has not been done in any systematic fashion. The development of tasks that capture the relevant adaptations required of child, parent, and the dyad at different ages and stages seems an important priority for longitudinal studies of parent–child interaction.

METHODS FOR THE ASSESSMENT OF
PARENT–CHILD INTERACTION

Why is it that statements such as "We observed mother–infant interaction in the home" or "We assessed parent–child interaction in the laboratory" convey such little meaning? While statements regarding the assessment of intelligence, temperament, depression, impulsivity, locus of control, and even personality, usually conjure up cognitive schemes encompassing a seemingly finite number of measurement operations, this is not so for statements concerning the assessment of "parent–child interaction." The methods that have been used to study parent–child interaction in both normal and maltreatment samples are almost as numerous as the studies in which they have been used.

Most of the measures used to study parent–child interaction have been unstandardized, and the manner in which specific constructs within measures have been operationalized has been highly idiosyncratic. Dimensions such as hostility, punitiveness, intrusiveness, mutuality, reciprocity, synchrony, and sensitivity, to name just a few, have been defined and measured in different ways from study to study. This state of affairs has made it extremely difficult to compare findings across studies and has led to inconsistencies in the literature that are likely a function of method variance.

It is important to recognize that many of the afore-mentioned constructs of parent–child interaction are themselves multidimensional. For example, the frequently used rating of "sensitivity" probably includes the mother's willingness to respond, her ability to read and understand the child's signals, her possession of effective caregiving strategies, and her recognition of the child as an individual who needs care (George & Solomon, 1989). A low sensitivity rating could indicate a deficit in any one or more of these areas, and the implications of particular deficits for intervention are quite different. Furthermore, from a longitudinal perspective changes in one or more of these areas could occur over time, and such qualitative changes in maternal sensitivity would be obscured by the global rating. There is need for the development of measures that are sensitive to the different elements of these global constructs. An example of such a potential measure with regard to maternal sensitivity was developed by Pederson and associates (1989). Their Maternal Behavior Q-set includes 90 items reflecting the mother's tendency to detect, respond promptly, and respond appropriately to her infant's signals. However, although the conceptual basis and content of this measure is multidimensional, the measure seems to yield a single sensitivity score.

Some General Comments

Multidimensional Approach

Measures of parent–child interaction in studies of maltreatment have almost always focused on the behavior of mothers in relation to their children (e.g., directiveness, disciplinary practices), frequently on children's responses to their mothers (e.g., reactions to separation, compliance), and far less frequently on the dynamic interactional behaviors of both partners (e.g., synchrony, simultaneous vocalizations, joint object play). As described earlier, the multidimensional nature of the parent–child construct itself has prompted the utilization of assessment strategies encompassing numerous interactional domains (Crittenden, 1988c; NCCIP, 1987). While measures of parent–child interaction have frequently included more than one scale, in most cases the statistical independence of these different scales has not been demonstrated.

Multimethod Approach

Parent–child interactions have been assessed in maltreatment populations utilizing rating scales, direct observations, interviews, and questionnaires. Measures have ranged from single ratings by caseworkers of the overall "quality" of the parent–child interaction, to complex multicategory coding systems requiring the direct observation of moment-to-moment interactional sequences by highly trained observers. In general, descriptions of parent–child interaction obtained by well trained and objective observers or raters are preferred to the more subjective accounts of parent–child interaction procured through questionnaires or interviews, and it is these measures that are the focus of the current discussion. However, as I have emphasized thus far, the suitability of any particular measure will depend on a complex set of factors (see Figure 10.1) and there can be no "preferred" measure(s) independent of the dimensions under consideration and/or the purposes of the research.

Furthermore, the growing recognition that all parent–child interactions encompass important cognitive and emotional/affective elements makes the use of subjective descriptions of interaction by parents and children a substantive as well as a methodological issue (Parke & Tinsley, 1987). Questionnaires, interviews, and other methods of verbal report must be used if we are to evaluate parents' and children's perceptions, expectations, interpretations, causal attributions, and subjective feelings toward one another in the context of their social interactions. Thus, for both methodological and conceptual reasons a multimethod approach has become the accepted norm for research on parent–child and family interactions (Bradbury & Fincham, 1990; Mash & Terdal, 1988).

Population-Specific Methods

In the discussion of methods to follow it will become evident that many of the measures used to study parent–child interactions in maltreatment samples were not developed specifically for these groups. More commonly, measures of parent–child or family interaction that were originally developed for use in developmental studies of normal, middle-class samples or in studies of other disturbed populations (e.g., conduct disordered children) have been applied to maltreatment samples. These measures have been used in either their original format or, using a rational approach, have been modified or adapted in ways that were presumed to make them more sensitive to specific characteristics associated with maltreatment samples.

This raises the rather complex issue of whether or not population-specific methods are needed for the study of parent–child interaction in research on maltreatment or whether parent–child measures developed for the study of other groups will suffice. There are obvious procedural needs associated with the study of low-functioning families that will require that measures used with other low-functioning nonmaltreatment samples or with middle-class families be adapted in one or more ways. However, the more important issues relate to whether or not the content and coverage characteristic of most measures of parent–child interaction are adequate to describe parent–child interactions in maltreatment populations. Are there qualitatively different organizations or expressions of behavior in maltreatment groups that require special coding categories? Or are interactions in maltreatment families to be viewed simply as quantitative aberrations that will be reflected in either higher or lower scores on the same dimensions of interaction that we observe in normal populations?

Procedures

Procedures for measuring parent–child interaction fall into two basic categories: those based on the reports of family members and those based on direct observation of parent–child or family interaction by trained raters or observers.

Report Procedures

Reports by family members represent their perceptions of family events and include perceptions of individuals (self or others), relationships, the family in general, or the connections between family and extrafamily influences (e.g., perceived social support). Most structured and semistructured interview schedules used in research with abusive parents have included items concerned with parent–child relationships (e.g., Ammerman, Hersen, & Van-Hasselt, 1989; McGee, Wolfe, & Wilson, 1990). Self-reports obtained through structured interviews or questionnaires have high face validity, are easy to administer and score, can be compared with group norms, and can be used to assess infrequently occurring, private, or covert events. On the negative side, such reports may represent biased, inaccurate, or seriously distorted views of family relationships.

There is now *sufficient* evidence to conclude that perceptual and cognitive distortions are common in both maltreating parents (e.g., Larrance & Twentyman, 1983; Newberger & White, 1989) and their children (e.g., Vondra, Barnett, Cicchetti, Shonk, & Toth, 1989), although the precise nature of such distortions is still in question. This creates a research dilemma in that we may want to develop research measures that are sensitive to these distortions (so that we can understand and modify them) at the same time that we wish to gather information about family relationships that are free from such bias and error. Identifying the types of reports about family functioning that are more likely to be characterized by such bias and inaccuracy than others is a worthwhile research goal.

Self-report measures do not provide the moment-to-moment descriptions of sequences of family interaction that are required for the study of family process. On the other hand, repeated measures of family perceptions taken over longer time intervals may provide process information at a more molar level concerning reorganizations in perceptions of family relationships in relation to ongoing development or changes in environmental conditions.

Researchers concerned with self-report measures must also reconcile the inevitable inconsistencies that are found in reports by different family members. Achenbach, McConaughy, and Howell (1987) reported that, across many studies, the mean agreement between parents and children was a dismally low +.22 for reports concerning children's behavior. In attempting to deal with such inconsistencies it is possible to use composite measures of agreements and disagreements to identify patterns of family agreement/disagreement. Understanding the sources of variance that may account for disparities in reports of different family members may also be important (e.g., motivation, interpretation, personality factors, etc.).

Some Illustrations. Report measures have encompassed parents' attitudes, behavioral intentions, beliefs, self-perceptions, and values in the context of childrearing. Common measures have included parents' descriptions of their reactions to hypothetical disciplinary situations (e.g., child drawing on the wall, hitting another child, or refusing to eat vegetables; Grusec & Kuczynski, 1980); parents' reports concerning their attitudes and views about childrearing and the parent–child interaction as assessed through a variety of questionnaires designed to tap dimensions such as consistency, organization, maturity demands, sensitivity, nurturance, involvement, and type and amount of control (e.g., Helfer, Hoffmeister, & Schneider, 1978; Slater & Power, 1987); and Q-sort measures designed to assess such childrearing attitudes and practices as control and discipline, expressions of affect, and achievement orientation (e.g., California Child-Rearing Practices Report Q Sort; Block, 1981). Q sorts have been used in longitudinal studies over long time periods and seem to have good predictive validity in this context. From a longitudinal perspective, the stability of childrearing attitudes may be much greater than the stability of specific parent–child interactional behaviors (e.g., Ianotti, Cummings, Pierrehumbert, Zahn-Waxler, & Milano, 1989).

A major recent focus has been on parents' views of themselves as parents as assessed with parenting efficacy questionnaires (e.g., Bugental, Blue, & Cruzcosa, 1989; Johnston & Mash, 1989) or using complex interviews directed at the parents' views of themselves as parents, the affective aspects of their relationship, and age- and attachment-related issues (e.g., Newberger & White, 1989). Such descriptions are an indirect measure of the parent–child relationship, in that parents are asked to indicate how they manage various childrearing issues or to describe what their interactions are like (e.g., Aber, Slade, Berger, Bresgi, & Kaplan, 1985; George & Solomon, 1989; Newberger & White, 1989).

An important emergent construct is reflected in parents' views of themselves as effective/ineffective and their children's behavior as being under/beyond their control (Mash & Johnston, 1990). Various terms have been used to describe this construct, including maternal self-efficacy, maternal effectance, perceived power, and helplessness. However, all seem to refer to a similar construct. Perceptions of efficacy have been shown to relate both to quality of attachments and to interactional behavior (Bugental et al., 1989). As has been the case for other constructs of parent–child interaction, the measurement operations that have been used to describe parenting efficacy are already quite diverse.

For a comprehensive discussion of parent report measures of childrearing attitudes the reader is referred to the recent review article by Holden and Edwards (1989). Although a neglected area, measures that assess children's perceptions of parent–child and family relationships are needed, especially for older children (e.g., Hazzard, Christensen, & Margolin, 1983).

Observation Procedures

Direct observations have been used to describe sequences of family interaction as well as family members' interactions in response to standardized assessment problems and tasks. While some studies have employed naturalistic home observations involving note taking without the use of pre-designed behavior codes (e.g., Crittenden, 1988b), there are numerous specific coding systems that are available for obtaining information about processes and patterns of interaction in maltreating families. In many instances interactions are videotaped and later summarized using (1) multicategory code systems that preserve the ordering of behaviors over time; (2) ratings of the component features or of the total interaction along dimensions of interest; or (3) recordings of family members' psychophysiological or physical responses during the interaction. Other, pseudo-observational measures have involved the use of parents' reports on the daily occurrence of specific child behaviors.

MultiCategory Code Systems

The rigorous use of observational coding procedures at all stages of research (e.g., recording, coding, summarization, analysis) provides a strong empirical base for understanding family interactional process in maltreatment populations. Technological advances such as automated data collectors and laboratory computers have greatly facilitated the ease with which observational procedures can be reliably employed (Fagot & Hagan, in press). Nevertheless, complex multicategory coding procedures continue to remain exceedingly costly from the standpoint of time, manpower, and resources. Research has shown that methodological difficulties, such as losses in reliability, are compounded by the complexity of the coding procedures used (Weinrott & Jones, 1984). As a result, where direct observational procedures were once viewed by some as the *sine qua non* of parent–child interaction assessment, current thinking would view their use as more a matter of *de gustibus non disputandum est* (Mash & Terdal, 1988).

There are numerous other methodological issues associated with direct observation. For example, the reactivity of family members to being observed may be of particular concern with low functioning parents who are suspicious and defensive. While studies have greatly enhanced our understanding of many of the methodological issues surrounding observational procedures (see Foster & Cone, 1986, and Bakeman & Gottman, 1987), virtually none of these studies have been conducted with maltreatment populations. Another issue, which is discussed later in this chapter, concerns the meaningfulness of highly specific behavioral codes in capturing some of the more global features of parent–child interaction, for example, relationship quality.

Some Illustrations. The work of John Reid and his colleagues (e.g., Reid et al., 1987) typifies the use of a multicategory code system with abusive families. This work follows from a social learning model, as have several of the other studies that have used multicategory code systems (e.g., Burgess & Conger, 1978; Mash et al., 1983). In several studies by Reid, abusive and control families have been observed by highly trained professional observers while interacting in their homes. Observations were conducted using the Family Interaction Coding System (FICS; Reid, 1978), an instrument that includes 29 behavior categories involving both prosocial and aversive family behaviors. Events are recorded in sequence so that the reactions of family members to one another can be evaluated.

Measures from this coding system have been used to describe interactional processes, develop theoretical models of abuse, and to evaluate the impact of intervention programs. For example, it has been found that the duration of coercive exchanges is longer in abusive families, that it is in these lengthier coercive exchanges that abusive incidents are most likely to occur, and that abusive parents have difficulty terminating their children's aversive behavior once it is initiated.

Since they apply to other multicategory code systems as well, a number of general points about the FICS can be noted for discussion:

1. The FICS was *not* developed specifically for maltreatment samples. This is true for a number of other coding procedures such as the Response-Class Matrix (Mash, Terdal, & Anderson, 1973), the Behavioral Coding System (Forehand & McMahon, 1981), Interactional Language (Bousha & Twentyman, 1984), and the Dyadic Parent–child Interaction Coding System (Robinson & Eyberg, 1981).
2. Although Reid has used the FICS in a number of studies, the FICS has *not* been used by other investigators in the area of maltreatment. This is true of almost all the multicategory codes mentioned in this section.
3. The FICS and most other multicategory code systems have been used predominantly to study physically abusive families, although some have been used to study neglect (e.g., Aragona & Eyberg, 1981), and others have compared abusive with neglectful family interactions (e.g., Burgess & Conger, 1978; Bousha & Twentyman, 1984).
4. Although the code categories in the FICS are extensive, it is often the case that sampling considerations necessitate the report of global summary measures such as "mean rate of aversive behavior" or "mean rate of positive behavior."
5. With the exception of the immediate social context, the FICS and similar code systems have been minimally sensitive to situational variations (e.g., task structure, social demands). As such, they tend to provide descriptions of how families interact "in general." One exception is the Interactive Behavior Code (Fagot, 1984), described in the study by Kavanagh and associates (1988), which included a variety of different context codes for describing play interactions.
6. Almost all of the multicategory behavioral code systems have been used with children older than 2 years.

With regard to this latter point, there presently exists an enormous conceptual and methodological gap between observational studies of mother–infant interaction in high-risk samples and observational studies of interaction in the maltreating families of older children. Obviously, this issue is of paramount importance for longitudinal studies, but it is not clear how best to resolve it. The progressive developmental reorganizations of both individuals and families would contraindicate the use of an omnibus code that could be used in the same format to describe parent–child interactions from cradle to grave. Such a code system Goliath would likely be both inefficient and insensitive to stage-salient parameters. On the other hand, the proliferation of idiosyncratic and methodologically diverse coding systems for families with children of different ages reduces the comparability of information concerning parent–child interactions over time, since it is not only the case that content categories vary but that the structural and procedural features of the coding systems do also. It would seem that the development of multicategory code systems that are sensitive to variations in content, but that maintain some structural consistency over time, is needed in longitudinal investigations. Ideally this should be done within the framework of a consistent theoretical approach. The FICS does not provide information regarding the "emotional tone" of the interactional event being described, whereas such other procedures as the Behavior Observation Scoring System (Burgess & Conger, 1978; Lahey et al., 1984), the Family Process Code (Dishion et al., 1984), and the INTERACT system (Dumas, in press) all do (see Bourdeau, 1986, and Wolfe & Bourdeau, 1987, for discussions of affective coding). In most cases, the emotional valence codes of positive, neutral, or negative have been attached to each behavioral code so that a response such as talking, for example, can be rated along this valence dimension. However, it is not known whether such emotional valence ratings can be done independently of code content.

The use of these types of valence ratings in multicategory code systems tends to reduce the differences between microanalytic behavioral codes and the more molar rating scales of interaction. This is also the case when observers who are employing multicategory codes make global ratings intended to describe an entire observation session, as occurs with the Observer Impressions Inventory developed by Weinrott, Reid, Bauske, and Brummett (1981).

Ratings

Numerous rating scales have been employed to observe parent–child and family interactions. The scales developed by Ainsworth, Bell, & Stayton (1971) are representative, and include 9-point rating scales for the maternal dimensions of acceptance-rejection, accessibility-ignoring, cooperation-interference, and sensitivity-insensitivity. Barnard, Eyres, Lobo, and Snyder (1983) describe scales involving binary ratings made during observations of teaching and feeding interactions. These scales are intended to measure maternal and child contributions to the "dyadic interactive quality." Child scores reflect such dimensions as clarity of cues and responsiveness to mother, and mother scores reflect ratings of sensitivity, alleviation of distress, and interactions fostering social-emotional growth and cognitive growth.

A variety of rating scales have been used to describe high risk mother–child interactions during infancy. For example, in a study of maltreated and nonmaltreated high risk infants, Lyons-Ruth and associates (1987) segmented a 40-minute videotaped infant-mother home interaction into ten 4-minute intervals. Within each 4-minute interval, maternal behavior was coded on twelve 5-point rating scales and one timed variable. Ratings were made of maternal sensitivity, warmth, verbal communication, quality and quantity of relational touching, quality and quantity of caretaking touching, interfering manipulation, covert hostility, anger, disengagement, and flatness of affect. It was found that covert hostility and interfering manipulation were the best group discriminators, and that negative dimensions seem to relate more to attachment classifications than do positive dimensions (e.g., sensitivity). In this study the same coders rated all variables so the possibility of halo effects cannot be dismissed, a problem that is pervasive with the use of ratings. Although the videotaped interaction was segmented into 4-minute intervals, it is not clear that the temporal aspects of ratings were considered in the analysis of this study. However, doing so might provide important information about the stability of ratings and about structural features of the interaction (e.g., fluctuations in ratings of affect over short time intervals), especially if the data were obtained by independent raters.

Crittenden (1988c) has described the Child–Adult Relationship Experimental Index (CARE Index) and its use with high-risk infants 1-36 months of age. The CARE Index uses a 3-minute sample of videotaped mother–infant play to categorize maternal and infant interaction patterns based on "categorical judgments of functionally equivalent behaviors." Fifty-two items are organized around seven aspects of interactional behavior (facial expression, vocal expression, position and body contact, expression of affection, pacing of turns, control, and choice of activity). For each of these aspects of behavior there are three items describing the quality of maternal behavior (controlling, unresponsive, sensitive) and four items describing the quality of child behavior (difficult, passive, cooperative, and compulsive compliant). Items are summed to yield scale scores. Crittenden has attempted to link these various maternal patterns to different types of maltreatment (e.g., controlling with abuse, unresponsive with neglect, inept with marginally maltreating mothers, and sensitive with adequate mothers).

Pseudo-Observational Procedures

A few studies have described measures of parent–child interaction derived from ongoing daily observations by parents (e.g., Chamberlain & Reid, 1987). For example, Trickett and Kuczynski (1983) trained abusive and matched-control parents to observe and immediately record naturally occurring disciplinary incidents in the home for five consecutive days.

Using this procedure it was found that abusive parents reported using punitive strategies more often and reasoning strategies less often than did the controls.

Level of Analysis

Molar versus Molecular

An issue that permeates most of the preceding discussion concerns the use of molar versus molecular units of measurement in research on child maltreatment. In part, the choice of measures has been related to the investigator's model of parent–child interaction. Those approaches that emphasize sequences of ongoing behavioral events—for example, the social learning approaches—have relied extensively on microanalytic observational strategies (e.g., Reid, Patterson, & Loeber, 1982). On the other hand, approaches to interaction as reflecting relationship dimensions that transcend individual response units—for example, attachment theories—have relied more heavily on macroanalytic ratings (e.g., Crittenden, 1988c). If "responsiveness" is believed to be a disposition that permeates all aspects of the parent–child relationship, for example, then global rating scales may constitute a more appropriate assessment than the recording of frequencies or sequences of minute behaviors (Bakeman & Brown, 1980).

In reality, this distinction is somewhat arbitrary in that most investigators acknowledge that interaction occurs at both the molar and molecular levels. Anyone who has used microanalytic observational strategies very quickly comes to recognize the need to aggregate information through the use of rationally or empirically derived decision rules. This need often emanates from methodological concerns, as when specific behavioral events (e.g., hitting) or event sequences (e.g., child cries mother hits) occur infrequently, and it becomes necessary that one or more supraordinate categories be constructed (e.g., physical negative, negative) in order to record and/or analyze information. At a conceptual level, the search for organizational structure or functions within parent–child interactional sequences also requires methods to aggregate molecular events into units that will capture these more molar features of interactional process.

In considering the use of molar versus molecular measures in longitudinal studies of parent–child interaction in child maltreatment, a number of considerations seem important: (1) Of special relevance for longitudinal studies are findings that molar ratings of parent–child interaction may show greater stability over time than molecular recordings (e.g., Jay & Farran, 1981); (2) studies have also found that macroanalytic ratings of early interaction may be better predictors of certain developmental outcomes, such as children's social competence, than microanalytic coding (e.g., Bakeman & Brown, 1980); (3) a cultural informants approach to social interaction suggests that molar ratings by human observers may be more sensitive to affective features of the interaction than molecular coding of discrete events; (4) a frequency count approach to measuring infrequently occurring events is not tenable; (5) global ratings may be less sensitive to minor variations in situational context than are frequency counts of specific behaviors; and (6) global ratings do not permit an examination of the specific time-dependent and context-specific dynamic processes that characterize mutual social adaptation. Fogel (1988) has cautioned that until these processes are clearly understood we must be careful not to prematurely employ summary measures of parent–child interaction that distort the observed social process.

Each level of analysis has its strengths and weaknesses, and generally speaking a measurement strategy that describes both micro- and macro-elements of parent–child interactions would seem advantageous. Some investigators have attempted to do this. For example, Pettit and Bates (1989) have developed a rather complex coding system (Social Events Coding) for obtaining and segmenting narrative descriptions of family social events. This approach employs highly trained and motivated observers to make narrative recordings of family social exchanges that in turn permit descriptions at the *global* (e.g., ratings of items such as "interactions in this home are characterized by respect and acceptance"), *molar* (e.g., types and proportions of events such as control events, teaching events, social contact events), and *molecular* (e.g., number of times child failed to comply) levels.

Quantitative versus Qualitative Measures

There is a need to assess both the quality and quantity of relationship difficulties in maltreatment samples. Groups of maltreating mothers may be equally insensitive to infant signals but one group may show hostile-controlling reactions while the other shows withdrawn and unresponsive behavior. Crittenden and DiLalla's (1988) findings suggest that as physically maltreated children grow older they may exhibit a form of pseudo or compulsive compliance. Such findings raise the question of whether or not simple behavioral measures such as the amount of child compliance are sufficient to capture these more qualitative features of the interaction. Perhaps the failure of a number of studies to discriminate between abused and nonabused children in the area of compliance is a reflection of the use of coding procedures that were insensitive to the qualitative features of this response.

SUMMARY AND RECOMMENDATIONS

The issues raised in this chapter suggest a number of conceptual and methodological recommendations with regard to the development and use of measures of parent–child interaction in longitudinal studies on child maltreatment.

1. The constructs describing parent–child interaction in maltreating families need to be better operationalized. To date, the manner in which the same constructs have been described and measured has varied greatly from study to study.

2. The fragmented and inconsistent manner in which measures of parent–child interaction have been employed in previous studies appears to be related to the lack of a consistent theoretical framework for organizing such measures in relation to child maltreatment. There is a need to develop measures of the interaction between the maltreating parent and his or her child that are based on more focused theoretical models of the behavior, as has been the case with measures of attachment.

3. There is a need for a greater "systems sensitivity" in the assessment of parent–child interaction (Emde, 1987). Such a sensitivity requires a recognition that multiple systems in determining behavior and development operate simultaneously and that assessment is therefore possible at many different levels. In this regard, we should select measures of parent–child interaction in a manner that will focus on understanding the system or subsystems needed to answer specific questions. Maltreating families should be viewed as polyadic interaction systems, and dyadic parent–child relations should be measured within the context of other family units. The use of measures of sibling relations, father–child relations, and whole family variables in maltreating families has been infrequent. There are now several extensive listings of family assessment measures. Although few of these measures have been used extensively with maltreating families, the expanded use of whole family measures in longitudinal studies is highly recommended if we are to understand family development and intergenerational continuities and discontinuities in the parent–child relationship (e.g., Widom, 1989a, 1989b).

4. Measures of parent–child and family interaction need to give greater recognition to the heterogeneity inherent in the child maltreatment label. The content and structure of our measures should be sensitive to the specific developmental and family issues associated with differing types of maltreatment.

5. As much as possible, we need to standardize the measures of similar constructs of parent–child interaction that are employed across studies, investigators, and laboratories. Unless a compelling case can be made for

the absence of an acceptable alternative, where psychometrically adequate established measures are available, they should be used.

6. There is a need to identify those parent–child interaction measurement issues that are uniquely important for longitudinal studies of child maltreatment. Low-frequency behaviors, family instability, parental defensiveness, reactions to being observed, and ongoing social service agency involvement are all potential areas of concern.

7. Social class exerts an important impact on family relationships. Numerous studies have shown parent–child interaction as well as maltreatment status to be related to family income (e.g., Herrenkohl, Herrenkohl, Toedter, & Yanushefski, 1984). Whenever possible, measures of parent–child interaction should be differentially sensitive to those interactional features associated with social class versus those associated with maltreatment. Unless our parent–child measures are sensitive to both sources of influence, it will be difficult to distinguish unambiguously between those developmental outcomes associated with maltreatment and those associated with low socioeconomic status and welfare dependency (Trickett, Aber, Carlson, & Cicchetti, 1991).

8. There is a need to develop and standardize specific measures and higher-order measurement operations that are sensitive to the structural organizations and functions of parent–child interaction.

9. A multimethod approach to the assessment of parent–child interaction is needed.

10. In light of the multitudinous number of ways that parent–child and family interaction can be described and coded, it would seem prudent in longitudinal studies on maltreatment to attempt, whenever possible, to videotape all observed parent–child interactions. Such a strategy will likely necessitate further study of the possible reactive effects in the populations of interest, and also of the possible loss in sensitivity that may occur in videotaped versus live codings (e.g., Kent, O'Leary, Dietz, & Diament, 1979). However, such archival videos will permit the recoding of similar data sets using new coding procedures, based on new information. It should be apparent that the same parent–child or family interaction can be coded in very different ways depending upon the questions one is asking and the available resources. Preservation of the "interaction" will mean that the same interactions could be coded at higher levels of complexity by researchers with sufficient resources. An archival approach will necessitate that greater attention be given to the representativeness of subjects and situations.

The availability of videotape archives also offers the promise of gaining a better understanding of continuities or discontinuities in parent–child relationships across generations. For example, we have been videotaping families for more than 20 years, and many of the children in our initial studies are themselves coming into the parenting years. We are hoping that we will be able to examine intergenerational continuities in parenting using direct observational methods.

11. We need to examine parent–child interactions in a much broader range of contexts than has previously been the case. The identification of stage-salient situations is critical in light of the aforementioned recommendation regarding videotaping. The establishment of stronger links between the contexts in which we observe parent–child interactions and our theories of development is needed, as has been the case for the link between attachment theory and the StS. We also need to construct a relevant taxonomy of situations, although it is not yet clear how this is to be done. Taxonomies should reflect both problem and nonproblem childrearing situations in terms of the meanings they have for both parents and children (e.g., Siebenheller, 1989).

12. Measures that examine parental and child cognitions and affect as part of the ongoing social interaction are needed. Procedures that ask parents to describe their reactions and feelings while they are observing videotapes of themselves interacting with their child offer some promise in this regard (Wolfe, 1988).

13. An impediment to the standardization and psychometric development of measures of parent–child interaction has been the lack of availability of many measures. Journal space often fails to provide the necessary detail needed for others to use particular measures, and the frequent modifications and adaptations that are made both within and across laboratories make it difficult to determine what procedure is being used by whom. Efforts to increase the general availability of measures of parent–child interaction in their entirety are needed.

14. There is a need for measures that better capture the dynamic interplay between parent and child or between larger social units such as the family. Many of the measures of parent–child interaction arbitrarily remove the interactional features of the relationship and substitute static descriptions of either the mother's behavior (e.g., sensitivity) or the child's (e.g., attachment). We need to develop measures that will better capture dynamic interactional processes as they develop over time.

15. There is a need for centralized resources and specialized laboratories that focus on the assessment of parent–child and family interaction. Many of the constructs and derived measures of parent–child interaction are too complex and too costly to be implemented by individual investigators. This is especially so when researchers are required to identify appropriate coding systems, train objective and blind observers, and develop the complex computer algorithms needed to summarize interactional data. In other areas, which are probably less complex than social interaction (e.g., the analysis of urine, blood, or semen), the reliance on specialized labora-

tories to provide the technology needed to carry out sophisticated analyses using procedures not available to on-line workers is commonplace. Would we ask all physicians to develop the methods and technologies for analyzing blood in their own office?

The aforementioned conceptual and methodological recommendations should lead to the development of more sensitive measures for describing parent–child interactions in maltreating families. Hopefully, as our understanding of these often dysfunctional interactions increases, so too will our ability to redirect and modify them.

REFERENCES

Aber, L., Slade, A., Berger, B., Bresgi, I., & Kaplan, M. (1985). *The parent development interview*, Unpublished manuscript, Barnard College, Columbia University, New York.

Achenbach, T. M., McConaughy, S. H., & Howell, C. T. (1987). Child/adolescent behavioral and emotional problems: Implications of cross-informant correlations for situational specificity. *Psychological Bulletin, 101*, 213–232.

Ainsworth, M. D. S., Bell, S. M., & Stayton, D. J. (1971). Individual differences in strange situation behavior of one-year-olds. In H. R. Schaeffer (Ed.), *The origins of human social relations* (pp. 17–57). London: Academic Press.

Ainsworth, M. D. S., Blehar, M. C., Waters, E., & Wall, S. (1978). *Patterns of attachment: A psychological study of the strange situation*. Hillsdale, NJ: Erlbaum.

Ammerman, R. T., Hersen, M., & Van Hasselt, V. B. (1989). *The Child Abuse and neglect interview schedule (CANIS), version IV*. Unpublished manual, Western Pennsylvania School for Blind Children.

Aragona, J. A., & Eyberg, S. M. (1981). Neglected children: Mothers' report of child behavior problems and observed verbal behavior. *Child Development, 52*, 596–602.

Azar, S. T. (1986). A framework for understanding child maltreatment: An integration of cognitive behavioural and developmental perspectives. *Canadian Journal of Behavioural Science, 18*, 340–355.

Bakeman, R., & Brown, J. V. (1980). Early interaction: Consequences for social and mental development at three years. *Child Development, 51*, 437–447.

Bakeman, R., & Gottman, J. M. (1987). Applying observational methods: A systematic view. In J. D. Osofsky (Ed.), *Handbook of infant development* (2nd ed., pp. 818–854). New York: Wiley.

Barnard, K. E., Eyres, S., Lobo, M., & Snyder, C. (1983). An ecological paradigm for assessment and intervention. In T. B. Brazelton & B. M. Lester (Eds.), *New approaches to developmental screening of infants* (pp. 199–218). New York: Elsevier.

Belsky, J., & Vondra, J. (1989). Lessons from child abuse: The determinants of parenting. In D. Cicchetti & V. Carlson (Eds.), *Child maltreatment: Theory and research on the causes and consequences of child abuse and neglect* (pp. 153–202). New York: Cambridge University Press.

Block, J. H. (1981). *The Child Rearing Practice Report (CRPR): A set of Q-items for the description of parental socialization attitudes and values.* Unpublished manuscript, University of California, Berkeley.

Bourdeau, P. (1986). *Quantifying the affective components of parent–child relationships in maltreating and high-risk families.* Unpublished manuscript, University of Western Ontario, London, Ontario.

Bousha, D. M., & Twentyman, C. T. (1984). Mother–child interactional style in abuse, neglect, and control groups: Naturalistic observations in the home. *Journal of Abnormal Psychology, 93,* 106–114.

Bradbury, T, N., & Fincham, F. D. (1990). Dimensions of marital and family interaction. In J. Touliatos, B. F. Perlmutter, & M. A. Straus (Eds.), *Handbook of family measurement techniques* (pp. 37–60). Newbury Park, CA: Sage.

Bronfenbrenner, U. (1986). Ecology of the family as a context for human development: Research perspectives. *Developmental Psychology, 22,* 723–742.

Bugental, D. B., Blue, J., & Cruzcosa, M. (1989). Perceived control over caregiving outcomes: Implications for child abuse. *Developmental Psychology, 25,* 532–539.

Bugental, D. B., Mantyla, S. M., & Lewis, J. (1989). Parental attributions as moderators of affective communication to children at risk for physical abuse. In D. Cicchetti & V. Carlson (Eds.), *Child maltreatment: Theory and research on the causes and consequences of child abuse and neglect* (pp. 254–279). New York: Cambridge University Press.

Burgess, R. L., & Conger, R. D. (1978). Family interaction in abusive, neglectful, and normal families. *Child Development, 49,* 1163–1173.

Carlson, V., Cicchetti, D., Barnett, D., & Braunwald, K. (1989a). Disorganized/disoriented attachment relationships in maltreated infants. *Developmental Psychology, 25,* 525–531.

Carlson, V., Cicchetti, D., Barnett, D., & Braunwald, K. (1989b). Finding order in disorganization: Lessons from research on maltreated children's attachments to their caregivers. In D. Cicchetti & V. Carlson (Eds.), *Child maltreatment: Theory and research on the causes and consequences of child abuse and neglect* (pp. 494–528). New York: Cambridge University Press.

Cassidy, J., Marvin, R., & the MacArthur Working Network on attachment. (1987). *Attachment organization in 3- and 4-year-olds: A classification system.* Unpublished scoring manual.

Chamberlain, P., & Reid, J. B. (1987). Parent observation and report of child symptoms. *Behavioral Assessment, 9,* 97–109.

Cicchetti, D. (1989). How research on child maltreatment has informed the study of child development: Perspectives from developmental psychopathology. In D. Cicchetti & V. Carlson (Eds.), *Child maltreatment: Theory and research on the causes and consequences of child abuse and neglect* (pp. 494–528). New York: Cambridge University Press.

Cicchetti, D., Cummings, M., Greenberg, M., & Marvin, R. (in press). An organizational perspective on attachment beyond infancy: Implications for theory, measurement, and research. In M. T. Greenberg, D. Cicchetti, & E. M. Cummings (Eds.), *Attachment in the preschool years: Theory, research and intervention.* Chicago: University of Chicago Press.

Cicchetti, D., & Todd-Manly, J. (1990). A personal perspective on conducting research with maltreating families: Problems and solutions. In G. Brody & I. Sigel (Eds.), *Methods of family research: Volume 2: Clinical populations* (pp. 87–133). Hillsdale, NJ: Erlbaum.

Cicchetti, D., & Rizley, R. (1981). Developmental perspectives on the etiology, intergenerational transmission and sequelae of child maltreatment. *New Directions for Child Development, 11,* 31–56.

Cicchetti, D., & Wagner, S. (1990). Alternative assessment strategies for the evaluation of infants and toddlers: An organizational perspective. In S. J. Meisels & J. P. Shonkoff (Eds.), *Handbook of early childhood intervention* (pp. 246–277). New York: Cambridge University Press.

Cohn, J. F., & Tronick, E. Z. (1987). Mother–infant face-to-face interaction: The sequence of dyadic states at 3, 6, and 9 months. *Developmental Psychology, 23,* 68–77.

Cohn, J. F., & Tronick, E. Z. (1988a). Mother–infant face-to-face interaction: Influence is bidirectional and unrelated to periodic cycles in either partner's behavior. *Developmental Psychology, 24,* 386–392.

Cohn, J. F., & Tronick, E. Z. (1988b). Discrete versus scaling approaches to the description of mother–infant face-to-face interaction: Convergent validity and divergent applications. *Developmental Psychology, 24,* 396–397.

Cole, P. M., & Woolger, C. (1989, April). *The role of emotion in the parenting difficulties of incest victims.* Paper presented at the meeting of the Society for Research in Child Development, Kansas City, MO.

Cole, P. M., & Woolger, C. (in press). Incest survivors: Their perceptions of their parents and their own parenting attitudes. *Child Abuse & Neglect.*

Connell, D. B. (1986). *Multivariate classification for Ainsworth Strange Situation.* Unpublished procedural manual, Abt Associates, Cambridge, MA.

Connell, J. P., & Thompson, R. (1986). Emotion and social interaction in the Strange Situation: Consistencies and asymmetric influences in the second year. *Child Development, 57,* 733–745.

Crittenden, P. M. (1981). Abusing, neglecting, problematic, and adequate dyads: Differentiating by patterns of interaction. *Merrill-Palmer Quarterly, 27,* 201–218.

Crittenden, P. M. (1985). Maltreated infants: Vulnerability and resilience. *Journal of Child Psychology and Psychiatry, 26,* 85–96.

Crittenden, P. M. (1988a). Distorted patterns of relationship in maltreating families: The role of internal representational models. *Journal of Reproductive and Infant Psychology, 6,* 183–189.

Crittenden, P. M. (1988b). Family and dyadic patterns of functioning in maltreating families. In K. Browne, C. Davies, & P. Stratton (Eds.), *Early prediction and prevention of child abuse* (pp. 161–189). New York: Wiley.

Crittenden, P. M. (1988c). Relationships at risk. In J. Belsky & T. Nezworski (Eds.), *Clinical implications of attachment* (pp. 136–174). Hillsdale, NJ: Erlbaum.

Crittenden, P., & Ainsworth, (1989). Child maltreatment and attachment theory. In D. Cicchetti & V. Carlson (Eds.), *Child maltreatment: Theory and research on the causes and consequences of child abuse and neglect* (pp. 432–463). New York: Cambridge University Press.

Crittenden, P. M., & DiLalla, D. L. (1988). Compulsive compliance: The development of an inhibitory coping strategy in infancy. *Journal of Abnormal Child Psychology, 16,* 585–599.

Cummings, E. M., & Cicchetti, D. (in press). Toward a transactional model of relations between attachment and depression. In M. T. Greenberg, D. Cicchetti, & E. M. Cummings (Eds.), *Attachment in the preschool years: Theory, research and intervention.* Chicago: University of Chicago Press.

Disbrow, M. A., Doerr, H., & Caulfield, C. (1977). Measuring the components of parents' potential for abuse and neglect. *Child Abuse & Neglect, 1,* 279–296.

Dishion, T., Gardner, K., Patterson, G., Reid, J., Spyrou, S., & Thibodeaux, S. (1984). *The family process code: A multidimensional system for observing family interactions.* Unpublished coding manual, Oregon Social Learning Center, Eugene, OR.

Donovan, W. L., & Leavitt, L. A. (1989). Maternal self-efficacy and infant attachment: Integrating physiology, perceptions, and behavior. *Child Development, 60,* 460–472.

Dowdney, L., Skuse, D., Rutter, M., Quinton, D., & Mrazek, D. (1985). The nature and quality of parenting provided by women raised in institutions. *Journal of Child Psychology and Psychiatry, 26,* 599–625.

Dozier, M., Bast, L., & Meston, J. (1989, April). *Individual differences in physiological responsiveness to the adult attachment interview.* Paper presented at the meeting of the Society for Research in Child Development, Kansas City, MO.

Dumas, J. E. (in press). INTERACT: A computer-based coding and data management system to assess family interactions: In R. J. Prinz (Ed.), *Advances in behavioral assessment of children and families* (Vol. 3). Greenwich, CT: JAI Press.

Egeland, B., & Farber, E. A. (1984). Infant–mother attachment: Factors related to its development and changes over time. *Child Development, 55,* 753–771.

Egeland, B., & Sroufe, L. A. (1981). Attachment and early maltreatment. *Child Development, 52,* 44–52.

Ekman, P., & Friesen, W. V. (1978). *Facial Action Coding System.* Palo Alto, CA: Consulting Psychologists Press.

Emde, R. N. (1987). Infant mental health: Clinical dilemmas, the expansion of meaning, and opportunities. In J. D. Osofsky (Ed.), *Handbook of infant development* (2nd ed., pp. 1297–1329). New York: Wiley.

Epstein, N. B., Rakoff, V., & Sigal, J. J. (1968). *Family categories schema.* Unpublished manuscript, Family Research Group, Department of Psychiatry, Jewish General Hospital, Montreal, Canada.

Fagot, B. I. (1984). *A training manual for the Fagot (1984) Interactive Behavior Code.* Unpublished manuscript, Oregon Social Learning Center, Eugene, OR.

Fagot, B. I., & Hagan, R. (in press). Coding of interactions: Is reliability really a problem? In E. Jacobs (Ed.), *Observing and recording procedures for research with young children.*

Fagot, B. I., & Kavanagh, K. (1990). The prediction of antisocial behavior from avoidant attachment classifications. *Child Development, 61,* 864–873.

Feshbach, N. D. (1989). The construct of empathy and the phenomenon of physical maltreatment of children. In D. Cicchetti & V. Carlson (Eds.), *Child mal-*

treatment: Theory and research on the causes and consequences of child abuse and neglect (pp. 349–373). New York: Cambridge University Press.

Field, T. (1987). Interaction and attachment in normal and atypical infants. *Journal of Consulting and Clinical Psychology, 55,* 853–859.

Fogel, A. (1988). Cyclicity and stability in mother–infant face-to-face interaction: A comment on Cohn and Tronick (1988). *Developmental Psychology, 24,* 393–395.

Fogel, A. (in press). The process of developmental change in infant communicative action: Using dynamic systems theory to study individual ontogenies. In J. Colombo & J. W. Fagen (Eds.), *Individual differences in infancy: Reliability, stability, prediction.* Hillsdale, NJ: Erlbaum.

Forehand, R. L., & McMahon, R. J. (1981). *Helping the noncompliant child: A clinician's guide to parent training.* New York: Guilford.

Foster, S. L., & Cone, J. D. (1986). Design and use of direct observation procedures. In A. R. Ciminero, K. S. Calhoun, & H. E. Adams (Eds.), *Handbook of behavioral assessment* (2nd ed., pp. 253–324). New York: Wiley.

Foster, S. L., & Robin, A. L. (1988). Family conflict and communication in adolescence. In E. J. Mash & L. G. Terdal (Eds.), *Behavioral assessment of childhood disorders* (2nd ed., pp. 717–775). New York: Guilford.

Frodi, A. M., & Lamb, M. (1980). Child abusers' responses to infant smiles and cries. *Child Development, 51,* 238–241.

Gaensbauer, T. J., & Harmon, R. J. (1982). Attachment behavior in abused/neglected and premature infants. Implications for the concept of attachment. In R. N. Emde & R. J. Harmon (Eds.), *The development of attachment and affiliative systems* (pp. 245–279). New York: Plenum.

George, C., Kaplan, N., & Main, M. (1984). *Attachment interview for adults.* Unpublished manuscript, University of California, Berkeley.

George, C., & Main, M. (1979). Social interactions of young abused children: Approach, avoidance, and aggression. *Child Development, 50,* 306–318.

George, C., & Solomon, J. (1989, April). *Internal working models of caregiving and security of attachment at age six.* Paper presented at the meeting of the Society for Research in Child Development, Kansas City, MO.

Giovannoni, J. (1989). Definitional issues in child maltreatment. In D. Cicchetti & V. Carlson (Eds.), *Child maltreatment: Theory and research on the causes and consequences of child abuse and neglect* (pp. 3–37). New York: Cambridge University Press.

Goldsmith, H. H., & Alansky, J. A. (1987). Maternal and infant temperamental predictors of attachment: A meta-analytic review. *Journal of Consulting and Clinical Psychology, 55,* 805–816.

Grotevant, H. D., & Carlson, C. I. (1989). *Family assessment: A guide to methods and measures.* New York: Guilford.

Grusec, J. E., & Kuczynski, L. (1980). Direction of effect in socialization: A comparison of the parent's versus the child's behavior as determinants of disciplinary techniques. *Developmental Psychology, 16,* 1–9.

Hartup, W. W. (1986). On relationships and development. In W. W. Hartup & Z. Rubin (Eds.), *Relationships and development* (pp. 1–26). Hillsdale, NJ: Erlbaum.

Hazzard, A., Christensen, A., & Margolin, G. (1983). Children's perceptions of parental behaviors. *Journal of Abnormal Child Psychology, 11,* 49–59.

Helfer, R. E., Hoffmeister, J. K., & Schneider, D. (1978). *MSPP: A manual for the use of the Michigan Profile of Parenting.* Boulder, CO: Test Analysis and Development Corporation.

Herrenkohl, E. C., Herrenkohl, R. C., Toedter, L., & Yanushefski, A. M. (1984). Parent–child interactions in abusive and nonabusive families. *Journal of the American Academy of Child Psychiatry, 23,* 641–648.

Hinde, R. A., & Stevenson-Hinde, J. (Eds.). (1988). *Relationships within families: Mutual influences.* Oxford, UK: Oxford University Press.

Hoffman, M. L. (1983). Affective and cognitive processes in moral internalization. In E. T. Higgings, D. N. Ruble, & W. W. Hartup (Eds.), *Social cognition and social development: A sociocultural perspective.* Cambridge: Cambridge University Press.

Holden, G. W., & Edwards, L. A. (1989). Parental attitudes toward child rearing: Instruments, issues, and implications. *Psychological Bulletin, 106,* 29–58.

Holden, G. W., & Ritchie, K. L. (1987, April). *Patterns of maternal behavior-revisited.* Paper presented at the meeting of the Society for Research in Child Development, Baltimore.

Hughes, H. M., & Haynes, S. N. (1978). Structured laboratory observation in the behavioral assessment of parent–child interactions: A methodological critique. *Behavior Therapy, 9,* 428–447.

Ianotti, R. J., Cummings, E. M., Pierrehumbert, B., Zahn-Waxler, C., & Milano, M. J. (1989, April). *Parental influences on prosocial behavior and empathy in early childhood.* Paper presented at the meeting of the Society for Research in Child Development, Kansas City, MO.

Izard, C. E. (1983). *The maximally discriminative facial movement coding system* (rev.). Unpublished manuscript, Department of Psychology, University of Delaware.

Jacob, T., & Tennenbaum, D. L. (1988). *Family assessment: Rationale, methods, and future directions.* New York: Plenum.

Jay, S., & Farran, D. C. (1981). The relative efficacy of predicting IQ from mother–child interactions using ratings versus behavioral count measures. *Journal of Applied Developmental Psychology, 2,* 165–177.

Johnston, C., & Mash, E. J. (1989). A measure of parenting satisfaction and efficacy. *Journal of Clinical Child Psychology, 18,* 167–175.

Kaplan, N., & Main, M. (1985). *A system for classifying children's drawings in terms of the representation of attachment.* Unpublished manuscript, University of California, Berkeley.

Kavanagh, K. A., Youngblade, L., Reid, J. B., & Fagot, B. I. (1988). Interactions between children and abusive versus control parents. *Journal of Clinical Child Psychology, 17,* 137–142.

Kent, R. N., O'Leary, K. D., Dietz, A., & Diament, C. (1979). Comparison of observational recordings in vivo, via mirror, and via television. *Journal of Applied Behavior Analysis, 12,* 517–522.

Kleinke, C. L. (1986). Gaze and eye contact: A research review. *Psychological Bulletin, 100,* 78–100.

Kobak, R. R. (1988). *Attachment Q-set.* Unpublished manuscript University of Delaware, Newark.

Kobak, R. R., & Sceery, A. (1988). Attachment in late adolescence: Working models, affect regulation, and representations of self and others. *Child Development, 59,* 135–146.

Kreppner, K. (1989a, April). *A longitudinal study of changes in socialization and interaction patterns in families.* Paper presented at the meeting of the Society for Research in Child Development, Kansas City, MO.

Kreppner, K. (1989b). Linking infant development-in-context research to the investigation of life-span family development. In K Kreppner & R. M. Lerner (Eds.), *Family systems and life span development* (pp. 33–64). Hillsdale, NJ: Erlbaum.

Lahey, B. B., Conger, R. D., Atkeson, B. M., & Treiber, F. A. (1984). Parenting behavior and emotional status of physically abusive mothers. *Journal of Consulting and Clinical Psychology, 52,* 1062–1071.

Lamb, M. E. (1987). Predictive implications of individual differences in attachment. *Journal of Consulting and Clinical Psychology, 55,* 817–824.

Lamb, M. E., Gaensbauer, T. J., Malkin, C. M., & Schultz, L. A. (1985). The effects of child maltreatment on the security of infant–adult attachment. *Infant Behavior and Development, 8,* 35–45.

Lamb, M. E., Thompson, R. A., Gardner, W., & Charnov, E. L. (1985). *Infant–mother attachment: The origins and developmental significance of individual differences in strange situation behavior.* Hillsdale, NJ: Erlbaum.

Larrance, D. T., & Twentyman, C. T. (1983). Maternal attributions and child abuse. *Journal of Abnormal Psychology, 92,* 544–547.

Lieberman, A., Weston, D., & Pawl, J. H. (1989, April). *Preventive intervention with anxiously attached dyads.* Paper presented at the meeting of the Society for Research in Child Development, Kansas City, MO.

Lorion, R. P. (1987). Methodological challenges in prevention research. In J. A. Steinberg & M. M. Silverman (Eds.), *Preventing mental disorders: A research perspective* (pp. 186–202). Washington, DC: Health and Human Services.

Lynch, M., & Wellborn, J. G. (1989, April). *Patterns of relatedness in maltreated and matched-control children: A look at mother–child relationships beyond infancy in high-risk groups.* Paper presented at the meeting of the Society for Research in Child Development, Kansas City, MO.

Lyons-Ruth, K., Connell, D. B., & Zoll, D. (1989). Maternal relations and infant attachment behavior at 12 months. In D. Cicchetti & V. Carlson (Eds.), *Child maltreatment: Theory and research on the causes and consequences of child abuse and neglect* (pp. 464–493). New York: Cambridge University Press.

Lyons-Ruth, K., Connell, D. B., Zoll, D., & Stahl, J. (1987). Infants at social risk: Relations among infant maltreatment, maternal behavior, and infant attachment behavior. *Developmental Psychology, 23,* 223–232. Lytton, H. (1980). *Parent–child interaction: The socialization process observed in twin and singleton families.* New York: Plenum.

Maccoby E., & Martin, J. (1983). Socialization in the context of the family: Parent–child interaction. In E. M. Hetherington (Ed.), *Handbook of child psychology* (Vol. 4, pp. 1–101). New York: Wiley.

Main, M., & Cassidy, J. (1988). Categories of response to reunion with parent at age 6: Predictable from infant attachment classifications and stable over a 1-month period. *Developmental Psychology, 24,* 415–426.

Main, M., & Goldwyn, R. (1984). Predicting rejection of her infant from mother's representation of her own experience: Implications for the abuse-abusing intergenerational cycle. *Child Abuse & Neglect, 8*, 203–217.

Main, M., & Goldwyn, R. (in press). Interview-based adult attachment classification: Related to infant–mother and infant–father attachment. *Developmental Psychology.*

Main, M., Kaplan, N., & Cassidy, J. C. (1985). Security in infancy, childhood, and adulthood: A move to the level of representation. *Monographs of the Society for Research in Child Development, 50* (Nos. 1-2, Serial No. 209, 66–104.

Main, M., & Solomon, J. (1986). Discovery of a disorganized disoriented attachment pattern. In T. B. Brazelton & M. W. Yogman (Eds.), *Affective development in infancy* (pp. 95–124). Norwood, NJ: Ablex.

Main, M., & Solomon, J. (in press). Procedures for identifying infants as disorganized/ disoriented during the Ainsworth Strange Situation. In M. T. Greenberg, D. Cicchetti, & E. M. Cummings (Eds.), *Attachment in the preschool years: Theory, research and intervention.* Chicago: University of Chicago Press.

Mash, E. J., & Johnston, C. (1990). Determinants of parenting stress: Illustrations from families of hyperactive and families of physically abused children. *Journal of Clinical Child Psychology, 19*, 313–328.

Mash, E. J., Johnston, C., & Kovitz, K. (1983). A comparison of the mother–child interactions of physically abused and non-abused children during play and task situations. *Journal of Clinical Child Psychology, 12*, 337–346.

Mash, E. J., & Terdal, L. G. (Eds.). (1988). *Behavioral assessment of childhood disorders* (2nd ed.). New York: Guilford.

Mash, E. J., Terdal, L. G., & Anderson, K. A. (1973). The Response-Class Matrix: A Procedure for recording parent–child interactions. *Journal of Consulting and Clinical Psychology, 40*, 163–164.

Mash, E. J., & Wolfe, D. A. (1991). Methodological issues in research on physical child abuse. *Criminal Justice and Behavior, 18*, 8–30.

Matias, R., Cohn, J. F., & Ross, S. (1989). A comparison of two systems that code infant affective expression. *Developmental Psychology, 25*, 483–489.

McGee, R. A., Wolfe, D. M. (in press). Psychological maltreatment: Towards an operational definition. *Development and Psychopathology.*

McGee, R. A., Wolfe, D. M., & Wilson, R. (1990). *A record of maltreatment experiences (ROME).* Unpublished instrument, University of Western Ontario, Department of Psychology, London, Canada.

Messer, D. J., & Vietze, P. M. (1988). Does mutual influence occur during mother–infant social gaze? *Infant Behavior and Development, 11*, 97–110.

NCCIP Program Evaluation Task Force. (1987). *Charting change in infants, families and services: A guide to program evaluation for administrators and practitioners.* Washington, DC: National Center for Clinical Infant Programs.

Newberger, C. M., & White, K. M. (1989). Cognitive foundations for parental care. In D. Cicchetti & V. Carlson (Eds.), *Child maltreatment: Theory and research on the causes and consequences of child abuse and neglect* (pp. 302–316). New York: Cambridge University Press.

O'Conner, M. J., Sigman, M., & Brill, N. (1987). Disorganization of attachment in relation to maternal alcohol consumption. *Journal of Consulting and Clinical Psychology, 55*, 831–836.

Oldershaw, L., Walters, G. C., & Hall, D. K. (1986). Control strategies and noncompliance in abusive mother–child dyads: An observational study. *Child Development, 57*, 722–732.

Oldershaw, L., Walters, G. C., & Hall, D. K. (1989). A behavioral approach to the classification of different types of physically abusive mothers. *Merrill-Palmer Quarterly, 35*, 255–279.

Parke, R. D., & Tinsley, B. J. (1987). Family interaction in infancy. In J. D. Osofsky (Ed.), *Handbook of infant development* (2nd ed., pp. 579–641). New York: Wiley-Interscience.

Pederson, D. R., Moran, G., Sitko, C., Campbell, K., Ghesquire, K., & Acton, H. (1989, April). *Maternal sensitivity and the security of infant–mother attachment: A Q-sort study.* Paper presented at the meeting of the Society for Research in Child Development, Kansas City, MO.

Pepler, D. J., & Moore, T. E. (1989, June). *Interparental violence and aggression between siblings: A test of the modelling hypothesis.* Paper presented at the meeting of the Canadian Psychological Association, Halifax, Nova Scotia.

Pettit, G. S., & Bates, J. E. (1989). *Describing family interaction patterns in early childhood*: A "social events" perspective. Unpublished manuscript, University of Tennessee, Department of Child and Family Studies, Knoxville, TN.

Pianta, R., Egeland, B., & Erickson, M. F. (1989). The antecedents of maltreatment: Results of the mother–child interaction research project. In D. Cicchetti & V. Carlson (Eds.), *Child maltreatment: Theory and research on the causes and consequences of child abuse and neglect* (pp. 203–253). New York: Cambridge University Press.

Plomin, R., McClearn, G. E., Pedersen, N. L., Nesselroade, J. R., & Bergeman, C. S. (1988). Genetic influence on childhood family environment perceived retrospectively from the last half of the life span. *Developmental Psychology, 24*, 738–745.

Plotkin, R. C., Azar, S., Twentyman, C. T., & Perri, M. G. (1981). A critical evaluation of the research methodology employed in the investigation of causative factors in child abuse and neglect. *Child Abuse & Neglect, 5*, 449–455.

Reid, J. B. (1978). *A social learning approach to family intervention: II. Observation in home settings.* Eugene, OR: Castalia.

Reid, J. B., Kavanagh, K., & Baldwin, D. V. (1987). Abusive parents' perceptions of child behavior problems: An example of parental bias. *Journal of Abnormal Child Psychology, 15*, 457–466.

Reid, J. B., Patterson, G. R., & Loeber, R. (1982). The abused child: Victim, instigator, or innocent bystander? In D. J. Bernstein (Ed.), *Response structure and organization: Nebraska Symposium on Motivation* (pp. 47–68). Lincoln, NE: University of Nebraska Press.

Reid, J. B., Taplin, P. S., Lorber, R. (1981). A social interactional approach to the treatment of abusive families. In R. B. Stuart (Ed.), *Violent behavior: Social learning approaches to prediction, management, and treatment* (pp. 83–101). New York: Brunner/Mazel.

Robinson, E. A., & Eyberg, S. M. (1981). The Dyadic Parent–child Interaction Coding System: Standardization and validation. *Journal of Consulting and Clinical Psychology, 49*, 245–250.

Rutter, M. (1989). Intergenerational continuities and discontinuities in serious parenting difficulties. In D. Cicchetti & V. Carlson (Eds.), *Child maltreatment: Theory and research on the causes and consequences of child abuse and neglect* (pp. 317–348). New York: Cambridge University Press.

Schaffer, H. R. (1984). Parental control techniques in the context of socialization theory. In W. Doise & A. Palmonai (Eds.), *Social interaction in individual development* (pp. 65–77). Cambridge, UK: Cambridge University Press.

Scherer, K. R. (1986). Vocal affect expression: A review and model for future research. *Psychological Bulletin, 99*, 143–165.

Schneider-Rosen, K., Braunwald, K. G., Carlson, V., & Cicchetti, D. (1985). Current perspectives in attachment theory: Illustrations from the study of maltreated infants. *Monographs of the Society for Research in Child Development, 50* (1–2, Serial No. 209).

Sedlak, A. J. (1989, April). *National incidence of child abuse and neglect.* Paper presented at the meeting of the Society for Research in Child Development, Kansas City, MO.

Seifer, R., Sameroff, A. J., Baldwin, C. P., & Baldwin, A. (1989, April). *Risk and protective factors between 4 and 13 years of age.* Paper presented at the meeting of the Society for Research in Child Development, Kansas City, MO.

Siebenheller, F. A. (1989). *Parental affective evaluations and discipline strategies in child rearing situations.* Unpublished manuscript, Catholic University, Institute of Family Studies, Nijmegen, The Netherlands.

Slater, M. A., & Power, T. G. (1987). Multidimensional assessment of parenting in single-parent families. *Advances in family intervention, assessment, and theory, 4*, 197–228.

Solomon, J., George, C., & Ivans, B. (1987, April). *Mother–child interaction in the home and security of attachment at age 6.* Paper presented at the meeting of the Society for Research in Child Development, Baltimore, MD.

Spieker, S. J., & Booth, C. (1988). Family risk typologies and patterns of insecure attachment. In J. Belsky & T. Nezworski (Eds.), *Clinical implications of attachment* (pp. 95–135). Hillsdale, NJ: Erlbaum.

Sroufe, L. A. (1988). The role of infant–caregiver attachment in development. In J. Belsky & T. Nezworski (Eds.), *Clinical implications of attachment* (pp. 18–38). Hillsdale, NJ: Erlbaum.

Sroufe, L. A., & Fleeson, J. (1986). Attachment and the construction of relationships. In W. Hartup & Z. Rubin (Eds.), *Relationships and development* (pp. 51–71). Hillsdale, NJ: Erlbaum.

Starr, R. H., Jr. (1987). Clinical judgment of abuse-proneness based on parent–child interactions. *Child Abuse & Neglect, 11*, 87–92.

Teti, D. M., & Ablard, K. E. (in press). Security of attachment and infant–sibling relationships. *Child Development.*

Teti, D. M., & Nakagawa, M. (in press). Assessing attachment in infancy: The strange situation and alternate systems. In E. D. Gibbs & D. M. Teti (Eds.),

Interdisciplinary assessment of infants: A guide for early intervention professionals. Baltimore: Paul H. Brookes.

Touliatos, J., Perlmutter, B. F., & Straus, M. A. (Eds.). (1990). *Handbook of family measurement techniques*. Newbury Park, CA: Sage.

Trickett, P. K., Aber, J. L., Carlson, V., & Cicchetti, D. (1991). The relationship of socioeconomic status to the etiology and developmental sequelae of physical child abuse. *Developmental Psychology, 27*, 148–158.

Trickett, P. K., & Kuczynski, L. (1983). Children's misbehaviors and parental discipline strategies in abusive and non-abusive families. *Developmental Psychology, 22*, 115–123.

Vasta, R. (1982). Physical child abuse: A dual component analysis. *Developmental Review, 2*, 164–170.

Verdonik, F., & Sherrod, L. R. (1984). *An inventory of longitudinal research on childhood and adolescence*. New York: Social Science Research Council.

Volkin, J. I. (1987). *Mother–child interaction in abusive, distressed, and normal families*. Unpublished doctoral dissertation, Department of Psychology, University of Pittsburgh.

Vondra, J., Barnett, D., Cicchetti, D., Shonk, S. M., & Toth, S. L. (1989, April). *Child maltreatment and perceived competence in school children*. Paper presented at the meeting of the Society for Research in Child Development, Kansas City, MO.

Wachs, T. D. (1987). Short-term stability of aggregated and nonaggregated measures of parental behavior. *Child Development, 58*, 796–797.

Waters, E. (1987). *Attachment behavior Q-Set, Revision 3.0*. Unpublished instrument, State University of New York at Stony Brook, Department of Psychology.

Waters, E., & Deane, K. E. (1985). Defining and assessing individual differences in attachment relationships: Q-methodology and the organization of behavior in infancy and early childhood. In I. Bretherton & E. Waters (Eds.), *Growing points of attachment theory and research: Monographs of the Society for Research in Child Development 50* (Nos. 1–2, Serial No. 209), 41–65.

Weinrott, M. R., & Jones, R. R. (1984). Overt versus covert assessment of observer reliability. *Child Development, 55*, 1125–1137.

Weinrott, M. R., Reid, J. B., Bauske, R. W., & Brummett, B. (1981). Supplementing naturalistic observations with observer impressions. *Behavioral Assessment, 3*, 151–159.

White, K. R., Taylor, M. J., & Moss, V. D. (1989, April). *Does research support claims about the benefits of involving parents in early intervention programs?* Paper presented at the meeting of the Society for Research in Child Development, Kansas City, MO.

Widom, C. S. (1989a). Does violence beget violence? A critical examination of the literature. *Psychological Bulletin, 106*, 3–28.

Widom, C. S. (1989b). The cycle of violence. *Science, 244*, 160–166.

Wolfe, D. A. (1987). *Child abuse: Implications for child development and psychopathology*. Newbury Park, CA: Sage.

Wolfe, D. A. (1988). Child abuse and neglect. In E. J. Mash & L. G. Terdal (Eds.), *Behavioral assessment of childhood disorders* (2nd. ed., pp. 627–669). New York: Guilford.

Wolfe, D. A., & Bourdeau, P. A. (1987). Current issues in the assessment of abusive and neglectful parent–child relationships. *Behavioral Assessment, 9,* 271–290.

Wolfe, D. A., Fairbank, J. A., Kelly, J. A., & Bradlyn, A. S. (1983). Child abusive parents' physiological responses to stressful and nonstressful behavior in children. *Behavioral Assessment, 5,* 363–371.

11

Assessment of Emotional Status among Maltreated Children

DAVID A. WOLFE
ROBIN McGEE
Institute for the Prevention of Child Abuse
and
The University of Western Ontario

Child maltreatment is a complex phenomenon that has proven hard to understand in terms of its causes and consequences. This is particularly true with regard to understanding the effects of maltreatment on the emotional development of children. We know from research that maltreatment does not lead to predictable developmental outcomes (see reviews by Ammerman, 1990; Shaw-Lamphear, 1985; Toro, 1982). In part, this complexity is related to the fact that maltreated children typically experience such additional environmental instabilities as parental marital discord and socioeconomic disadvantage. However, there are a number of attractive theoretical explanations as to the mechanisms by which maltreated children may become "at-risk" for developmental impairments or delays. In particular, research on child development and psychopathology provides guidelines for studying child development in context that can help in developing an understanding of the putative effects of child maltreatment.

Theory and research are thus shifting away from the study of child maltreatment and its specific effects on childhood adjustment and toward examining maltreatment as one component in the life-span context of child and adult development (Cicchetti, 1989; Rutter, 1989). Such study of developmental sequelae is guided by the principle stating that issues at one developmental period lay the groundwork for subsequent issues

(Sroufe & Rutter, 1984). That is, a child who may fail to develop secure attachments to others or to learn self-control has missed important social-ization experiences that can interfere with his or her competency in ado-lescence or adulthood. From the perspective of the child's development, this viewpoint argues that physical consequences of maltreatment are typi-cally overshadowed by the associated disruption in critical areas of psy-chological development. It is these disruptions and deviations in socialization practices and learning opportunities—(that is, "adaptational failure" (Sroufe & Fleeson, 1987)—that may be primarily responsible for the observed adjustment problems among abused and neglected children.

The importance of children's emotional development as a marker of overall child development constitutes the focal point of this chapter. We begin by discussing aspects of developmental theory that bear upon the functioning of the parent–child relationship, and then turn to explanations regarding the role of emotions in child development. We demonstrate through laboratory findings and field studies how children's emotional and social-cognitive development can be used as valuable indicators of their rate and style of developmental progress. A strategy for identifying and measuring critical aspects of emotional and social-cognitive develop-ment amongst maltreated children of different ages is then presented, accompanied by examples of currently available assessment methods.

DEVELOPMENTAL ISSUES PERTAINING TO CHILD AND ADULT FUNCTIONING

From our understanding of child development in normal families, it is believed that children's sense of self and their development of emotional expression stem from important early experiences involving significant members of their families. It is not surprising, therefore, that abused and neglected children are overrepresented in clinical and criminal justice pop-ulations. Yet the mechanisms by which family members may influence the child's ongoing development require a careful understanding of the trans-actional processes occurring between children and their caregivers over time. As discussed by Cicchetti and Aber (1986), the transactional model of development argues that the factors operating in normal or pathologi-cal conditions do not occur in isolation but, rather, contribute to the child's development in a reciprocal, dynamic fashion. Over time, the mul-tiple interactions between child and caregiver begin to shape the develop-mental consequences to the child, as well as the parent's behavior and the environmental context.

Pursuing this model, researchers have begun to investigate child mal-treatment from the perspective of developmental-maturational differences, rather than pathological differences (e.g., Zigler & Hall, 1989). This emphasis requires divergent methodologies aimed at detecting developmental differences that appear among maltreated children across the life span, while de-emphasizing unitary explanations for observable symptomatology. In effect, there is a movement away from a static, psychopathology model of abuse and more toward a process model emphasizing the developmental nature of parenting and the interactive nature of the parent– child relationship. This movement, moreover, can be recognized regardless of theoretical framework. For example, theories of attachment (e.g., Bowlby, 1973; Sroufe & Fleeson, 1986) note that the early parent–child relationship sets the stage for the child's future development of relationships. If the early relationship is characterized by trust, reciprocity, consistency, and child-centered nurturing activities, the child's propensity to develop positive, desirable relations with peers and other adults is greatly enhanced. In a similar vein, social learning theorists (e.g., Dumas & Wahler, 1985; Patterson, 1986) raise as a central assumption the formation of a parent–child relationship that is built upon consistent parental responses to the child's prosocial and undesirable behavior, such as praising attempts at compliance and effectively punishing the child's coercive, disruptive behaviors.

We contend that the influence of developmental theories and the movement toward the study of interactive processes between parent and child have led to many significant modifications in approaches to studying child maltreatment. Most notably, the literature reflects a decrease in the study of parent and child psychopathology per se, and a concomitant increase in research designs aimed at assessing the developmental changes amongst parents as well as children who are deemed "high-risk" (see, for example, Cicchetti & Carlson, 1989). In this regard, renewed interest in parent and child characteristics that are developmentally relevant and affect their interactive process has emerged. To understand the developmental consequences and contributing causes of maltreatment, it is argued, one must identify the stage-relevant issues (pertaining to both adults and children) that influence these phenomena (Cicchetti, Toth, & Bush, 1988).

The following discussion offers a framework for studying the emotional development of maltreated children and begins by looking at the degrees of parental caregiving from normal to abusive and the degrees of child development from adaptive to pathological. By addressing some of the similar processes influencing the parent–child relationship, from the direction of parent as well as child roles, we hope to highlight some of the more important developmental themes that warrant careful assessment planning.

Stages of Parenting

Newberger and Cook (1983) have proposed that parenting behaviors and attitudes follow a pattern of stages in which the parent gradually recognizes the child as a unique person and his or her own responsibilities in the parental role. Parenting, according to this developmental perspective, is a process of adaptation in which the person may possess some degree of competence interspersed with lower functioning. Applying this perspective to abusive parents, Zigler and Hall (1989) suggest that when lower functioning individuals encounter stress, their methods of coping resemble those of an immature person, such as striking out at the threat. Individuals who possess higher levels of competency and skill, in contrast, are more inclined to express their interactions with their offspring through more verbal means (Patterson, 1986; Zigler & Hall, 1989).

Extending this perspective on parenting, we can conceptualize child abuse as a pattern that *develops* within the family context and that is dynamically influenced by individual (e.g., intelligence, anger-control), situational (e.g., unemployment, marital conflict), and cultural factors (e.g., acceptance of severe corporal punishment). Wolfe (1987) describes the process that changes aspects of the parent–child relationship gradually over time into more aversive and high-risk interactions in terms of three progressive stages, each of which represents a transformation from mild to more harmful interactions. The first stage of abusive parenting begins with the parent's own socialization (in terms of psychological and social resources and modeling and similar learning experiences from childhood), as one determinant of his or her current style of coping with the daily competing demands of childrearing. Problems surfacing during this stage may then lead to poor management of acute crises and stressful events, which serve to heighten parental anger, arousal, and level of discomfort. In the second stage, when this point of reduced tolerance for stress is reached, the parent may become easily overwhelmed by the amount and intensity of uncontrollable events. The child's current behavior or characteristics serve as a "trigger" that unleashes a flood of anger and frustration (or, alternatively, withdrawal and neglect). Finally, during the third stage, a habitual pattern of irritability, arousal, and/or avoidance of responsibility may become established, which may serve to perpetuate the use of power-assertive or neglectful childrearing methods.

Presumably, inadequacies in parental caregiving behavior can occur during any time in the child's development, and therefore the impact of maltreatment on the child will depend to a large extent upon the prominent childrearing methods used by the parent during important transitional stages of child development. Accordingly, the study of the impact of abuse on the child's development must take into consideration the full arena of socialization activities prescribed by the parent. These activities, in turn, are largely a function of the parent's own developmental maturity.

Stage-Salient Issues for Maltreated Children

Until very recently, child development has been primarily approached from the perspective of the normal child, with a focus on the child's mastery of different presumed stages of cognitive, behavioral, and emotional development. Psychopathology, in contrast, has long been studied on a parallel plane that infrequently intersected with information pertaining to normal development. These independent approaches were of limited usefulness, however, due to the unrecognized importance of the mutual benefits to be gained from sharing a similar paradigm and information. Child maltreatment, due to its far-reaching developmental and clinical consequences, was soon recognized as a topic that bridged the areas of normal and abnormal development and required simultaneous consideration of both approaches (Cicchetti, 1989). The quickly growing field of developmental psychopathology (Sroufe & Rutter, 1984) provided a promising strategy for placing the problems of maltreated children within the context of normal developmental stages and adaptive abilities.

One comprehensive framework for understanding the problems of maltreated children that emerged from this union of normal and abnormal developmental has been recently proposed by Cicchetti and associates (1988). These investigators review the stage-salient issues for maltreated children (as well as for other clinical populations, such as children with Down syndrome, nonorganic failure to thrive, and depressed parents) and present convincing data indicating how these issues, because they are chronic and unresolved, can lead to developmental psychopathology. Their stage-salient issues are reviewed in reference to child maltreatment to provide a developmental framework for deciding on assessment goals for this population.

The period of infancy and toddlerhood (ages 0–3 years), according to Cicchetti and associates (1988), includes three stage-salient issues that are unsuccessfully resolved by children from abusive and neglectful families. The first issue of importance is the formation of attachment to the caregiver (6–12 months), a phenomenon that has been strongly related to subsequent adaptation and development (Crittenden & Ainsworth, 1989; Sroufe & Fleeson, 1986). Cicchetti and associates (1988) find that the vast majority of maltreated infants form insecure attachments with caregivers (70% - 100% across studies), which over time tend to become anxious avoidant patterns of attachment. Similarly, the issue of the development of an autonomous self (18–24 months), in which the infant gains a well-differentiated sense of functioning as an independent entity, is often unsuccessfully resolved among samples of maltreated children. These researchers report that nearly 80% of maltreated toddlers show neutral or negative affect during visual self-recognition experiences. Furthermore, in problem-solving tasks requiring autonomy, these toddlers are more aggressive, frustrated, and noncompliant than comparison children. Symbolic representation and further self-other differentiation (24–36 months) which pertains to their ability to construct more differentiated mental representations of animate and inanimate objects, is the third issue identified by Cicchetti and associates for this period. Not surprisingly, they review studies indicating that maltreated children use proportionately fewer "internal state" words representing their mood or affect, their language relating more to their immediate activity and context.

The developmental framework of Cicchetti and associates continues into early childhood, when maltreated children, they note, show unsuccessful resolution of issues related to peer relations and school functioning. In particular, they report that maltreated children show evidence of avoidance of and aggression toward peers, even in response to friendly overtures. In the classroom they function more poorly on cognitive tasks and are reported more often for behavioral difficulties by teachers.

From the perspective of the child's ongoing development, it is clear that maltreatment has implications considerably beyond physical injuries or a lower standard of care. In effect, maltreatment can be viewed from a psychological perspective in terms of the degree to which it impairs or alters the child's developmental progression over the short or long term. It is not surprising, therefore, that reviews of studies of maltreated children are unable to identify a consistent pattern of psychopathology that is congruent with existing diagnostic criteria relating to other childhood disorders (Shaw-Lamphear, 1985; Toro, 1982; Wolfe, 1987). Child maltreatment represents only the visible aspects of a more endemic process affecting child development, and thus should be viewed in relation to its significance to the parent–child relationship. Moreover, these findings argue for the continued expansion of investigations to include the more subtle yet critical aspects of child behavior that constitute the mechanisms by which developmental psychopathology operates. We now turn to the literature on children's emotional development that provides a foundation for our assessment methods.

DEVELOPMENTAL EXPLANATIONS CONCERNING THE ROLE OF EMOTIONS

The maltreated child's psychological adjustment includes aspects of internal functioning that do not lend themselves readily to scientific observation and understanding. However, guided by advances in theoretical understanding and developmental knowledge, many reliable inferences can be drawn as to the relationship between the child's observed behavioral expression of emotion and the child's cognitive and emotional "processing" of information that preceded such expression.

In pursuing an understanding of emotions, developmental theorists have proposed a "functionalist perspective" of human emotions to the study of emotional development in infants and children. This perspective explains how young children learn from the emotional expressions of others owing to the adaptive, functional nature of emotional reactions (Bretherton, Fritz, Zahn-Waxler, & Ridgeway, 1986). According to this view, the critical functions of emotions include their adaptive, survival-promoting processes, such as the infant's fear of heights or strangers. Emotions also serve as important internal monitoring and guidance systems that are designed to help the child appraise events as being beneficial or dangerous, and provide motivation for action. Similarly, emotions serve interpersonal regulatory functions, as demonstrated by a person's ability to gain access to another's emotional state by reading facial, gestural, postural, and vocal cues. This latter function permits "social referencing," a process whereby an inexperienced person, such as a child, may rely on a more experienced person's affective interpretation of an event.

Developmental evidence (reviewed in Bretherton et al., 1986) suggests that children begin to learn the importance of emotions for communication and regulation early in the first year of life. By the second year, they are beginning to develop rudimentary attempts to attribute cause to emotional expression. Of most significance to the present discussion is the finding that children look to the emotional expression and cues of their caregivers to provide them with the information needed to formulate a basic understanding of "what's going on." In the context of child maltreatment and family violence, it is not difficult to imagine how an arousing, emotion-laden situation can challenge children's preconceived notions of their parents with conflicting new information—that is, parents who care about their children are engaging in highly fearful and threatening behavior toward the child or another family member (Jaffe, Wolfe, & Wilson, 1990). Children look for guidance on how to respond, and see it in the faces of their parents: fear, apprehension, and anger. In a similar manner, older children look for explanations for parental behavior and may utilize the additional information provided by verbal cues, tone of voice, gestures, and expressions.

Mechanisms by which children's emotional arousal and expression may be affected by adult interaction were suggested by the results of a series of studies by Cummings and his colleagues (Cummings, 1987; Cummings, Zahn-Waxler, & Radke-Yarrow, 1981; Cummings, Iannotti, & Zahn-Waxler, 1985). Through laboratory manipulation of an unfamiliar adult's anger and cooperation in the presence of the target child and his or her peer, these researchers discovered that preschool children responded to the angry adult with significantly greater displays of distress and subsequent increases in aggression with their peers. Moreover, among slightly older children, the researchers were able to identify three types of response patterns on the basis of their behavioral reactions to the observed arguments (Cummings, 1987). "Concerned" emotional responders (46% of the sample) showed negative emotions concurrent with exposure, and later reported feeling sad and wanting to leave. "Unresponsive" children (19%) showed no immediate evidence of emotion, yet later reported that they were angry. "Ambivalent" responders (35%) showed high emotional arousal during exposure and reported feeling happy later on; however, this latter group was most likely to become physically and verbally aggressive later on with their peers.

Cummings (1987) proposed two explanations to account for these findings regarding children's emotional reactions to adult conflict. The first explanation, termed "contagion of emotion," accounts for the child's emotional distress on the basis of being exposed to a stressful situation (i.e., the child reflects the distress shown by the adult actor). Alternatively, they cite the "transfer of excitation" premise, namely, that emotional arousal occurs as a function of witnessing strong emotions and that such arousal leads to undercontrolled (e.g., aggressive) behavior. From this line of research, therefore, we have persuasive evidence of the importance of emotional experiences in the lives of children, and some indication of how these experiences are transferred into behavioral expression. The role of emotions in the development of maltreated children, although rarely studied specifically, is implied by these findings as well. That is, the emotional atmosphere that these children frequently encounter poses a challenge to their developing coping and adaptational abilities. Not surprisingly, researchers often encounter elevated symptomatology among this population of children; however, some of the functional explanations for such reactions, beyond those that focus on the more proximal aspects of deviant behavior, have been typically overlooked. As our understanding of children's emotional development progresses, we need to consider more carefully the stage-salient issues that require identification and assessment.

A STRATEGY FOR ASSESSING EMOTIONAL AND SOCIAL–COGNITIVE DEVELOPMENT OF MALTREATED CHILDREN

The preceding discussion concerning the developmental nature of behavior problems displayed by maltreated children leads us to a strategy of assessment and research that is more developmental and less clinical in nature. This strategy is a reflection of the belief that our primary concern is the measurement of alterations or delays in development, rather than the measurement of an end-product, such as a psychopathologic syndrome. Consequently, current trait-based instruments designed to assess particular diagnostic patterns (e.g., anxiety, depression, anger, aggression) have limited utility, because they fail to distinguish the deviant developmental process as it unfolds and tend to identify only the more extreme cases.

Only recently have researchers focused on the cognitive processes underlying emotional adjustment in children. Because child maltreatment represents a stressful event that requires attribution and appraisal on the part of the child, the child's *interpretation* of traumatic life events is presumed to influence his or her adaptive or maladaptive coping responses. Current researchers have argued for an assessment strategy that investigates children's "internal working models,"—that is, their expectations, beliefs, and conceptions that are shaped (or misshaped) by their socialization experiences (Mueller & Silverman, 1989).

We advocate an assessment approach that prescribes a thorough investigation of a maltreated child's development and social behavior across different settings, which will more reliably permit conclusions as to his or her current needs (Wolfe, 1988). Because the task of assessing all potentially relevant areas can be overwhelming, we have formulated the present strategy around several stage-salient issues and milestones that, in the aggregate, reflect the child's ongoing emotional status. For the sake of clarity, we discuss these issues in relation to both emotional and social-cognitive development, for these two dimensions are interrelated and form the foundation of the child's "internal" maturation. To explore this issue of social-cognitive and socioemotional development in relation to child maltreatment, we begin by discussing social-cognitive factors that have a bearing on emotional and behavioral adjustment in these children: their attribution for maltreatment and their aggressive attributional bias toward peers. We present throughout some assessment ideas that have been explored in the literature concerning children's attributions and social sensitivity to others. Implications for longitudinal research form the concluding summary.

Children's Attributions Regarding Parental Behavior

Attribution is a broad term that, unfortunately, has been employed indiscriminately in much research on victimization (Shaver & Drown, 1986). In particular, social psychologists have noted important distinctions between different forms of attribution that may play a role in children's long-range adjustment. Whereas attribution of *cause* refers to the subject's perception of causal locus and causal stability, attribution of *responsibility* involves judgments of accountability and/or personal control. Attribution of *intent* refers to a judgment regarding whether the behavior was intentional and consciously deliberated or accidental. Finally, attribution of *blame* is an evaluative response that occurs after the perceiver has assessed the behavior and does not accept the validity of the offending person's justification or excuse for an effect that the perceiver believes was *intentionally* brought about (Shaver, 1985; Shaver & Drown, 1986).

The theoretical manner in which the process of attributional formation occurs and leads to behavioral outcomes can be summarized briefly.

When exposed to the aversive behavior of another person, an individual engages in a process of appraisal. First, the individual seeks to determine the causes for the perpetrator's behavior. Explanations of causality can be made on several dimensions (e.g., situational versus dispositional, global versus specific, stable versus unstable). Next, the individual attempts to determine whether the perpetrator is responsible for his or her behavior. According to Shaver (1985), attributions of responsibility are tied to the subject's appraisal of the degree to which the offending person causally contributed to the event, was aware of the consequences of his or her action, intended to bring about the event, acted on his or her own volition (in the absence of external coercion), and appreciated the moral wrongfulness of his or her behavior. Thus, causal attributions constitute a necessary condition for holding the person responsible for his or her action (Fincham, Bradbury, & Grych, 1990). Similarly, an attribution of intent is necessary for an attribution of blame. In turn, attribution of blame is believed to be responsible for the emotional arousal instigated by interpersonal conflict (Fincham et al., 1989).

Previous work examining the attributions of child victims of child maltreatment has not focused on the victim's attributions regarding the *perpetrator's* behavior. Rather, the literature has examined the child's self-directed attributions. This approach has been based on the "learned helplessness" model of victimization that guided much of the early research (Peterson & Seligman, 1983). Essentially, this theory posits that victims interpret victimization as their "failure" experience, and seek attributional explanations accordingly. Emotional maladjustment will occur if the child attributes the abuse to his or her own internal, stable, and global factors. However, this framework has been shown to lack adequate explanatory power in at least one empirical study with victims of sexual abuse (Gentile, 1988). We propose that the learned helplessness conceptualization of children's adjustment following maltreatment is incomplete in that it does not take into account the reciprocity and interpersonal dynamic underlying conflict and maltreatment in close relationships. That is, the victim will make attributions for the behavior of the perpetrator, as well as for his or her own behavior. The circumstances motivating the perpetrator's behavior may impinge on the victim's assessment of the maltreatment, and may in turn influence the victim's emotional reaction to it. For example, the child who attributes physical maltreatment to his or her parent's mean character would be expected to fare worse than the child who sees the same behavior as caused by external circumstances (e.g., job stress).

Research on attributions for physical maltreatment suggests that child victims do indeed make simultaneous self- and perpetrator-directed attributions. For example, Herzberger, Potts, and Dillon (1981) conducted interviews with 14 abused and 10 nonabused boys in residential care regarding their explanations for parental behavior. Subjects were asked, "When your parent hit you, was it because you did something bad?" and also "Was it because (s)he was mean?" Both abused and nonabused children attributed responsibility for punishment to themselves. As the severity of the abuse increased, so did the likelihood of attributing the punishment to parental meanness, particularly for fathers. Unfortunately, the researchers did not clarify what was meant or understood by "cause," "responsibility," "intent," or "blame." Also, they did not attempt to establish any connection between attributional patterns and current behavioral adjustment.

Findings by Herzberger and associates (1981) suggest that the dimensions of maltreatment (e.g., severity, chronicity) may influence the nature of the child's attributions for such events. As the severity of the maltreatment increases, attributions of blame to the perpetrator increase. This finding is congruent with studies involving adult victims of wife assault (Holtzworth-Munroe, 1988), and furthermore suggests that researchers should carefully quantify the dimensions of maltreatment (e.g., severity, chronicity, frequency) in order to assess their impact on the attributional process. If attributions of blame result from the maltreatment (either to self or the perpetrator), emotional reactions of sadness or anger will be more likely to result.

A recent reformulation of the learned helplessness model of depression (Abramson, Metalsky & Alloy, 1989) deemphasized causal attributional processes and instead emphasizes many other factors, including perceptions of controllability for aversive events. Some recent work has been done on children's cognitions of the controllability of various domains of their lives (Connell, 1985). These studies suggest that children's *expectancies*, as well as their attributions, may influence emotional and behavioral expression. Perceptions of control over parent behavior and maltreatment, in particular, may mediate adjustment. Another potentially profitable area of exploration may be the way in which coercive interchanges act as a means of control over parental behavior for some children (Whaler & Dumas, 1986). That is, some youngsters may evade a sense of helplessness and noncontingency in their lives by engaging in acting-out behavior, which serves as an effective mechanism for aversive control of parental behavior.

Cicchetti and associates (1988) have also addressed the relationship between child maltreatment and children's social–cognitive development, and have suggested some promising assessment approaches. They contend that maltreatment interferes with children's development of a success-based orientation, that is, with the degree of control they perceive having over the impact of their actions. For this reason, these researchers suggest an assessment strategy that documents both children's school performance and their level of social (i.e., social problem-solving and coping skills). For example, Aber and associates (1989) measured children's "effectance motivation" (i.e., the child's tendency to perceive some control over the effect of his or her actions) by having them interact with an unfamiliar adult. Effectance motivation was measured on the basis of the child's curiosity, variability seeking, and level of aspiration while engaging in games with the adult. Maltreated children significantly differed from a matched sample of nonmaltreated children in terms of displaying less "secure readiness to learn" and less "outer directedness," two factors that were derived from the researchers' theoretical domains of social-cognitive and emotional development.

Aggressive Attributional Bias toward Peers

Several authors (Dodge & Richard, 1985; Parke & Slaby, 1983; Rubin & Krasnor, 1986) have suggested that behavior problems in children may develop as a function of the ways in which children process social information. According to the social information processing model of social competence (Dodge, 1986), social problem-solving proceeds in a series of stages. First, the child must encode and interpret the social cues displayed by others. In cases of social conflict, this involves making an attribution regarding the other party's intent. Second, the child must engage in a response search and decision stage. He or she must generate possible solutions to the conflict, evaluate their potential effectiveness, and decide on an initial solution. The third stage requires enactment of the selected problem-solving method, subsequent monitoring of the outcome, and potential reinitiation of earlier stages in the process.

Current theory in adult conflict problem-solving suggests that attribution of blame instigates an immediate affective reaction (e.g., anger, sadness) which, in turn, may influence response selection (Fincham et al., 1989). Affect, therefore, is also likely to be implicated in the social problem-solving process, although this is not addressed in Dodge's (1986) model. Specifically, aggressive behavior is potentiated by anger, whereas withdrawal is potentiated by sadness.

Using hypothetical scenarios, videotaped stimuli, and confederate peers, Dodge and his colleagues have demonstrated that aggressive, rejected children are biased in their attributions of others' intentions and that this attributional pattern is directly related to their decision to retaliate aggressively (Dodge, 1980; Dodge & Frame, 1982; Dodge, 1986; Dodge, Murphy, & Buchsbaum, 1984; Steinberg & Dodge, 1983; Nasby, Hayden, & de Paulo, 1980). Specifically, aggressive children are most likely to attribute hostile intent when exposed to an ambiguous provocation by a peer (e.g., being hit in the back by a ball). Aggressive children also demonstrate deficits in problem-solving ability, such as a tendency to generate fewer and lower-quality solutions to hypothetical problems.

Dodge and Richard (1985) speculate on the origins of attributional biases and problem-solving deficits among maladjusted children. Cultural norms, television violence, direct instruction, and direct reinforcement (e.g., attainment of possessions) are all possible influences. These researchers also suggest that "early trauma, such as that which occurs in physical abuse" may also contribute to cognitive distortion. "Such an event", they write, "may leave a lasting impression on a child by shaping the child's perception of future events . . . [and] may increase the probability that the child will be perceptually ready to interpret hostility and aggression in his or her world in the future" (p. 53). Thus, attributions regarding original victimization may influence attribution for the "aggressive" behavior of peers. A disrupted parent–child relationship, therefore, may lead to a cognitive distortion. Generalization of this bias to peer contexts may contribute to social failure later in the child's development.

Assessment of Children's Social Sensitivity

Researchers have been very interested in how the developing parent–child relationship may be affected by the adverse conditions of emotional rejection, harsh treatment, insensitivity, and verbal and physical assaults (Aber & Cicchetti, 1984). The two predominant approaches to understanding the socioemotional development of maltreated children have focused on assessment of attachment formation with infants and toddlers and on preschool and school-age maltreated children's ability to empathize with their peers and form positive peer relationships. In the following paragraphs we address some of the assessment implications arising from these studies, with particular reference to recognition of emotions in others.

Due to the significance of relationship development, researchers have investigated maltreated children's initial manifestations of sensitivity to others' emotions and their early prosocial behavior. This area of research has been a particularly difficult one in which to establish firm relationships between concepts, because a number of individual, parental, familial, and cultural factors influence the expression of empathy and prosocial behavior (Radke-Yarrow, Zahn-Waxler, & Chapman, 1983).

The assessment strategies used by researchers primarily reflect a preference toward direct observation of child behavior under contrived and naturalistic situations. Several researchers have used the Affective Situation Test (Feshbach & Roe, 1968) to elicit and measure children's social sensitivity to hypothetical situations. This procedure involves a picture story in which children's social sensitivity is measured in terms of how they label specific affect-laden situations. By far the most preferred assessment strategy, however, involves parent–child or peer interactions (Feshbach, 1989). For example, Main and George (1985) studied abused toddlers in a naturalistic setting in which they could observe their reactions to distress in their playmates. They discovered that the target children not only failed to show concern toward others but actively responded to distress in others with fear, physical attack, or anger (reactions that are not dissimilar to those of their parents). Thus, the important study of maltreated children's developmental progress in the area of social sensitivity suggests the crucial nature of this concept. The assessment of this developmental ability, moreover, can be conducted by relying on naturalistic observations with children and adults (see also procedures used by Cummings, 1987, and by Hinchey & Gavelek, 1982).

However, results of studies to date that have attempted to link deficits in social-cognitive functioning to maltreatment have been inconclusive, which may be due in part to the choices of assessment methodology. For example, Rosenberg (1986) compared children exposed to family violence (aged 5 to 8) to children from nonviolent families on a measure of social-cognitive problem-solving abilities (Social Problem Situation Analysis Measure (SPSAM). When responding to hypothetical scenarios portrayed in pictures, the wife assault sample scored lower on interpersonal sensitivity to the feelings of the actors. Also, relative to control subjects, they were more likely to choose aggressive or passive solutions to resolve interpersonal conflict, and less likely to choose assertive strategies. Groisser (1986) replicated these results using videotaped scenarios as stimuli. Barahal, Waterman, and Martin (1981) compared 6- to 8-year-old abused and control children on measures of locus of control, social sensitivity, cognitive perspective taking, and moral judgment. After adjusting for IQ, these researchers found that abused children displayed greater external locus of control and less comprehension of complex social roles than did controls.

In contrast, Frodi and Smetana (1984) found no differences between abused, neglected, and low-IQ nonmaltreated preschoolers on tests of social sensitivity, although the maltreated groups differed significantly from high-IQ nonmaltreated children. Similarly, Smetana, Kelly, and Twentyman (1984) found few differences in moral reasoning among matched abused and control subjects aged 3 to 6 after controlling for IQ. More recently, Downey and Walker (in press) found no correlation between maltreatment (defined categorically) and interpersonal problem-solving skills or aggressive attributional bias. Results from their correlational study indicated that the relationship between maltreatment and maladjustment was not mediated by aggressive attributional bias or interpersonal problem-solving skills. Rather, these variables appeared to have a compensational role: as social-cognitive skills increased, peer rejection, as measured by select items on the Child Behavior Check List (CBCL; Achenbach & Edelbrock, 1983)—decreased. Finally, Pettit, Dodge, & Brown (1988) found that exposure to family aggression was not associated with interpersonal problem-solving ability in young economically disadvantaged children.

These contradictory findings may be explained in part by methodological differences between the studies. In the social problem-solving research, the child's attributions with respect to the hypothetical problems are assessed through interviews. The child is asked why the peer behaved in that manner, how he or she would feel in the situation, and how he or she would respond to the peer. Unfortunately, most studies examining attributional bias in this manner do not describe the content of the hypothetical situation, making it difficult to compare results across studies. Because methodological work in social psychology indicates that the content of vignettes and the wording of subsequent questioning can influence results (Fishbein & Ajzen, 1975), this research area would clearly benefit from some standardization in the content of the hypothetical vignettes and assessment techniques. The role of intelligence and social class must also be controlled for, given the evidence of their pervasive influence on child adjustment (e.g., Sandler, 1980). Finally, future research examining the link between maltreatment and social cognition with peers should specifically address the hypothesis that attributions for parent behavior are generalized to others (e.g., my parents are hostile to me, so others must be, too). Accordingly, attributional measures must be used in reference both to peer and parent behavior.

IMPLICATIONS FOR LONGITUDINAL RESEARCH

This brief review of issues and findings regarding maltreated children's emotional status has revealed several important trends in the literature that have implications for planning and conducting longitudinal research. Most notably, the quantification of maltreatment experiences should respect the various forms of maltreatment (e.g., sexual abuse, physical abuse, etc.) the child may have experienced. An unfortunate tendency in maltreatment research in recent years has been the drift toward categorical yet somewhat arbitrary distinctions between the different forms of maltreatment (see discussions by Giovannoni, 1989; Erickson, Egeland, & Pianta, 1989; McGee & Wolfe, 1991). In principle, such a categorical approach may assist in research design, yet it oversimplifies the concept of maltreatment. A categorization methodology obscures differences in the severity of abuse and ignores the co-occurrence of many forms of maltreatment in the lives of children (McGee & Wolfe, 1991). Moreover, the need to develop precise conceptual and operational definitions of each of the various forms of maltreatment has been identified as a major methodological concern (Besharov, 1981; Plotkin, Azar, Twentyman, & Perri,

1981). In particular, we have argued that these definitions must not be redundant with respect to each other (McGee & Wolfe, 1991). The unique, additive, and/or interactive effects of the various forms of child maltreatment (i.e., physical abuse, sexual abuse, exposure to family violence, psychological maltreatment, and neglect) can be determined only by defining and measuring these constructs as distinct entities.

Furthermore, researchers are discovering that the specific pattern and type(s) of maltreatment a child has been exposed to may influence the attributional set he or she adopts toward parents and, subsequently, toward peers. For example, physical abuse often occurs in the context of discipline (Herrenkohl, Herrenkohl, & Egolf, 1983). The nature of the situation increases the likelihood that children will attribute the cause of the abuse to themselves. Moreover, in discipline situations the parent is likely to tell the child that he or she is at fault. In contexts of overt parental aggression (e.g., physical abuse, wife assault), where the behavior is often spontaneous, the child has the opportunity to attribute the violence to uncontrollable and unintentional factors (e.g., "bad moods"). In contrast, the topography of sexual abuse is likely to lend itself to a different attributional analysis by the child. That is, the sexual abuse victim may perceive the perpetrator's behavior as planned and intentional. Neglect, which by definition refers to a chronic pattern of inadequate parenting, is also likely to favor a different explanation in the child's mind than other forms of maltreatment (e.g., patterns of neglect may be perceived as having global, stable causes). According to this theoretical premise, therefore, the exact nature of an attribution (for cause, intent, responsibility, and blame) will vary with the scenario in which the child finds himself or herself. If researchers wish to determine the mediating role of attributions for maltreatment, it is critical to know the precise nature of the child's maltreatment history.

Finally, we see that the measurement of maltreated children's emotional and social-cognitive development has not kept pace with the theoretical advances on these topics. Developmentalists are noting the important role of emotions in organizing the child's adaptive responses to novel stimuli, and social psychologists and others are stressing the importance of studying attributions as a means of understanding children's coping reactions to stressful and traumatic events. The current state of the literature calls for a renewed effort to develop standardized, interview-based techniques for assessing children's and adolescents' attributions for traumatic events across the life span. As well, this review has revealed a paucity of assessment strategies aimed at evaluating children's internal mood states and self-regulation of emotion, a weakness that will undoubedly merit considerable attention in future studies.

REFERENCES

Aber, J. L., Allen, J. P., Carlson, V., & Cicchetti, D. (1989). The effects of maltreatment on development during early childhood: recent studies and their theoretical, clinical, and policy implications. In D. Cicchetti & V. Carlson (Eds.), *Child maltreatment: Theory and research on the causes of child abuse and neglect* (pp. 579–619). New York, NY: Cambridge University Press.

Aber, J. L., & Cicchetti, D. (1984). The socio-emotional development of maltreated children: An empirical and theoretical analysis. In H. Fitzgerald, B. Lester, & M. Yogman (Eds.), *Theory and research in behavioral pediatrics* (Vol. 2, pp. 147–199). New York: Plenum.

Abramson, L. Y., Metalsky, G. I., & Alloy, L. B. (1989). Hopelessness depression: A theory-based subtype of depression. *Psychological Review, 96,* 358–372.

Achenbach, T., & Edelbrock, C. S. (1983). *Manual for the Child Behavior Checklist and Child Behavior Profile.* Burlington: University of Vermont.

Ammerman, R. T. (1990). Etiological models of child maltreatment: A behavioral perspective. *Behavior Modification, 14,* 230–254.

Barahal, R. M., Waterman, J., & Martin, H. P. (1981). The social-cognitive development of abused children. *Journal of Consulting and Clinical Psychology, 49,* 508–516.

Besharov, D. J. (1981). Toward better research on child abuse and neglect: Making definitional issues an explicit methodological concern. *Child Abuse & Neglect, 5,* 383–390.

Bowlby, J. (1973). *Attachment and loss: Vol. 2. Separation.* New York: Basic Books.

Bretherton, I., Fritz, J., Zahn-Waxler, C., & Ridgeway, D. (1986). Learning to talk about emotions: A functionalist perspective. *Child Development, 57,* 529–548.

Cicchetti, D. (1989). How research on child maltreatment has informed the study of child development: Perspectives from developmental psychopathology. In D. Cicchetti & V. Carlson (Eds.), *Child maltreatment: Theory and research on the causes and consequences of child abuse and neglect* (pp. 377–431). New York: Cambridge University Press.

Cicchetti, D., & Aber, J. L. (1986). Early precursors of later depression: An organizational perspective. In L. Lipsett & C. Rovee-Collier (Eds.), *Advances in infancy* (Vol. 4, pp. 87–137). Norwood, NJ: Ablex.

Cicchetti, D., & Carlson, V. (Eds.). (1989). *Child maltreatment: Theory and research on the causes and consequences of child abuse and neglect.* New York: Cambridge University Press.

Cicchetti, D., Toth, S., & Bush, M. (1988). Developmental psychopathology and incompetence in childhood: Suggestions for intervention. In B. B. Lahey & A. E. Kazdin (Eds.), *Advances in clinical child psychology* (Vol. 11, pp. 1–77). New York: Plenum.

Connell, J. (1985). A new multidimensional measure of children's perceptions of control. *Child Development, 56,* 1018–1041.

Crittenden, P. M., & Ainsworth, M. D. S. (1989). Child maltreatment and attachment theory. In D. Cicchetti & V. Carlson (Eds.), *Child maltreatment: Theory and research on the causes and consequences of child abuse and neglect* (pp. 432–463). New York: Cambridge University Press.

Cummings, E. M. (1987). Coping with background anger in early childhood. *Child Development, 58,* 976–984.

Cummings, E. M., Iannotti, R. J., & Zahn-Waxler, C. (1985). Influence of conflict between adults on the emotions and aggression of young children. *Developmental Psychology, 21,* 495–507.

Cummings, E. M., Zahn-Waxler, C., & Radke-Yarrow, M. (1981). Young children's responses to expressions of anger and affection by others in the family. *Child Development, 52,* 1274–1282.

Dodge, K. A. (1980). Social cognition and children's aggressive behavior. *Child Development, 51,* 162–170.

Dodge, K. A. (1986). A social information processing model of social competence in children. In M. Perlmutter (Ed.), *Minnesota symposium on child psychology* (Vol. 18, pp. 77–125). Hillsdale, NJ: Erlbaum.

Dodge, K. A., & Frame, C. L. (1982). Social cognitive biases and deficits in aggressive boys. *Child Development, 53,* 620–635.

Dodge, K. A., Murphy, R. R., & Buchsbaum, K. (1984). The assessment of intention-cue detection skills in children: Implications for developmental psychopathology. *Child Development, 55,* 163–173.

Dodge, K. A., & Richard, B. A. (1985). Peer perceptions, aggression, and the development of peer relations. In J. B. Pryor & J. D. Day (Eds.), *The development of social cognition* (pp. 35–58). New York: Springer-Verlag.

Downey, G., & Walker, E. (in press). Social cognition and adjustment in children at risk for psychopathology. *Child Development.*

Dumas, J., & Wahler, R. G. (1986). Indiscriminate mothering as a contextual factor in aggressive–oppositional child behavior: "Damned if you do, damned if you don't." *Journal of Abnormal Child Psychology, 13,* 1–17.

Erickson, M. F., Egeland, B., & Pianta, R. (1989). The effects of maltreatment on the development of young children. In D. Cicchetti & V. Carlson (Eds.), *Child maltreatment: Theory and research on the causes and consequences of child abuse and neglect* (pp. 647–684). New York: Cambridge University Press.

Feshbach, N. D. (1989). The construct of empathy and the phenomenon of physical maltreatment of children. In D. Cicchetti & V. Carlson (Eds.), *Child maltreatment: Theory and research on the causes and consequences of child abuse and neglect* (pp. 349–373). New York: Cambridge University Press.

Feshbach, N. D., and Roe, K. (1968). Empathy in six- and seven-year olds. *Child Development, 39,* 133–145.

Fincham, F. D., Bradbury, T. N., & Grych, J. H. (1990). Conflict in close relationships: The role of intrapersonal phenomena. In S. Graham & V. Folkes (Eds.), *Attribution theory: Applications to achievement, mental health, and interpersonal conflict* (pp. 161–184). Hillsdale, NJ: Erlbaum.

Fishbein, M., & Ajzen, I. (1975). *Belief, attitude, intention, and behavior: An introduction to theory and research.* Reading, MA: Addison-Wesley.

Frodi, A., & Smetana, J. (1984). Abused, neglected, and nonmaltreated preschoolers' ability to discriminate emotions in others: The effects of IQ. *Child Abuse & Neglect, 8,* 459–465.

Gentile, C. (1988). *Factors mediating the impact of child sexual abuse: Severity of abuse, attributional style, and learned helplessness.* Unpublished master's thesis, The University of Western Ontario, London, Ontario, Canada.

Giovannoni, J. (1989). Definitional issues in child maltreatment. In D. Cicchetti & V. Carlson (Eds.), *Child maltreatment: Theory and research on the causes and consequences of child abuse and neglect* (pp. 3–37). New York: Cambridge University Press.

Groisser, D. (1986). *Child witnesses to interparental violence: social problem-solving skills and behavioral adjustment.* Unpublished master's thesis, University of Denver, Denver, CO.

Herrenkohl, R., & Herrenkohl, E., & Egolf, B. (1983). Circumstances surrounding the occurrence of child maltreatment. *Journal of Consulting and Clinical Psychology, 51,* 424–431.

Herzberger, S., Potts, D., & Dillon, M. (1981). Abusive and nonabusive parental treatment from the child's perspective. *Journal of Consulting and Clinical Psychology, 49,* 81–90.

Hinchey, F. S., & Gavelek, J. R. (1982). Empathic responding in children of battered mothers. *Child Abuse & Neglect, 6,* 395–401.

Holtzworth-Munroe, A. (1988). Causal attributions in marital violence: Theoretical and methodological issues. *Clinical Psychology Review, 8,* 331–344.

Jaffe, P., Wolfe, D. A., & Wilson, S. (1990). *Children of battered women.* Newbury Park, CA: Sage.

Main, M., & George, C. (1985). Responses of abused and disadvantaged toddlers to distress in agemates: A study in the daycare setting. *Developmental Psychology, 21,* 407–412.

McGee, R. A., & Wolfe, D. A. (1991). Psychological maltreatment: Towards an operational definition. *Development and Psychopathology, 3,* 3–18.

Mueller, E., & Silverman, N. (1989). Peer relations in maltreated children. In D. Cicchetti & V. Carlson (Eds.), *Child maltreatment: Theory and research on the causes and consequences of child abuse and neglect* (pp. 529–578). New York: Cambridge University Press.

Nasby, W., Hayden, B., & de Paulo, B. M. (1980). Attributional bias among aggressive boys to interpret unambiguous social stimuli as displays of hostility. *Journal of Abnormal Psychology, 89,* 459–468.

Newberger, C. M., & Cook, S. (1983). Parental awareness and child abuse: A cognitive–developmental analysis of urban and rural samples. *American Journal of Orthopsychiatry, 53,* 512–524.

Parke, R. D., & Slaby, R. G. (1983). The development of aggression. In E. M. Hetherington (Ed.), *Handbook of child psychology* (Vol. 4, pp. 547–641). New York: Wiley.

Patterson, G. R. (1986). Performance models for antisocial boys. *American Psychologist, 41,* 432–444.

Peterson, C., & Seligman, M. E. (1983). Learned helplessness and victimization. *Journal of Social Issues, 39,* 103–116.

Pettit, G., Dodge, K., & Brown, M. (1988). Early family experience, social problem solving patterns, and children's social competence. *Child Development, 59*, 107–120.

Plotkin, R. C., Azar, S., Twentyman, C. T., & Perri, M. G. (1981). A critical evaluation of the research methodology employed in the investigation of causative factors of child abuse and neglect. *Child Abuse & Neglect, 5*, 449–455.

Radke-Yarrow, M., Zahn-Waxler, C., & Chapman, M. (1983). Children's prosocial dispositions and behavior. In E. M. Hetherington (Ed.), *Handbook of child psychology* (Vol. IV, pp. 469–545). New York: Wiley.

Rosenberg, M. S. (1986, August). *Children of battered women: The effects of witnessing violence on their social problem–solving abilities*. Paper presented at the annual convention of the American Psychological Association, Washington, DC.

Rubin, K. H., & Krasnor, L. R. (1986). Social–cognitive and social behavioral perspectives on problem solving. In M. Perlmutter (Ed.), *The Minnesota symposia on child psychology* (Vol. 18, pp. 1–68). Hillsdale, NJ: Erlbaum.

Rutter, M. (1989). Intergenerational continuities and discontinuities in serious parenting difficulties. In D. Cicchetti & V. Carlson (Eds.), *Child maltreatment: Theory and research on the causes and consequences of child abuse and neglect* (pp. 317–348). New York: Cambridge University Press.

Sandler, I. N. (1980). Social support resources, stress, and maladjustment in poor children. *American Journal of Community Psychology, 8*, 41–52.

Shaver, K. G. (1985). *The attribution of blame: Causality, responsibility, and blameworthiness*. New York: Springer-Verlag.

Shaver, K. G., & Drown, D. (1986). On causality, responsibility, and self-blame: A theoretical note. *Journal of Personality and Social Psychology, 50*, 697–702.

Shaw-Lamphear, V. S. (1985). The impact of maltreatment on children's psychosocial adjustment: A review of the literature. *Child Abuse & Neglect, 9*, 251–263.

Smetana, J. G., Kelly, M., & Twentyman, C. T. (1984). Abused, neglected, and nonmaltreated children's concepts of moral and social–conventional transgressions. *Child Development, 55*, 277–287.

Sroufe, L. A., & Fleeson, J. (1987). Attachment and the construction of relationships. In W. W. Hartup & Z. Rubin (Eds.), *Relationships and development* (pp. 51–72). Hillsdale, NJ: Erlbaum.

Sroufe, L. A., & Rutter, M. (1984). The domain of developmental psychopathology. *Child Development, 55*, 17–29.

Steinberg, M., & Dodge, K. A. (1983). Attributional bias in aggressive adolescent boys and girls. *Journal of Social and Clinical Psychology, 1*, 312–321.

Toro, P. A. (1982). Developmental effects of child abuse: A review. *Child Abuse & Neglect, 6*, 423–431.

Wahler, R., & Dumas, J. (1986). Family factors in childhood psychopathology: Toward a coercion–neglect model. In T. Jacob (Ed.), *Family interaction and psychopathology: Theories, methods and findings*. (pp. 581–627). New York: Plenum Press.

Wolfe, D. A. (1987). *Child abuse: Implications for child development and psychopathology*. Newbury Park, CA: Sage.

Wolfe, D. A. (1988). Child abuse and neglect. In E. J. Mash & L. G. Terdal (Eds.), *Behavioral assessment of childhood disorders* (2nd ed., pp 627–669). New York: Guilford.

Zigler, E., & Hall, N. W. (1989). Physical child abuse in America: Past, present, and future. In D. Cicchetti & V. Carlson (Eds.), *Child maltreatment: Theory and research on the causes and consequences of child abuse and neglect* (pp. 38–75). New York: Cambridge University Press.

12

The Impact of Child Maltreatment on Health

HOWARD DUBOWITZ
University of Maryland School of Medicine

The immediate and serious injuries suffered by victims of child abuse have been the focus of considerable media and professional attention. The less dramatic and long-term health consequences of child maltreatment, however, have been largely ignored. A comprehensive appreciation of the ramifications of child abuse and neglect requires a better understanding of both the long-term and short-term consequences of child maltreatment.

Child maltreatment involves harm to the physical or psychological health of a child. Depending on the specific incident and circumstances, a wide array of effects on the child's health can ensue. These effects may be brief, lasting hours or days, or long-term and perhaps permanent. This chapter focuses on the long-term physical health outcomes of child maltreatment, and in particular, on the measurement of these outcomes.

How frequently do maltreated children suffer long-term impairment of their physical health? Unfortunately, the paucity of longitudinal research in this area means that hypotheses are based primarily on speculation. However, studies indicate that children in foster care, most of whom experienced abuse or neglect, tend to suffer from poor health (Hochstadt, Jaudes, Zimo, & Schachter, 1987; Kavaler & Swire, 1983; Schor, 1982); this suggests that maltreatment is associated with impaired health.

There are a few issues that need to be considered when extrapolating from reports of children in foster care. These reports have generally been based on clinical assessments of foster children without any comparison groups (Hochstadt, Jaudes, Zimo & Schachter, 1987; Kavaler & Swire, 1983; Schor, 1982). Another limitation is the problem of separating the effects of maltreatment from those of foster care. This is particularly important given the serious shortcomings that have been identified in the foster care system (Fanshel & Shinn, 1978). Further, it is not possible to randomly assign maltreated children to be placed in foster care or to remain in their homes. Because those children who have been most seriously maltreated are more likely to be removed from their biological families, the comparison with children who remain at home is not methodologically ideal.

Despite these limitations, assessments of foster children provide useful insights into the health problems that may be associated with maltreatment. In general, these assessments reveal an increased incidence of a wide array of health problems, including impaired growth, dental caries, neuromuscular and visual disorders, psychological problems and developmental delays (Fanshel & Shinn, 1978; Kavaler & Swire, 1983; Schor, 1988).

DEFINITIONAL AND CONCEPTUAL ISSUES

At the outset it needs to be stated that the distinction between physical and mental health is arbitrary and theoretically problematic. For example, Engel has argued for a broadened conceptual framework of health and illness, proposing that the traditional biomedical model be replaced by a biopsychosocial model (Engel, 1977). Simply stated, this perspective holds that physical and mental health are not discrete phenomena, but that there exists an important interplay between physical, psychological, and social factors, all of which affect health and disease. This model is central to recent efforts aimed at assessing health status; these will be discussed later in this chapter. An example is seen in nonorganic failure to thrive, a condition in which infants fail to grow adequately primarily because of psychosocial problems, and yet in which subtle organic factors are frequently contributory and can influence the parental approach to the infant (Bithoney & Dubowitz, 1985). However, for research purposes, it is useful to disentangle the components of health status; therefore, the focus of this chapter is on physical health, and the long-term health effects resulting from child maltreatment.

In order to examine the health outcomes of child maltreatment, it is necessary to clearly define health status and to be able to operationalize the definition. However, this is a new area of research and there is no single agreed upon approach. For example, ideas range from a view of health outcome as "recovery, restoration of function, and survival" (Donabedian, 1966) to the broader conceptualization of the World Health Organization, which was used in the Rand Health Insurance Study: "health is a state of complete physical, mental and social well-being and not merely the absence of disease or infirmity" (World Health Organization, 1978).

HEALTH ISSUES ASSOCIATED WITH
DIFFERENT TYPES OF MALTREATMENT

There appears to be an emerging consensus as to the need for a holistic view of health and illness, and the current challenge is how to best assess health and illness from this viewpoint. For example, Starfield has proposed that a profile of seven aspects of health status be developed (Starfield, 1988). This chapter reviews those measures of health status that have been applied to children. First, there are specific aspects of physical health related to the different forms of child maltreatment; they will be considered separately.

Physical Abuse

Physical abuse can result in a wide array of injuries, ranging from transient redness and tenderness of the skin to fractures, serious internal damage, and death. Medical texts on child maltreatment illustrate that almost any manifestation of trauma to any part of the body *can* be inflicted (e.g., Ellerstein, 1981). Data from the major incidence studies in recent years (American Humane Association, 1988; U.S. Department of Health and Human Services, 1988) indicate that serious trauma, including fractures and internal head injuries, occurs in approximately 3% of all reports for child maltreatment. Minor trauma such as bruising or a superficial abrasion occurs in about 14% of reports. A further 11% have been found to have unspecified injuries. The remaining 72% of reports, constituting other forms of maltreatment, do not include signs of any physical injury.

Of course, different injuries lead to varied outcomes. In fact, even the same injury might have rather different results in different children, influenced by such factors as the child's prior health, the immediate medical care received or not received, and subsequent care and rehabilitative interventions. This means that the outcome of a physically abusive incident is not simply related to the injury per se but also to additional factors. It is therefore difficult to fully attribute a particular health outcome to the injury alone; the surrounding circumstances also need to be considered.

There is a long list of minor injuries that can be inflicted, including bruises, abrasions, redness, and superficial lacerations (cuts). Such injuries result from a minor to moderate degree of trauma. Almost always, in an otherwise healthy child, these injuries heal well without any residual impairment. For example, a superficial laceration that is not properly cleansed could become infected, but when treated this will generally heal within a few weeks. Perhaps a scar will be left that might have cosmetic implications. It seems likely that in these instances of minor trauma, the possible psychological sequelae of the abuse might last long after the bruises have faded.

As with minor injuries, a wide array of major injuries can result from maltreatment. For example, fractures, damage to internal organs or bleeding around the brain could result from moderate to severe trauma. Among major injuries, the greatest mortality and morbidity is incurred by trauma to the head and abdomen, and the probability of a long-term physical handicap is substantial. As mentioned earlier, the health outcome is influenced by several factors besides the actual injury.

Given the considerable variation in injuries, it is not easy to generalize about their long-term outcomes. Even within one type of injury, such as head trauma resulting in a subdural hematoma (bleeding around the brain), there is marked variability in both the short- and long-term outcomes. For this particular type of injury, some prognostic guidance is provided by a rating scale, such as the Glasgow Coma Score, which is derived from functional disturbances associated with a brain injury (Teasdale & Jennett, 1974).

For many injuries, particularly the more common ones, there is ample evidence of the likely course to expect. For example, an orthopedic surgeon can usually give a good estimate of what to expect from a particular fracture. Similarly, outcome data are available for trauma that causes bleeding in the front part of the eye. Most injuries are not unique to abuse, and therefore longitudinal research in this area should be conducted on populations of adequate sample size and not necessarily limited to abused children. It is important to add that even the majority of major injuries are likely to result in few long-term physical impairments, particularly if good medical care is obtained in a timely fashion. However, delay in seeking medical care is often a substantial problem in child abuse, thereby aggravating the outcome.

Sexual Abuse

There is almost no longitudinal research in the area of physical health outcomes of child sexual abuse. Most studies of sexually abused children have found that the majority of children, particularly boys, have *no* signs of injury, and of those who do, the trauma is mostly minor and superficial, such as redness, bruising, or abrasions (Emans, Woods, Flagg, & Freeman, 1987; Herman-Giddens & Frothingham, 1987). Follow-up evaluations of these children suggest that complete healing of superficial injuries is the rule. With deeper and more substantial injury, scarring is likely to result, although this might be rather subtle and bear little resemblance to the original injury (Finkel, 1989). It is unknown, although it seems unlikely, whether such minor physical changes have any functional significance or result in long-term disability. It should be noted that the violent sexual assault resulting in major internal injuries and requiring gynecological repair is extremely unusual. Under such circumstances, long-term sequelae appear much more likely.

Children who have been repeatedly molested might present with unique physical findings. For example, anal sodomy may cause laxity of muscle tone, resulting in gaping of the anus and thickening of the surrounding skin folds. Although longitudinal data are not available, it seems probable that within months the anatomy would gradually revert to normal. Scarring or altered pigmentation might persist, but these are unlikely to have functional importance. It has been suggested that the trauma of anal sodomy might be associated with stool withholding and encopresis (soiling); however, this association has not been demonstrated.

Sexually transmitted diseases are another consequence of sexual abuse, and studies indicate that up to 13% of sexually abused children are infected (White, Loda, Ingram, & Pearson, 1983). These diseases often cause symptoms such as genital pain and itching and a persistent vaginal discharge, particularly if treatment is not obtained. More serious complications can ensue, such as pelvic inflammatory disease in pubertal girls, which can lead to infertility. It is difficult to estimate the extent to which these problems result from sexual abuse, partly due to the frequency of unreported abuse. Still, it seems unlikely that serious long-term physical complications affect more than a very small minority of sexually abused children. Another consideration is HIV infection and the development of AIDS. At this time, there have been only a handful of cases reported where the mode of transmission is believed to have been via sexual abuse, but it is probable that this will be an increasing concern (Gellert, Durfee, & Berkowitz, 1990). Finally, another important, although infrequent, consequence of sexual abuse is pregnancy.

It is evident that longitudinal research is needed to delineate the long-term physical effects of sexual abuse. Extended medical follow-up is also warranted, since some of the sexually transmitted diseases such as virus induced anal and genital warts or HIV infection have long incubation periods and may take months or years before manifesting.

Child Neglect

The ramifications of child neglect on physical health might be less obvious and dramatic, but they can be substantial and long-term. The majority of fatalities caused by child maltreatment result from neglect (National Committee for the Prevention of Child Abuse, 1987). Usually this is a consequence of inadequate supervision; for example, when young children are left unattended and die in a house fire. The outcomes of neglect deserve more attention, since most reports of child maltreatment are for neglect (American Humane Association, 1988; U.S. Department of Health and Human Services, 1988).

It is not easy to attribute health outcomes to neglectful behavior by the parent or caretaker. Frequently, neglect is identified in a context of poverty, and it is clear that poverty per se is associated with impaired health (Parker, Greer, & Zuckerman, 1988). A landmark follow-up study of abused children found few psychological differences compared to an equally impoverished comparison group (Elmer, 1977). The author suggested that the abuse had little apparent deleterious impact *beyond* the problems associated with poverty.

Access to health care is correlated with socioeconomic status (Anderson & Aday, 1978). Poor children are less likely to receive high quality primary pediatric care by a single provider or clinic. Even if a primary care clinic is available, it may be open only during regular working hours, requiring the use of an emergency room at other times of the day. This discontinuity in care is considered to be inferior to having one provider and might contribute to poor outcomes, particularly in a high risk population. Therefore, if one is to study the effects of neglect, it is necessary to use comparison groups matched for socioeconomic status and access to health care.

Failure to thrive (FTT) is one example of possible neglect where longitudinal research has been conducted. FTT refers to impaired growth in infancy and has generally been classified either as organic (due primarily to an identified medical problem) or nonorganic (due primarily to psychosocial factors). Within the nonorganic FTT group, multiple and interacting etiological factors exist and the role of neglect is not always clear. This is particularly difficult if the definition of neglect focuses on parental behavior. For example, a misunderstanding of how to mix the infant formula might be responsible for the child's poor growth, but would probably not lead to a report for neglect. In contrast, if the primary criterion concerns the crucial unmet needs of the child, then most infants with nonorganic FTT can be said to have had their nutritional needs neglected. I suggest that the definition of neglect be based on such unmet needs, and the response should be based on a comprehensive assessment and weighing of the possible alternatives.

Longitudinal data on the normative growth of children have been developed, which allow for the monitoring of growth trends. Follow-up studies of children with nonorganic FTT reveal that their subsequent growth frequently does *not* reach the expected patterns for their age and sex (Sturm & Drotar, 1989). In mild undernutrition, weight is the first growth parameter to be affected, and if the inadequate nutrition becomes more severe and chronic, height is also impaired. In severe undernutrition, particularly in infancy, brain growth reflected by head circumference is also retarded. These three growth parameters—weight, height, and head circumference—are useful but relatively crude markers of undernutrition, because they are also influenced by genetic factors. This makes it difficult to distinguish normally small infants from those who are undernourished. A number of anthropometric measures (e.g., triceps and subscapular skin-folds) and laboratory tests (e.g., hemoglobin as a marker of iron deficiency) provide a more accurate assessment of undernutrition and are recommended for research purposes (Waterlow, 1984).

Another aspect of child neglect involves the failure to seek necessary health care, that is, medical neglect. What is the impact on health of poor compliance with recommendations for medical care? An example is asthma; appropriate treatment could keep a child relatively free of symptoms and out of the hospital, whereas noncompliance might lead to frequent wheezing, admissions to hospital, and school absence. Asthma is particularly amenable to study because tests for blood levels of one of the commonly used medications are readily available.

Other areas of medical neglect are more problematic to examine. For example, iron deficiency anemia or dental caries might be more common in neglected children, but parental level of understanding, poverty, and access to care need to be considered. Another example is the teenager whose diabetes is under poor control. The parent could be trying valiantly to supervise care, but a teenager denying his or her disease might pose a challenge to the most competent of parents. Probably, and appropriately, this would not be construed as neglect by a child protective agency. However, it is also the case that the parent could be inadequately responsive to the child's medical needs. It is therefore important that the underlying circumstances in the relationship between neglect of a child's health needs and the impact on health status be clearly determined.

Another area that might include child neglect is that of so-called accidents. Recently, the use of the term *accidents* has been replaced by the term *unintentional injuries*. This latter term implies that abuse *is* intended; I prefer the term *noninflicted injuries*. This shift in terminology is based on substantial epidemiological research demonstrating that injuries are often not simply the unpredictable random events that the term *accident* suggests (Rivara & Mueller, 1987). In a household that contains toxic substances, a dangerous ingestion is more likely to occur if there is poor supervision of a toddler. At some point it is reasonable to consider such circumstances as neglectful. If noninflicted injuries are associated with child neglect, then monitoring the incidence of such injuries and ingestions and their health effects should be a useful outcome measure for longitudinal research in this area.

Psychological Maltreatment

All forms of maltreatment can include an emotional or psychological component. Indeed, even when there are physical problems, these are often minor compared to the possible effects on the child's mental health. The anxiety a child might experience could manifest in many different ways, including psychosomatic conditions. Stomach aches, chest pain, headaches, enuresis, and encopresis are among the more commonly encountered presentations in children. Although these problems are not specific to maltreatment, it is likely that an association does exist. However, no controlled study has examined whether maltreated children have an increased incidence of psychosomatic disorders.

MEASURES OF HEALTH STATUS

The assessment of health status of maltreated children is similar to the measurement of health status in general. Therefore, it is useful to review the literature in this area and to consider what might be applied to the study of child maltreatment.

Since early in this century, there has been interest in measuring child health. Family interviews were used to determine the extent of illness due to communicable disease and how school absence was a result of illness and disability (Balinsky & Berger, 1975). In the mid-1950s the National Health Survey was first conducted, incorporating a variety of approaches to ascertain child health: checklists of chronic conditions, assessments of the limitations of activity due to chronic illness, and determinations of the number of days of restricted activity (days in bed, days absent from school) associated with acute illnesses (National Center for Health Statistics, 1963).

In the last two decades, efforts have been made to operationalize an expanded perspective of health status, as discussed earlier (National Center for Health Statistics, 1971). Several projects evaluating the impact of health services or aspects of health not previously assessed have led to the development of new measures, for example, the RAND Health Insurance Experiment added mental and social health status to the assessment of overall health status (Eisen, Donald, Ware & Brook, 1980).

One straightforward measure is to ascertain which diagnoses or conditions apply to a child. In this way, for example, asthma or stunted growth or cerebral palsy are identified as problems. Longitudinal research should primarily focus on chronic health conditions, although acute recurrent problems such as noninflicted injuries might also be of interest as markers of neglect. Frequent injuries also suggest possible ongoing abuse. In addition, recurrent injuries or acute illnesses can substantially impair a child's health and limit functioning over time. In a sense, this is similar to having a chronic condition. Research by Diaz and colleagues suggests that the *number* of conditions an individual has yields a good aggregate measure of morbidity for either an individual or a population group (Diaz et al., 1986). This research also indicates that a child with one condition is likely to continue to have that condition, and that one type of morbidity tends to be associated with other types of morbidity. The latter point suggests that one problem either predisposes a child toward or at least is associated with other problems.

There are other relatively crude measures of health status. These include the assessment of health care seeking behavior, although this behavior is confounded by the subjective perception of the need for care and by access to care. More objective measures might include the number (and length) of hospitalizations over a given period, although physician practice can vary markedly, and the severity of the condition is not the only consideration when admitting a patient to the hospital. Another reflection of health status could be the need for, or use of, medications. For example, a mild asthmatic might only need a single medication when wheezing starts, whereas one who is more severely afflicted might require continuous treatment with two medications. This principle, however, does not apply to most conditions. For example, a child with cerebral palsy might be seriously handicapped, but not require any medication. It is apparent that these proxy measures have serious shortcomings, and they are not recommended for general research purposes or in most areas of study.

For certain conditions, a narrowly focused outcome measure can be appropriate, meaningful, and useful. This approach might be particularly applicable to those types of maltreatment that affect a limited part of the body or affect a circumscribed aspect of health. One example would be the longitudinal study of undernutrition in infants with failure to thrive. The primary health outcome of interest might be the growth pattern in subsequent years, and the rate of growth and other anthropometric measures are very useful to assess outcome. Another example is that of sexual abuse, complicated by a sexually transmitted disease from which infertility might result. An advantage of a narrowly focused outcome measure is that it can be more readily attributed to the maltreatment, although potential confounding still must be carefully excluded.

Another approach has been to have a group of pediatricians rate the health status of a child by reviewing the medical records. This approach was used in a study of foster children (White & Benedict, 1985). No clear criteria were established and it appears that a general gestalt was used by the pediatricians; nevertheless, adequate interrater reliability was obtained.

It appears that a general measure, based on the collective subjective opinions of health professionals, might capture the general health status of the individual. However, this approach presents a conceptual problem; how can one reasonably compare vastly different conditions that affect health status in very different ways? For example, it seems impossible to compare on a single continuum the outcomes of infertility and paraplegia, other than to crudely assess them both as "very serious." Although this method might be relatively convenient, assuming the medical records are available and legible, there are invariably significant gaps in what is documented, and more direct and comprehensive measures of health status are preferable.

The major research efforts in recent years have conceptualized health status broadly, integrating physical, psychological, and social health, while remaining primarily concerned with the functioning of the individual. The level of functioning appears essential since almost any condition can have a very wide range of effects on a child's health. For example, a healed fracture of a leg might only leave a minor deformity noticeable only under close observation, but growth of the limb could be impeded, resulting in a marked and permanent limp. Similarly, serious head trauma could leave one child with a seizure disorder that is well controlled by medication and another child with a permanent hemiplegia without the use of one side of the body. These examples illustrate the importance of functioning in the assessment of health status.

In order to determine limitations in functioning, the most commonly used approach is to assess how major functions of the child are limited due to the health problem. For example, going to school, being able to play sports or games, and being able to be up and around are important basic functions. The parent or child can be asked on how many days in a given period these functions were not manageable and why not. Variations of this approach are included in the measures discussed below.

The RAND Health Insurance Study

The RAND Health Insurance Study operationalized health status as including physical, mental, and social health as well as general health perceptions (Eisen et al., 1980). Physical health was conceptualized in terms of functional status, and five categories of activities were examined: self-care, mobility, physical activity, role activity, and leisure. General health perceptions included prior and current health, resistance and susceptibility to illness, and parental health-related concerns about the child. (Extensive data on the measures of mental and social health are available, but will not be presented here.)

Questionnaires were developed for two age groups—children 4 years and under and those 5 to 13 years old—and were usually completed by the mother. The sample included 679 children in the younger age group and 1,473 older children who were being enrolled in one of various health plans. The items in the questionnaire were adapted from research with older children and adults.

The functional status in the younger age group involved three categories of limitations: physical activity, role activity (involving play), and self-care activity (e.g., eating, dressing). In addition to these domains, mobility was assessed in the sample of older children. The duration of any limitation was also obtained. The data analyses for the development of the scales and the testing of reliability, homogeneity and validity are presented in the report by Eisen and associates (1980). The internal consistency reliability estimates for the combined-site samples were satisfactory ($\alpha > .65$) for some of the scales and marginal ($\alpha > .50$) for others. Although considerable effort was made to ascertain content validity, face validity and construct validity, the authors acknowledged the need for additional research in these areas. Nevertheless, they concluded that their measures of child health (1) apply to general populations, (2) are able to detect differences in health status, (3) are generally reliable, and (4) have validity.

In the younger age group, only 1% to 3% of children had any of the functional limitations, with the vast majority described as being in excellent health. The small number of children with limitations restricted the analyses that could be done and the authors were careful to indicate the preliminary nature of the results. Items were scored dichotomously, without capturing severity of the limitations; while the crudeness of this approach is acknowledged, the conclusion is drawn that children who were scored as "limited" were worse off physically than those who were not.

As with the younger children, very few of the older children had any limitation (0.3% to 3%), and this again restricted the data analyses. Efforts to combine items into aggregate scales did not succeed; instead, a total limitations score was computed, based on one or more physical, mobility, self-care, or role activity limitations. Again, the authors state the preliminary nature of these results, since it is not clear that the relationship between items is cumulative.

The results of the RAND study were in agreement with other surveys of the functional limitations of children in the general population; 91% to 93% of children under age 16 appear to have no functional limitations (Eisen, Ware, Donald, & Brook, 1979). The basic issue of measurement precision remains to be resolved, because the measure probably identifies only those children who are significantly impaired.

Functional Status Measure

Stein and Jessop, in their research on children with chronic illnesses, have developed a useful measure for examining health status (Stein & Jessop, 1982). Their efforts have been guided by an interest in the generic, rather than the disease-specific, impact of different conditions on the functioning of children. Their Functional Status Measure assesses impairment in physical, psychological, and social functioning.

The authors acknowledge difficulties in this line of research. There is limited agreement on the normal roles and functions of children of different ages, both within and between contexts. In addition, the dynamic interaction between biological and environmental influences makes it difficult to attribute limited functioning in one area to a normal developmental process, fostered dependency, or an illness. Further, it is not clear that the normal sequences of development apply to significantly handicapped children. Despite these difficulties, efforts have been made to measure functional status. Whereas the RAND measure distinguishes between normal children and those with significant disabilities, Stein and Jessop's measure attempts to discern differing degrees of impaired functioning.

In developing the Functional Status Measure, child health was defined as the capacity to perform age-appropriate roles and tasks. Behavioral responses to illness that interfere with performing normal social roles are measured: communication, mobility, mood, energy, sleeping, eating, and toileting patterns. Behavior in the home, neighborhood, and school is measured and leisure, work, and rest activities are included. Different behavioral items were selected for infants, toddlers, preschoolers, and school-age children. Depending on the child's age, the measure has 23 to 55 items and is administered to a parent, taking about 30 minutes to complete.

The psychometric properties of the Functional Status Measure have been investigated on children with and without chronic illnesses (Stein & Jessop, 1982, 1986). Factors with good reliability were derived for each of the four age groups. Construct validity was demonstrated in children older than 9 months by the significantly better scores of the healthy children, who also showed less variability. Satisfactory criterion validity was shown by the significant correlations between scale scores and traditional health indicators such as days absent from school and number of hospitalizations.

In summary, the Functional Status Measure appears to have adequate psychometric properties. It distinguishes healthy from ill children and it is moderately sensitive in discerning degrees of impairment.

A modified version of the Functional Status Measure, named the Functional Status Questionnaire—Specific (FSQ-S), has been recently reported (Lewis, Pantell, & Kieckhefer, 1989). The main aim of this effort was to test a shorter measure that could be completed by parents in 10 minutes. To do this, the authors selected only the 14 items from the Functional Status Measure (FSII-R) that apply to the entire age range (0-16 years). The sample consisted of parents of 113 children, mainly asthmatics.

The construct and criterion validity were partially demonstrated by moderately significant correlations with the RAND study's parents' global ratings of their children's health and susceptibility to illness and with other traditional indicators of health status such as number of days hospitalized. Acceptable reliability was shown, similar to that of the longer version. The authors did not find the measure to be stable across time, but attribute this to the fluctuating nature of asthma.

The FSQ–S appears to be an easily administered, reliable measure, convenient for researchers and clinicians who wish to use brief measures of child health status. However, the authors acknowledge that the data showing reliability and construct validity are preliminary, and their sample is small and consists mainly of children with a single chronic illness. Further research on the measure is required.

The Child Health and Illness Profile (CHIP)

Starfield has proposed a model of health status composed of seven categories of outcome, each of which is a vector with both magnitude and direction (Starfield, 1988). In this theoretical construct, health status is described as a profile consisting of these components: longevity, activity, comfort, satisfaction, disease, achievement, and resilience. Although each of these components is conceptually distinct, somatic, psychological, and social manifestations of health are considered interrelated within the different domains.

Longevity involves an estimate of life expectancy expressed directly in numbers or as a percentage of normal life expectancy. Because it is usually difficult to predict premature death, estimates could be based on proxy measures such as life expectancy based on social class or family history of premature death.

Activity includes measures of functional health as manifested by interruption or altered performance of major social roles. One such rating scale is the Activities of Daily Living, which is used in adults with chronic illness. Another example is from the National Center for Health Statistics National Health Interview Survey, which assessed restriction to bed and restriction of "usual activities," defined differently for different age groups (Sullivan, 1971). Attending school serves as the "usual activity" for children over age 5, but obviously is not applicable to infants and preschoolers. One study found that eating and sleeping problems and unusual irritability were useful markers for younger children, but mainly for assessing the effects of *acute* illness.

Comfort includes a variety of physical and mental symptoms, with the psychological section adapted from the RAND Health Insurance Study (Eisen et al., 1980).

Satisfaction incorporates perceptions of well-being and general perceptions of personal health and attitudes toward it. Starfield notes that satisfaction should refer to satisfaction with one's health status and *not* with the structure or process of medical care.

Disease is represented by an index of the number of each type of illness experienced during a specified period, including asymptomatic but detectable, and temporary, diseases. Both physical and mental health conditions are considered, but not their severity; severity is reflected in other domains.

Achievement represents the level of development as measured by intelligence quotients and achievement tests in the cognitive realm, and by the Denver Developmental Screening Test (Frankenberg & Dodds, 1967) for motor or social abilities.

Resilience includes factors known to increase or reduce the risk of subsequent ill health, and those likely to enhance future health. Some examples are immunizations, drug abuse and smoking, and seat belt use.

The seven aspects of health status described constitute the Child Health and Illness Profile (CHIP), an instrument that is currently being developed (Starfield, 1988). This measure has the primary purpose of ascertaining current health status and aspects of prior health that are thought to bear on current and future health. Starfield has stated that it will be different from the National Health Interview Survey Child Health Supplements and the National Health and Nutrition Examination Surveys by being much shorter and targeting current and future health and functional ability.

It is expected that child health status measures will soon be available for primary school children aged 6 through 10 years and for youth aged 11 through 17 years. Initially, parents will report on the health of the younger children, whereas the older group will be questioned directly. The goal is to develop child and parent measures for both age groups and also a measure for preschoolers. Work on the psychometric properties of the measures is in progress and at a preliminary stage.

CONCLUSIONS

Little is currently known about the long-term physical health effects of child maltreatment. It seems likely that a small but significant minority of maltreated children suffer serious injuries and will have lasting physical handicaps. However, more subtle problems such as impaired growth or increased complications of diabetes due to poor care may be more likely. It is important that these health ramifications be studied. First, this knowledge would help guide optimal medical care for these high-risk children. Second, the information is needed to inform social policies and the allocation of resources. In this time of budgetary constraints and interest in cost-effectiveness, the hidden costs of child maltreatment should be demonstrated.

How should we measure the health effects of maltreatment? Several measures are available, but no single measure fully captures the complexity of health status. The traditional indices of health status, such as number of days absent from school, are useful albeit crude proxies of impaired health and functioning. Recent work in the field of measuring health status has been guided by a broad conceptualization that integrates the physical, psychological, and social aspects of health. This is a more comprehensive and useful approach. Further, Starfield's suggestion that health status be reflected in a profile, rather than by a summary score, is a promising idea.

At this time, there is no consensus as to which measure of health status is optimal. Some of the more recent measures require further research on their psychometric properties. It therefore seems prudent that the longitudinal study of child maltreatment include more than one of these newer measures in addition to the traditional indices of health status. This approach will yield optimal data on the health outcomes of child maltreatment.

Acknowledgments. The author thanks Susan Feigelman, M.D., Ray Starr, Ph.D., Eli Newberger, M.D., Barbara Starfield, M.D., and Diana Zuckerman, Ph.D., for their thoughtful reviews of this paper.

REFERENCES

American Humane Association. (1988). *Highlights of official child neglect and abuse reporting—1986.* Denver, CO: American Association for Protecting Children.

Anderson, R., & Aday, L. A. (1978). Access to medical care in the U.S.: Realized and potential. *Medical Care, 16*(7), 533–546.

Balinsky, W., & Berger, R. (1975). A review of the research on General Health Status Indexes. *Medical Care, 13*(4), 283–293.

Bithoney, W. G., & Dubowitz, H. (1985). Organic concomitants of non-organic failure to thrive: Implications for research. In D. Drotar (Ed.), *New directions in failure to thrive* (pp. 47–68). New York: Plenum Press.

Diaz, C., Starfield, B., Holtzman, N., Mellits, E. D., Hankin, J., Smalky, K., & Benson, P. (1986). Ill health and use of medical care: Community-based assessment of morbidity in children. *Medical Care, 24*, 848–856.

Donabedian, A. (1966). Evaluating the quality of medical care. *Milbank Memorial Fund Quarterly, 43*(3), 166–206.

Eisen, M., Donald, C. A., Ware, J. E., Jr., & Brook, R. H. (1980). *Conceptualization and measurement of health for children in the Health Insurance Study.* Santa Monica, CA: RAND Corporation.

Eisen, M., Ware, J. E., Donald, C. C., & Brook, R. H. (1979). Measuring components of children's health status. *Medical Care, 12*(9), 902–921.

Ellerstein, N. S. (1981). *Child abuse and neglect: A medical reference.* New York: Wiley.

Elmer, E. (1977). A follow-up study of traumatized children. *Pediatrics, 59*, 273–279.

Emans, S. J., Woods, E. R., Flagg, N. T., & Freeman, A. (1987). Genital findings in sexually abused, symptomatic and asymptomatic girls. *Pediatrics, 79,* 778–785.

Engel, G. L. (1977). The need for a new medical model: A challenge for biomedicine. *Science, 196,* 129–136.

Fanshel, D., & Shinn, E. G. (1978). *Children in foster care: A longitudinal investigation.* New York: Columbia University Press.

Finkel, M. A. (1989). Ano-genital trauma in sexually abused children. *Pediatrics, 84,* 317–322.

Frankenberg, W. K., & Dodds, J. B. (1967). The Denver Developmental Screening Test. *Journal of Pediatrics, 71,* 181–191.

Gellert, G. A., Durfee, M. J., & Berkowitz, C. D. (1990). Developing guidelines for HIV antibody testing among victims of pediatric sexual abuse. *Child Abuse & Neglect, 14,* 9–17.

Herman-Giddens, M. E., & Frothingham, T. E. (1987). Pre-pubertal female genitalia: Examination of evidence of sexual abuse. *Pediatrics, 80,* 203–208.

Hochstadt, N. A., Jaudes, P. K., Zimo, D. A., & Schachter, J. (1987). The Medical and psychosocial needs of children entering foster care. *Child Abuse & Neglect, 11,* 53–62.

Kavaler, M., & Swire, F. (1983). *Foster child health care.* Lexington, MA: D. C. Heath.

Lewis, C. C., Pantell, R. H., & Kieckhefer, G. M. (1989). Assessment of children's health status: Field test of new approaches. *Medical Care, 27*(3s), S54–S65.

National Center for Health Statistics. (1971). *Children and youth: Selected health characteristics* (DHEW Publication No. 1000, Series 10, No. 62). Rockville, MD: U. S. Department of Health, Education, and Welfare.

National Center for Health Statistics. (1963). *Origin, program and operation of the U. S. National Health Survey.* Washington, DC: Author.

National Committee for the Prevention of Child Abuse. (1987). *Deaths due to maltreatment soar: The results of the 8th semi-annual fifty state survey.* Chicago: Author.

Parker, S., Greer, S., & Zuckerman, B. S. (1988). Double jeopardy: The impact of poverty on early child development. *Pediatric Clinics of North America, 35*(6), 1227–1240.

Riviara, F. P., & Mueller, B. A. (1987). The epidemiology and causes of childhood injuries. *Journal of Social Issues, 43,* 13–31.

Schor, E. L. (1982). The foster care system and health status of foster children. *Pediatrics, 69,* 521–528.

Schor, E. L. (1988). Foster care. *Pediatric Clinics of North America, 35,* 1241–1252.

Starfield, B. (1988). Measuring health status in children. *Quality of Life and Cardiovascular Care, Winter,* 147–150.

Stein, R. E. K., & Jessop, D. J. (1982). A non-categorical approach to chronic childhood illness. *Public Health Reports, 97,* 354–362.

Stein, R. E. K., & Jessop, D. J. (1986). *Tables documenting the psychometric properties of the functional status II(R) measure.* New York: Albert Einstein College of Medicine.

Sturm, L., & Drotar, D. (1989). Prediction of weight for height following intervention in three-year-old children with early histories of nonorganic failure to thrive. *Child Abuse & Neglect, 13*, 19–28.

Sullivan, D. (1971). *Disability components for an index of health* (National Center for Health Statistics, U.S. DHEW, Public Health Service 1000, Series 2, No. 42). Washington, D.C.: U.S. Government Printing Office.

Teasdale, G., & Jennett, B. (1974). Assessment of coma and impaired consciousness. *Lancet, 2*, 81–84.

U.S. Department of Health and Human Services. (1988). *Study findings: study of national incidence and prevalence of child abuse and neglect—1988.* Washington, DC: National Center on Child Abuse and Neglect, Children's Bureau, Administration for Children, Youth and Families, Office of Human Development Services.

Waterlow, J. C. (1984). Current issues in nutritional assessment by anthropometry. In J. Brozed & B. Schurch (Eds.), *Malnutrition and behavior: Critical assessment of key issues* (pp. 77–90). Lausanne, Switzerland: Nestle Foundation.

White, R., & Benedict, M. (1985). *Health status and utilization patterns of children in foster care.* Final report submitted to the Department of Health and Human Services, Office of Human Development Services, Administration of Children, Youth and Families.

White, S. T., Loda, F. A., Ingram, D. L., & Pearson, A. (1983). Sexually transmitted diseases in sexually abused children. *Pediatrics, 72*, 16–21.

World Health Organization. (1978). Constitution. In *Basic Documents*. Geneva, Switzerland: Author.

Index